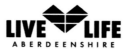

LIVE LIFE

A B E R D E E N S H I R E

livelifeaberdeenshire.org.uk

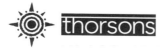

thorsons

Thorsons
An imprint of HarperCollins *Publishers*
77–85 Fulham Palace Road
Hammersmith, London W6 8JB
The website is www.thorsonselement.com

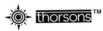

and *Thorsons* are registered trademarks of
HarperCollins *Publishers* Ltd

First published by Thorsons 2003

10 9 8 7 6 5 4 3

© Master John Ding 2003

Master John Ding asserts the moral right to be
identified as the author of this work

Photography by Guy Hearn

A catalogue record for this book is
available from the British Library

ISBN 0 00 714592 6

Printed and bound in Great Britain by
Martins the Printers Ltd, Berwick upon Tweed

This book is dedicated to

Grandmaster Ip Tai Tak,

5th Generation of Yang Family Tai Chi Chuan
First disciple of Great Grandmaster Yang Sau Chung

whose lifetime study and practice of Tai Chi Chuan
has given him a unique depth of knowledge and
an inexhaustible source of experience.
He is one of the few remaining forefront figures in
Yang Style Tai Chi Chuan and without his selfless dedication
to the discipline of Tai Chi Chuan,
the art would not be as rich as it is today.

Contents

Acknowledgements

My son and I would like to thank the following students – Sara Muldowney, Philippa Kennedy, Bob Thomas, Liz Welch, Chris Davala, Richard Mechen, Ken Young, Robert Appleton, Sue and Richard Kale, Michael Velsey – and many others who have contributed in one way or another to the publication of this book.

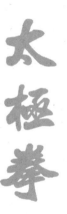

Preface

It has always been an aspiration of mine to preserve, promote and disseminate the true teachings of Tai Chi, or more correctly, Tai Chi Chuan. The first time I embarked upon writing a full-length manuscript about the art was to bring to light and share the immense knowledge and understanding of my mentor and *Sifu*, Grandmaster Ip Tai Tak, fifth generation of the Yang Family Lineage, who had recorded his thoughts on traditional Tai Chi Chuan in his diaries for over half a century. The project centred on the organization, translation and interpretation of these memoirs. Several years' hard work resulted in the publication of the first volume of *Tai Chi Chuan Revelations* – over two hundred pages focused solely on the art's principles and concepts.

The creation of *Tai Chi Chuan Revelations: Principles and Concepts* involved meticulously dissecting the diaries and grouping texts into defined themes, so that subject matter was prioritized above chronology. The approach of depth rather than breadth was taken so that I could focus specifically on principles and concepts. But whilst this format provides a powerful source of reference for the more experienced Tai Chi practitioner, this theoretical approach lends itself less well to the Tai Chi novice, and makes it difficult for them to get started. Traditional Tai Chi Chuan is a vast discipline taking time and commitment to practise, refine and develop. But *Tai Chi Chuan Revelations: Principles and Concepts* represents only one aspect of this multi-faceted traditional system.

To provide a balanced introduction to Tai Chi Chuan would therefore need a new approach that would bring together its diverse elements. The emphasis would be different to that of its predecessor and instead be directed towards the needs of the beginner and those who seek an introduction to the *traditional* art. But more than just giving a balanced overview, it was important to me that this new book would present Tai Chi Chuan in a way that would be accessible to a wider audience, and even to those who have the busiest of lifestyles.

Therefore, by regrouping the team that were the backbone to the publication of *Tai Chi Chuan Revelations*, work began on a book that would provide both concise and easy-to-follow theoretical and practical instruction, yet at the same time remain true to the traditional teachings of Tai Chi Chuan. The result is *15-Minute Tai Chi*, which attempts to encapsulate the essence of what is normally taught in a much longer traditional Tai Chi lesson, which may last one or two hours.

By carefully selecting some of the most important elements of the traditional system of Tai Chi (Chi Kung, the Tai Chi Chuan form and breathing exercises), while at the same time preserving the fundamental principles of the art, it is hoped that even after a short period of time, substantial benefits in health and well-being may be gained. Although this book does not explicitly focus upon the martial aspects of Tai Chi Chuan, the method outlined here, if correctly practised, can become the foundation of what can later be developed into an effective form of self-defence, as each posture of the form has potent martial applications.

My aim is that through this specially designed training programme, readers will be given a good grounding in the art, one that will also serve as a stepping-stone towards greater understanding and the development of traditional Tai Chi Chuan. My hope is that even more people will be able to benefit from and have fun with this wonderful art.

How To Use This Book

This book has been specifically written and designed for those who have an interest in learning authentic Tai Chi Chuan, and is divided into four parts: Overview, The Basics, The Practice and Daily Life. Each of these four parts is a self-contained section that provides you with a methodical approach to different aspects of the art. Tai Chi Chuan, although outwardly a practical discipline, encompasses elements of theory as well as practice. Hence, this is a book that consolidates many of the fundamental aspects of the art and presents them in a fashion that focuses equally on the practical and the theoretical.

Theory provides the foundations from which we can build the practical aspects of the art. Without theory, our foundations are weak and practice becomes only an empty shell. The essence of Tai Chi Chuan is not simply aimlessly choreographed movements but something much deeper; it focuses upon the harnessing and circulation of the vital energy, Chi, within the body. With this in mind, the book begins by laying out the basic theory behind Tai Chi Chuan in its first two sections.

Part One gives an overview of Tai Chi Chuan, and will hopefully leave you with a true representation of the art. Part Two further consolidates and extends this theme by concentrating on the fundamental theoretical aspects. It is best to read, understand and focus upon these sections first before you embark on to the practical section. In doing so, you will gain better understanding to the elements that lie behind Tai Chi's movements, so that the future practice you do will be more meaningful and beneficial.

The practice of Tai Chi Chuan is set out in Part Three. It introduces you to an easy-to-follow, step-by-step guide to learning its method. There are 10 chronological 15-minute sessions. Each routine will take you on a journey that starts with Zhan Zhang Chi Kung, guides you through a shortened, concise Tai Chi form and ends with settling breathing exercises. These sessions are specially designed so that they are as safe to learn (regardless of your age or ability) as they are effective. Try to work within your own limits and at your own pace, learning a few postures at a time. Don't try to learn too much too quickly. Instead, spend time in getting the movements correct, so that you develop your skills in a constructive way.

Tai Chi Chuan is an art that has an abundance of potential that can extend far beyond the 15-minute session. Hence, Part Four introduces you to the diverse ways in which Tai Chi Chuan can be brought into our daily lives. The crossover of Tai Chi Chuan into our everyday lives can occur at all levels. Tai Chi Chuan will balance, inform and enrich your life experience by developing both the mental and the physical. Here we explain how the principles of Tai Chi Chuan can be encompassed in the physical activities of daily living, as well as examining how it can help to prevent and treat illness. Stress has become a modern-day epidemic and Tai Chi Chuan can play a large role in helping us find ways in which we can manage stress. Eastern and Western models of stress are described, with particular reference to how Tai Chi Chuan can be applied to relieve it.

Use this book from beginning to end and you will find that it will bring you a wealth of indispensable knowledge. Tai Chi Chuan is a complete and holistic system of training. The method laid out here will allow you to realize your true potential on a physical and non-physical level, and provide you with the tools by which you can ultimately improve your quality of life in mind, body and spirit.

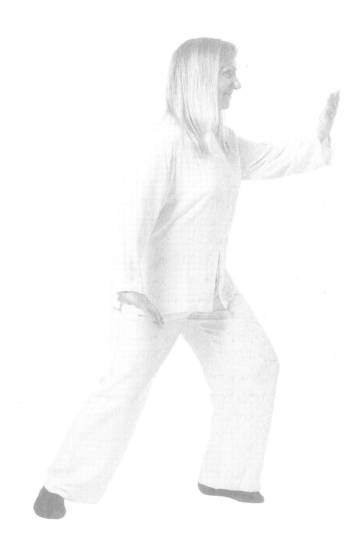

PART ONE

Introduction to the book

Moving slowly under the trees
Without pause, without break
The breath is quiet, soft and slow
As is the heart content and at peace

An exactingly majestic motion through space and time
Stillness within motion
Motion within stillness
Akin to the tranquil water of a slow flowing stream

The un-wavered focus of mind
The fluid movements of body
The purity of spirit
United as one entity
Wrapped and entwined by the surrounding morning mist
Man and nature harmoniously merged as one

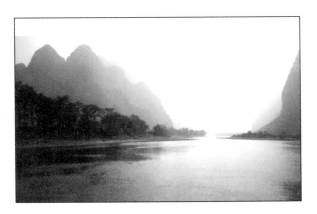

A poetic expression of Tai Chi. Yet these words still fail to convey the true spirit and experience of a Tai Chi performance.

For hundreds of years from the days of the earliest explorers to the East, the West has been puzzled at seeing the Chinese from all walks of life practise the effortless looking, ballet-like exercise they call Tai Chi Chuan. These unhurried, measured, relaxed and soft movements manage to encapsulate the essence of calm and tranquillity. In the familiar surroundings of a public courtyard or park, performers would shift seamlessly from one motion to another, unperturbed by the perplexed frown of the foreign traveller looking on. Visitors to China would take home stories of strange but wonderful images of Tai Chi to their friends and families, adding to its mystic charms. With the advent of modern travel, many more have since discovered first hand the magic of Tai Chi Chuan in its homeland, China.

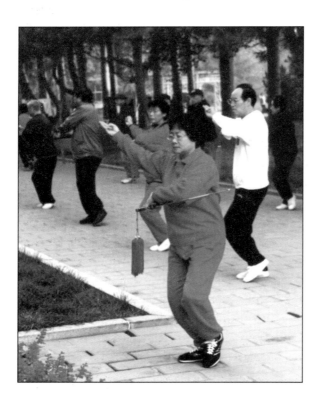

Yet this is only one side of the coin. Since the world started to become a smaller place, with greater accessibility of travel bringing the corners of every continent closer together, pockets of Chinese communities began to migrate, grow and thrive all over the world. The Chinese took with them their food, their culture, their heritage and also their Tai Chi. Soon Tai Chi Chuan could be seen being practised as close as next door's back garden. Tai Chi had travelled successfully across China's borders, and slowly but surely has been disseminated throughout the world. Perhaps this serves to illustrate how important Tai Chi Chuan is to the Chinese, and how closely linked it is to their culture. Certainly cultural stereotyping and its links with Tai Chi added that air of mystery that has intrigued the West for many years.

Today Tai Chi Chuan is no longer a fringe activity and has moved into the mainstream. People from all walks of life – doctors, nurses, waiters, actors, carpenters, mechanics, athletes – practise Tai Chi. It is mutually inclusive to all and extends beyond the boundaries of race, religion and creed. The marvel is that anyone can practise Tai Chi, regardless of age or ability. There are no physical or mental barriers. Millions of people have now caught the Tai Chi bug, and its popularity has risen exponentially. It has become fashionable. Tai Chi Chuan is not only part of the individualism of those of us who practise it but has also become part of modern living. Seeing Tai Chi in commercial advertising, movies and health promotion has become commonplace. Gone is the day that kept Tai Chi Chuan behind closed cultural doors.

The popularity of Tai Chi Chuan in the West today reflects an increasing awareness of what the art has to offer. Tai Chi Chuan is in high demand because its benefits outweigh those of many other forms of exercise. It has the unique ability to enrich the mind as well as invigorate the body. Whilst the outward expression of Tai Chi's methods may be mainly physical, its effects are not. Through its softness and relaxation, it is able to harmonize the mind, body and spirit bringing about both physical and mental well-being. There are few other training activities that are so holistic. Its process is also a simple one. Tai Chi Chuan in its purist form requires no specialized

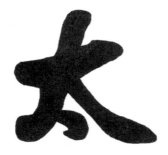

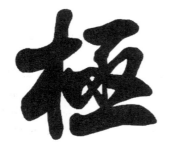

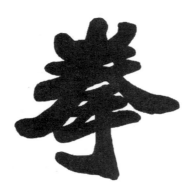

equipment or devices. Its only prerequisites are that you have a body, a mind, time, motivation and a little floor space. The Chinese believe that once Tai Chi Chuan is practised correctly you will gain the pliability of a child, the health of a lumberjack and the peace of mind of a sage. Little wonder, then, that Tai Chi Chuan is one of the fastest growing, most sought after exercise systems available.

WHAT IS TAI CHI CHUAN?

Tai Chi Chuan, or Tai Chi, as it is more commonly referred to in the West, is a discipline about which there are many preconceptions. Ask a dozen people what Tai Chi is, and sure enough you will get a dozen different answers. Some will claim it is a potent martial art, whilst others will suggest it is an exercise system for health, or even a spiritual discipline. Often these answers will reflect what a particular person wants from the art. However, none of these labels can exclusively claim to describe the art. It can be all of the above. Tai Chi Chuan, of its very nature, offers a wide range of attractions, all mysteriously interlinked: health, meditation, self-healing, self-defence, fitness and so on. It is this holistic approach to mind and body that attracts so many to Tai Chi.

Together, the three Chinese words 'Tai Chi Chuan' literally translate to 'The Great Ultimate Fist'

However, the wealth of differing views and the assortment of different classes to cater for them mean that the absolute Tai Chi beginner can become overwhelmed with disjointed information. Tai Chi is broad-based and multifaceted, and perhaps the danger is that the beginner can too easily be coerced into a skewed view of what the art can really offer. The most important consideration for anybody starting Tai Chi Chuan is to do some research beforehand to get an unbiased view of the art.

Tai Chi Chuan is a complete discipline. It is a training method that allows you to discover your true potential on a physical and non-physical level. It is able to integrate the mind, body and spirit, and thus improves both physical and mental well-being. Tai Chi Chuan allows you to grow both in body and in mind, and hence its associations with health are the most well known of its attributes.

The soft, relaxed, flowing series of movements that are unique to Tai Chi Chuan allow the body to be used in a very precise and definite way. Muscles, bones and joints are all utilized in a meticulous fashion that increases our awareness of ourselves and of those around us. Muscles gently tone and strengthen as balance and posture improve. However, the benefits are felt not only in the musculoskeletal system, and go far beyond simply developing fitness. The Tai Chi process also works from within on a much more profound level.

By practising Tai Chi Chuan, the body's internal energy (known to the Chinese as *Chi* or *Qi*) can be harnessed and is able to circulate freely within the body. As a result the internal organs become healthier and both the mind and body become stronger and more robust from the inside. Even with a small amount of practice Tai Chi Chuan will invigorate you from within, and provide you with a powerful antidote to stress. It will make you will feel more relaxed, refreshed and revitalized, as well as more tolerant, self-confident and, above all, happier with life.

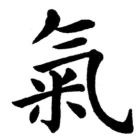

Chi, the body's internal energy

Because Tai Chi is often regarded as only a health exercise in the West, there have been many misconceptions about the practical use of Tai Chi Chuan for self-defence. This is a mistaken view. Indeed, Tai Chi Chuan's origins stem from the martial arts. It is well recognized in the East for its potent martial abilities. Hidden within every Tai Chi movement is a logical and practical combat application. Tai Chi Chuan is an internal martial art and hence very different to those more established, 'external' martial arts found in the West. Internal martial arts not only cultivate the internal energy, *Chi,* for health but also utilize Chi for self-defence and it is this emphasis that makes Tai Chi an internal martial art. To use Tai Chi Chuan for self-defence requires a lot of dedication and persistent correct practice with the help of an able instructor. Men and women can achieve equal proficiency in this discipline, as expertise is not dependent on size, physical strength or speed. At a high level, Tai Chi Chuan has the ability to use Chi in self-defence applications to achieve the apparent paradox of effortlessness and tremendous power simultaneously. The subtlety of such expertise cannot be adequately described, only felt.

Tai Chi is a training process, not a religion. You are not required to have any special beliefs, ideals or desires in order to practise and benefit from it. However, Tai Chi draws on many beliefs and theories from its parent Chinese culture, and its background is much influenced by Taoist ideas. Taoism is an ancient Chinese philosophy based on observations of the natural world around us. Taoism describes a way, path or method to maintain harmony and balance with the natural order. Tai Chi Chuan provides a vehicle to facilitate this process, and thus some practitioners use the art as a form of spiritual discipline to further develop their study in Taoism. You do not have to go into an in-depth study of Taoist thought to benefit from Tai Chi. However, to ignore these aspects would be to close the doors on understanding the art's Taoist roots and those Tai Chi principles associated with them. Spiritual or personal growth must be taken one small step at a time, and in this respect the art is an excellent way of discovering yourself. Tai Chi necessitates time, patience and determination, but it is completely self-imposed. It demands you to look inside yourself as well as out for sources of stability and strength. Through time Tai Chi will change you, and whilst you may be doing it for other reasons, personal development is inevitable.

Tai Chi is so much to so many. It is a martial art, a health exercise, a spiritual discipline. It offers all these aspects and more. *15-Minute Tai Chi* will hopefully provide you with a balanced view of the art, and empower you to find your own reasons to start Tai Chi Chuan. Some beginners start Tai Chi Chuan wanting to learn how to fight. In so doing they may also find that they become stronger and healthier, and discover new ways to look upon life. Some, who are looking for its health benefits, are often surprised to find that they enjoy testing postures and pushing hands – those aspects of the art that are associated with the martial. Whilst others, drawn by the philosophy, find that they also enjoy the challenge of the physical discipline as much as the mental. Tai Chi Chuan is as diverse as the people who practise it, and whilst you may start Tai Chi for one particular reason, you might just find it takes you on a pleasant journey that you didn't expect.

THE HISTORY OF TAI CHI CHUAN

Whilst millions of people openly practise Tai Chi Chuan today, the origin of the art is far more elusive. The history of Tai Chi Chuan spans many centuries, much of which has gone unrecorded, especially in the earlier years when word of mouth rather than written texts were relied on to propagate the discipline. This disjointed chronology, coupled with the secrecy and mysticism that once were associated with Tai Chi Chuan, has meant that there is now much uncertainty as to the art's true beginnings. Consequently today, conjecture and speculation have spawned a number of hypotheses to account for Tai Chi Chuan's earliest origins, each with its own mix of theories, legends and folklore.

Certainly Tai Chi Chuan's ties with traditional Chinese medical theories and Taoist beliefs are strong. Many stories of the origin of Tai Chi Chuan and the exercise systems that may have been its precursors are often linked to famous historical figures within the fields of Traditional Chinese Medicine and Taoism. However, perhaps the most famous myth about Tai Chi Chuan's creation is that of the Taoist sage, Chang San Feng, of the Sung Dynasty (960–1278).

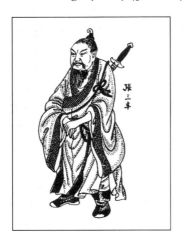

Chang San Feng

Chang San Feng was the son of a government official. Well educated, he followed in his father's footsteps by taking up an official position in government. But with little taste for the political arena of the time, upon the death of his parents, Chang San Feng relinquished his official role and instead became a hermit. He travelled the length of ancient China in search of enlightenment and reason from elders who were scattered throughout the country. In so doing he was able to study and develop meditation, Taoist health disciplines and martial arts, most notably during his travels into the Wu Tang Mountains.

It is said that on one such occasion while Chang San Feng was meditating, he was disturbed by an unusually strange and intense sound. Unfamiliar with the noise that had broken his thoughts, Chang San Feng was curious to discover its origin. He rose from his place and cautiously followed the sound back to its source. Led to a nearby courtyard, he was startled to find an agitated commotion of cranes. As he approached closer, the cause for this discord became clear. The group of birds surrounded a solitary snake, seething and staring at it fiercely, as if in contempt and anger. A battle was about to begin.

The threatened snake rattled its tail in preparation for combat, and lifted its fore-body away from the ground, hissing in challenge. In doing so, one of the eager encircling cranes dived at speed to attack the snake with its dagger-like beak. Without panic or fear, the lone snake kept its composure and circular shape, eyes fixed upon the incoming strike. Curiously, however, it did not confront the impulsive crane's attack head on. Instead it simply, smoothly and effectively shifted its body, turning to one side to evade the attack. The crane, unable to change the direction of its full-blooded attack in time, shot past the snake missing its target. Worse still, and to the snake's advantage, the crane's long neck was exposed, and without hesitation the snake lunged forward to counter. But as soon as the snake began its attack, the crane raised its wing to shield the slender neck. With its wings up as protection, the snake had to find an alternative opening to strike, and swiftly weaved and turned to move between the crane's legs. The crane looked down to see its enemy sliding beneath it. Fearful of an assault from below, the crane lifted its leg to flick the snake away. But in anticipation of this, the snake relaxed its hind body and as the crane struck its leg forward, the relaxed snake wrapped itself around the leg of the crane, like a piece of string around an upturned hook.

Chang San Feng watched with rapt attention, intrigued as the contest continued back and forth. Each attack was countered with an equal defence. Neither had the advantage over the other, and before long fatigue took over. The bird, tired and frustrated, and unable to penetrate the reptile's defences, flew off and perched on a nearby tree, while the snake slithered between boulders away from the open.

Chang San Feng reflected upon his observations. Fascinated by how softness and circular motions could overcome an attack, he began to develop a system of movements based upon what he had seen, incorporating them into his daily routine. Before long Chang San Feng had integrated his knowledge of Taoist meditation and breathing into the movements, and adapted the martial aspects to form a new type of exercise system that had never been seen before. It is this holistic system of exercise that is now known as Tai Chi Chuan.

Surprisingly, the popularity of Tai Chi Chuan did not begin until the eighteenth century. Before this time, much like the other martial arts, Tai Chi Chuan was a very strictly guarded discipline, kept firmly closed behind family doors. Outsiders were not welcome to share the knowledge, and to teach them was an uncommon event. Tai Chi Chuan of this era had been passed down from one generation down to the next, within small selective circles, mainly consisting of family members and clansmen. However, perhaps one of the earliest influential figures to initiate Tai Chi Chuan's popularity was Yang Lu Chan (1799–1872).

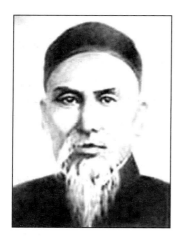

Yang Lu Chan

Prior to Yang Lu Chan's teachings in Peking (Beijing), Tai Chi Chuan was little heard of, being only discreetly taught amongst members of the Chen clan village. Yang Lu Chan came from Yong Nian District, Hubei Province and, as an outsider, was very fortunate and one of the rare few 'strangers' to become accepted as a disciple of Chen Chang Hsing (1771–1853). Yang mastered the teachings of early Tai Chi Chuan in his teacher's home in Chen Chia Kou (Chen Village), Wen District, Henan Province, and finally settled in Peking where he gained even wider recognition after being appointed as an instructor to the local noblemen. Today, most of the major styles of Tai Chi Chuan practised (i.e. Chen, Yang and Wu) can be traced back to the Chen Village. However it was Yang Lu Chan and his descendants who spread Tai Chi Chuan across the country. Hence, the Yang Style of Tai Chi Chuan created by Yang Lu Chan is the most widely practised around the world today.

Whatever particular version of Tai Chi Chuan's earliest origins you believe, most people accept that Tai Chi Chuan evolved as it was passed down from one generation to another. Successive heirs not only preserved and sustained the art, but also enhanced it with new ideas and philosophies. It was initially developed as a martial art, and in the volatile climate of ancient China, contests and challenges between the different martial arts were quite common. Tai Chi undoubtedly played a part in these proceedings, and through natural selection, slowly but surely over the centuries Tai Chi Chuan became more refined and developed, eventually becoming something similar to the holistic art that we practise today.

TAI CHI CHUAN AND MODERN SOCIETY

Modern society is dynamic. Since industrialization and its aftermath have served to initiate the acceleration of social change, society has evolved at an exponential rate. Society and its environment are linked in a complex interdependent relationship. Today, our environment is continually changing, and we face an overwhelming need to adapt and accommodate ourselves to its new demands. We evolve and adapt ourselves in all aspects of our daily living – be it at work or at play – to meet the changes.

Our work lives demand that we constantly have to meet deadlines and targets, while the nature of our work itself is continually changing. Without reservation we readily accept this phenomenon in the work place, find methods to adapt and call it a 'challenge'. We learn new skills, giving freely of our time to master our chameleon-like job descriptions, and finally, when the challenge is met, we feel satisfied at the completion of the task at hand. Challenge in our work lives is thus an important ingredient for healthy and productive work, energizing us both physically and psychologically. However, as the speed of change increases, demands from the work environment grow more and more. Regardless of the willingness and determination to adapt and mould ourselves, challenges will not always be met. Requirements surpass capabilities, resources and needs in the same way that unlimited demand outstrips limited supply. Compromises set in. The feeling of satisfaction turns into exhaustion, and the sense of accomplishment turns into failure and stress. In short, the stage is set for illness, injury and job failure.

In leisure, too, we have become tainted by the same pattern of unforgiving persistent change. The modernization of society has meant that our supposed wants and needs are fulfilled with increasing efficiency and speed. We have become used to the idea of instant panaceas. Happiness is the unspoken promise of a thousand products that make up the reality of our every day. We consume in order to be happy, since it is advertising that assures us that youth, glamour, health and sexual attraction are all derivatives of our consumption. As we increasingly neglect ourselves for our occupations, consumption becomes the mainstay of our limited social relations, and our individualism is replaced by generic templates dreamed up by the corporate machine. Modern society is on the road to becoming a global monoculture, dominated by a consumerism that constantly replaces achievable if relatively meaningless goals with different ones, to ensure that we continue to chase the newest objects of our desire.

Society and social change march on, hand in hand, regardless of those who are left behind in their wake. As our environment evolves and the fabric of our society changes, there is a perpetual expectation for us to adapt with it. The luxury of being in equilibrium with our environment is long gone. Instead rapid continuous change in our everyday environment generates disequilibrium. Many sociologists believe that this disequilibrium and people's maladaptation to change are the root causes of illness in today's modern society. Western medicine fails us too, often by disregarding this model, and looks only upon the pathological processes for sources of disease, neglecting both the psychological and the social state of the individual. Often it is dissatisfaction with both the physical and mental manifestations of modern lifestyles that turns our eyes eastwards. It may be comforting to latch on to some Eastern alternative such as Tai Chi Chuan in an effort to find stability and fixity in a foreverchanging environment. But although Tai Chi Chuan does represent an alternative, we do not always treat it as such.

Tai Chi Chuan's image as a product of the Western market is indeed intriguing, and perhaps skewed. Far from the forefront are the art's martial origins and abilities. Instead we are induced by cultural stereotyping, if not by genuine insight, to consider the East as the spiritual half of the materialistic West. Thus Eastern religions and philosophies appeal to what seems to be missing from our lives. Furthermore, the lack of concise public information on Tai Chi Chuan lends it an air of mystery, certainly compared to more established martial arts such as Karate or Judo. Tai Chi Chuan, of its very nature, offers a wide range of attractions, all bewilderingly interrelated to the innocent bystander. It can combine health, meditation, spiritual enlightenment, self-healing, self-defence, fitness and so on. This no doubt adds further to the art's mystic charms.

Too often the Westerner drawn to this 'product profile' only takes a short-term approach. Liking the Tai Chi basket of attractions, he or she is all too tempted to walk off with it. This attitude can easily lead to frustration when progress seems slow. Intangible advances may seem like no advance at all. It is easier to buy Tai Chi-related products (like this book!), or to chop and change instructor, than to persist towards a goal that cannot be bought. Instead, this goal is one that necessitates effort, commitment and concentration.

So Tai Chi Chuan demands of us qualities which we as Westerners are often lacking: patience, persistence, application and a willingness to look inside as well as out for sources of stability. It necessitates trust in your chosen instructor. If you have started on a long road and cannot quite see the way, it is much easier to trust in your guide, and much more helpful if you can also extend a hand to help others too. The absence of competitiveness, the need for cooperation, the willingness to concede a part of yourself to others, as well as to trust yourself with others, is a high hurdle. As Westerners instilled with a sense of individual needs and necessities, it may be a hard one to jump. But it is essential to realize that this is not a race with a definable end, but a process that is its own reward. Through it you do not *possess* something new, but *become* something new.

TAI CHI CHUAN AND HEALTH

Tai Chi Chuan's association with health is perhaps its most well known benefit. Whether you are part of the new wave of Tai Chi enthusiasts, or part of the traditionalist camp who practise Tai Chi Chuan in its full entirety, the art's health benefits are universal to all. Tai Chi Chuan has a multifaceted approach to health. Its medicinal purposes go beyond the treatment of illness, taking also a role in disease prevention. The principles and concepts behind the slow, relaxed, fluid movements of Tai Chi Chuan are central to its healing ability. Tai Chi may at first seem only to work on the external body. Its precise and particular use of muscles, bones and joints serve to enhance their tone and strength as well as improve balance, coordination and posture. However, the benefits of Tai Chi Chuan are not only apparent on the superficial musculoskeletal component, and they go beyond simply developing fitness. The Tai Chi process operates on a much deeper level, working from within.

Tai Chi Chuan draws on many beliefs and theories of its parent Chinese culture. One fundamental and universal concept is that of *Chi* or *Qi*. The Chinese believe that Chi is the force that lies behind the biological function of all living tissues. Chi brings with it life and without it we die. Hence Chi represents little less than the vital energy of all life. It circulates and flows through each of us in predetermined channels and meridians within the body. The resulting complex interaction between the circulating internal energy, the channels through which it travels, and its effects on the body's organs is of central importance in the balance of a person's Chi, and hence in the maintenance of good health. It is through the regulation and management of Chi and its circulation that Tai Chi Chuan and Traditional Chinese Medicine directly derive many of their health benefits.

The concept of balance is essential in the Chinese approach to health. Chinese physicians will advocate moderation in all things, be it alcohol, food or even exercise. Substances or actions that are taken or done in excess will disrupt the balance of Chi, resulting in illness and, ultimately, death. Thus the ability to avoid both excess and deficiency is also vital in managing the balance of Chi in order to achieve both mental and physical well-being. The Chinese believe implicitly that it is the delicate balancing act or homeostasis of Chi that brings and retains good health. This is the balance between *yin* and *yang*.

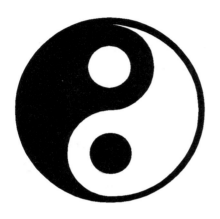

Yin Yang

The essence of Yin Yang Theory describes the dual, co-existing relationship between yin and yang within nature. Yin and yang represent two opposites to a whole, yet one cannot exist without the other. Whilst yin may take the form of night, cold or sadness, yang will correspond to their opposites; that is day, heat or happiness. But without first having the understanding of sadness, how would we appreciate the experience of happiness? Though they are opposites, there is also an inter-dependent, inter-consuming, inter-supporting and inter-transforming relation between the two forces. Pure yin and pure yang form the two ends of an infinite spectrum, which can never be reached. Thus inside each force must remain an element of the other, and as the end extremes are approached so the desire to return to a state of balance becomes greater, creating the natural flowing oscillation that is the dynamic interplay between yin and yang. It is only by harmonizing these forces so that they fluctuate within the norm, away from the realms of extremes, that we are able to create equilibrium and balance.

The ancient Chinese text, the *I Ching*, states that nature is always in motion and that mankind should follow nature, and exercise and strengthen itself continuously. It also stresses that the balance of yin and yang energies – physically, mentally and emotionally – are essential to mankind's well-being. All Chinese health disciplines apply this theory to their practice. Our bodies, and each of our organs, have within them elements of yin and yang. Both internal and external factors have a bearing on their balance. In some instances these organs may become more yang than yin. In others they may be more yin than yang. However, the consequence is the same: an imbalance of Chi, which, if prolonged, may lead further on to illness and disease. Treatment in the form of needles (Acupuncture), oral remedies (Herbal Medicine), massage (Tui Na) and movement (Tai Chi Chuan) all have a common theme, which is to re-establish and maintain the balance of Chi.

One of the main principles of Chinese health disciplines is to observe imbalances as they arise and address them before they develop into more serious illnesses or pathologies. For many of us, too often we start Tai Chi Chuan late with the imbalance of Chi already well established for years. Perhaps this imbalance may take the form of an illness, a weak constitution, destructive lifestyle habits, bad posture or even certain negative ways of thinking. However, it is through the Tai Chi Chuan process that the whole system of mind, body and spirit will start to recover and prevent further disease or emotional problems from arising. Even with a small amount of regular practice, you will find beneficial effects to your health.

The consistent and regular practice of the slow, flowing, circular movements that are particular to Tai Chi Chuan allows the Chi energy within the body to be harnessed and regulated to once again achieve balance and harmony. Tai Chi Chuan has the ability to improve the strength and quality of these energies to cure illness, maintain health and prevent disease. Blockages in the channels through which Chi flows to the body's organs are said to be one of the chief factors that cause imbalance, and hence mental and physical illness. Tai Chi Chuan allows these channels to regain their patency, and recover their confluence with one another. Then Chi is able to flow and circulate freely again within these meridians and channels, invigorating the mind and body to improve, and in some cases cure, the ill.

Tai Chi Chuan does not make a distinction between physical and mental illness, as the root to an illness's pathology ultimately lies in the same reasoning. Thus Tai Chi Chuan and other Chinese health disciplines may seem like the 'magic bullet' that cures all. In fact it is simply putting right what is going wrong. Initially Tai Chi Chuan will remove blockages in the energy system caused by incorrect body alignments or tension, to enable you to move with suppleness, poise, lightness and speed. Then through persistent, regular, correct practice Tai Chi will improve many cardiovascular, respiratory and digestive disorders. Indeed, the lack of reliance on tension and speed makes Tai Chi Chuan uniquely applicable to anyone suffering from such disorders.

Tai Chi Chuan also helps many mental and psychological disorders. Tai Chi principles can enhance your performance in all areas, stripping away the tension and anxiety that inhibit you from giving your best. Being able to be totally relaxed and concentrated at the same time is just one of the art's innumerable effects. Little wonder, then, that Tai Chi also acts as an effective revitalizer, improving the quality of life, and is thus used by many people as a tool to combat the stresses and pressures of modern society.

Research into Tai Chi Chuan's health benefits has been slow. Whilst Tai Chi Chuan offers many claims, evidence-based medicine is needed to substantiate them. The West is perhaps realizing at last the diverse treatment potential that Tai Chi Chuan and other Chinese medical disciplines have to offer. Despite the lack of substantial evidence-based research, it is clear that Tai Chi Chuan is beneficial to a significant number of practitioners. The studies that have been carried out point to Tai Chi Chuan's range of benefits, from slowing post-menopausal bone loss, to reducing falls among the elderly, to improving cardiorespiratory function and reducing stress. Some of these studies are listed in the Further Reading section on p.174.

Closed doors are beginning to be opened. In the UK, for example, some doctors and health practitioners are adopting and recommending Tai Chi Chuan as a safe exercise for the elderly to reduce the incidence of falls. More funding, and perhaps less scepticism by fellow professionals, is needed so that larger and more diverse studies can be performed. Their potential results should help us determine an interesting future role of Tai Chi and Traditional Chinese Medicine.

The Basics

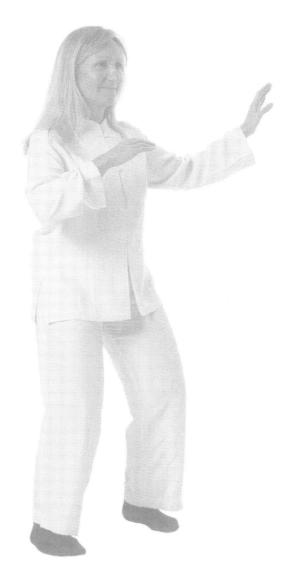

PART TWO

INTRODUCTION

It is the basics within Tai Chi Chuan that are perhaps the most important element to the art. They form the foundations from which we can learn and grow. Strong foundations allow us to build upon them consecutive layers of knowledge, one level at a time, so that we can develop and mature in a constructive fashion. By this process we can be sure that we harvest the art's benefits in the most advantageous way available. Weak foundations, however, have quite the opposite effect. Without a solid grasp of the Tai Chi Chuan fundamentals, practice will yield little return and reap no benefit. Only a genuine understanding of the basics can help you to make sure that Tai Chi Chuan is as safe and effective a discipline as possible.

It is for this reason that I have dedicated one whole section to the basics of Tai Chi Chuan. By the early disbandment of misconceptions and erroneous beliefs, healthy practice can hopefully prevail and provide you with a holistic art from which you will be able to benefit.

This section will attempt to answer many of the common questions that are asked by the complete Tai Chi Chuan beginner, and allow you to gain confidence before you stride forward to begin your first class. Tai Chi Chuan involves the body as well as the mind, and whilst some other sections of this book may have given you food for thought, this section will provide you with the more practical side of the art. It will look at the universal suitability of Tai Chi Chuan, and examine what the complete art actually involves. This book, however, does not offer the complete art – no book can. Instead it offers an outline of what can be provided and achieved within the structure of 10 15-minute sessions. Your first few attempts at practice will undoubtedly throw up many simple practical problems, and some of the most common of these are described here.

Perhaps the most important part of this section is that given to the Tai Chi principles and concepts. The principles and concepts lie behind the movements of the Tai Chi method, and it is only through them that we are able to derive the art's benefits. They are thus paramount to our understanding. They give us guidance on how best to approach the art as well as providing the fundamental elements needed for growth and development. However, I do not intend to focus solely on them. Instead, what is described are some of the essential factors that will aid beginners to enjoy and gain from the art that is Tai Chi Chuan.

WHO CAN DO TAI CHI CHUAN?

Stereotypical images of the art are usually associated with Chinese elderly folk practising in parks at dawn and dusk. Undeniably, many elderly people do practise in this fashion. It provides them with gentle exercise that will not only increase tone, balance and flexibility but also aid in the improvement and prevention of illness. However, the art is not restricted to this section of the population. Neither is Tai Chi Chuan exclusively for those who are fit, or eager to learn about the internal martial arts; nor is it only accessible to those who follow Taoism as their primary religion. All these images, although applicable, do not represent the whole of what the art can offer. Ultimately, too often it is our own preconceived ideas that hinder the unlocking of the hidden potential that can be achieved from Tai Chi Chuan.

In fact Tai Chi Chuan's doors are open to all who wish to pursue its method. It precludes nobody. It does not distinguish between the social classes, and is available to all, irrespective of race, religion and creed. Builders, architects, doctors, nurses, teachers, students, computer experts, martial artists, clergymen, spiritualists, housewives, circus clowns, all can and do practise Tai Chi Chuan.

The Tai Chi method is multifaceted, and whilst there may be myriad reasons why you may want to start, it is the mental and the physical health benefits that are universal to all. Good exercise leads to good health, high spirits and rational thinking. However, many forms of exercise and sports have built-in limitations. Your own fitness, age, strength, speed and gender can hinder participation and the achievement of the full benefits. Tai Chi Chuan is different – with a skilled instructor who can adapt Tai Chi to your needs, even the most severe disabilities will not exclude you. The marvel is that truly anybody can profit from the art regardless of age, ability or disability. There are simply no physical or mental barriers.

WHAT DOES TAI CHI CHUAN INVOLVE?

Tai Chi Chuan is a complete system. Its roots historically stem from the martial arts, with traditionalists categorizing the Tai Chi system as part of the 'internal' arts. Martial arts are separated into two distinct camps – the internal and the external martial arts – each with a different approach to self-defence. The external arts rely on muscular power, strength, speed and use of technique for their fighting potential. However, it was by combining the theories of Chinese medicine, fighting applications and Taoist philosophy that the importance of training both the mind and body, together with the spirit, was recognized, and hence a potent new internal system of combat developed. It was this internal system that was called Tai Chi Chuan – the Great Ultimate Fist.

In Tai Chi Chuan the aim is not to increase physical muscular strength, but instead is to cultivate, develop and apply our internal energy or Chi. However, the use of the internal energy is not limited to the improvement of health. Instead, through the correct development of Chi, a potent penetrating power can be generated that can be used effectively for self-defence. No matter how strong you are in muscle power, at some stage you will always be met by someone who is stronger. There is only one method that can surmount the power of muscle and that is the power of the mind and Chi. It is the relentless power of Chi, used in conjunction with the infinite diversity of soft and supple Tai Chi techniques that will overcome the hard and aggressive power of muscle. Thus the Tai Chi method creates tremendous power, which, when used by a Master, is irresistible and potentially fatal.

The applications of the art today, however, are much more varied and passive, with an outlook more geared towards health. Self-defence in Tai Chi's modern-day profile tends to take a back seat, and is often not in the curriculum of many schools. Whilst less emphasis may be placed on its combat applications, what must not be forgotten is that the art's traditions of self-defence sprang from the same traditional training system that produced Tai Chi Chuan's multifaceted benefits. Purists thus argue that to achieve the complete and traditional Tai Chi Chuan that encompasses all that the art has to offer, a traditional approach must be taken. Traditional Tai Chi Chuan needs a traditional training method. The old Masters maintained that the art consisted of three fundamental elements. Thus, traditional Tai Chi Chuan training consists of a triad of form practice, Chi Kung and pushing hands, which are all vital for a student's development. Here we take a look at each.

Forms

At the heart of Tai Chi Chuan is a series of coordinated and linked movements known as a *form*. The art is perhaps most famous for its forms. Almost everyone who sees their movements associates them correctly with Tai Chi Chuan. They are as distinctive as they are unique, and few mistake them for being anything else. When a form is performed accurately, it radiates an image of perpetual motion within a circular frame. Practitioners are deeply engaged with their practice, oblivious to any distractions, and in this sense many that watch the movements of the art often describe them as a moving state of meditation. But whilst Tai Chi Chuan certainly does have its meditative aspects, the forms play a much greater role to the Tai Chi practitioner.

Forms are usually slow in nature; however, some schools will teach faster forms within their curriculum to more senior students. Beginners to the art often start by learning a slow empty-handed form so that a concise and methodical approach can be taken. Forms vary in length from school to school. A short form will take around four to five minutes to complete, whereas a long form will take anything up to fifteen minutes. Whatever type of form you start to learn, it is this that becomes the backbone of your Tai Chi practice. The form contains within it flowing circular movements. Carrying them out with a relaxed body devoid of muscular tension not only allows the internal energy to be harnessed, but also gives Chi direction, so that it can flow naturally within the body.

Forms, especially those of the empty-handed type, provide the ideal skeleton from which large amounts of detailed information can hang. All Tai Chi Chuan forms are learned in fine detail. However, throughout every exacting movement that is learnt, there are underlying common principles and concepts that apply throughout. Tai Chi principles and concepts are fundamental for progress. It is only through them that you can grow and develop, and hence gain Tai Chi's benefits. Conversely, learning movements without learning the principles and concepts gives you only a shell of the whole and will hence yield little return. The empty-handed forms create the perfect platform from which these common principles and concepts can be learned and applied.

Perhaps second to the knowledge of your instructor, 'posture testing' is the most useful tool in consolidating knowledge from the form. It is said that once the principles and concepts are integrated well within our forms, Chi will flow freely within us. It is through this unblocked flow of internal energy that our movements and postures will derive natural strength and intrinsic stability. Posture testing is thus an important method through which you can assess your posture's strength and stability by means of a push or external force applied by a partner. This will give you a direct measure of your ability to apply the Tai Chi principles. Postures that are strong and stable to testing should reassure you that the posture is correct and that you have applied the principles well. However, postures that are weak and unstable should alert you that the posture is incorrect and may need further attention. Posture testing is an integral part of Tai Chi Chuan form practice, and by methodically focusing on particular postures and movements from the form, and then 'testing' them, you can ensure that your forms are using the Tai Chi principles to the best of your ability.

Whilst we put much emphasis on Tai Chi Chuan's principles and concepts, we must always remember the art's martial origins. Hidden within every Tai Chi movement of the form is a logical and practical combat application. Thus those who preach a traditional method of teaching should also be able to demonstrate that Tai Chi Chuan is not simply aimless arm waving, but that each movement can be effectively used as a potent form of self-defence. If any movement cannot be used in combat then clearly the movement is incorrect. In the hands of a true Master, Tai Chi Chuan is little less than the ultimate of martial arts, uniquely able to apply in combat the potent power generated from Chi energy.

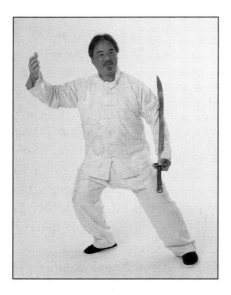

Martial content may be less obvious in Tai Chi's empty-handed forms but the art clearly maintains this element in its weapon forms. The various weapons used in Tai Chi are seen as extensions of the body. As such, a sound grasp of the knowledge contained within the empty-handed form must be gained before progressing to the weapon forms. Sword forms, broadsword forms and staff forms are just a few examples that are in Tai Chi Chuan's armoury. Each weapon demands different skills and each brings with it its own set of benefits. However, apart from each individual weapon's merits, what is often forgotten is that the weapon forms are also adjuncts to the empty-handed forms. Whilst the latter applies the core principles and concepts with the hand, the former applies those same principles through and with the weapon. Hence Tai Chi Chuan weapon forms not only provide us with new skills but also further help to consolidate and extend our existing knowledge of Tai Chi Chuan.

Chi Kung (or Qigong)

Chi Kung is a form of meditation. All forms of meditation, though similar in concept, are very different in practice. Buddhists see their meditation as essentially a spiritual process seeking mental liberation and enlightenment. However in Tai Chi, meditation takes the form of Chi Kung exercises and is focused on the training of consciousness and the development of the vital energy Chi. Chi Kung is the second part of the triad that is traditional Tai Chi Chuan. It is said that whilst the Tai Chi Chuan forms give Chi energy direction and speed, it is Chi Kung that stimulates, concentrates and develops the Chi in the first place.

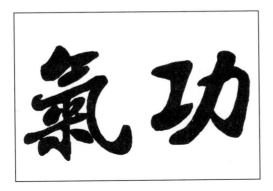

Chi Kung

'Chi Kung' is made up of two Chinese characters – 'Chi' and 'Kung'. Whilst the literal translation of 'Chi' is life energy, force or breath, the meaning behind 'Kung' is far less obscure and is usually used to represent work and the work place. Thus together Chi Kung can be taken to mean a system that works with Chi.

Although Chi Kung is part of Tai Chi Chuan, it is also a separate discipline in its own right, with its own set of Masters who focus exclusively on Chi Kung exercises and their applications. There are many styles of Chi Kung. Whilst the outward expression of some are dynamic and contain movement, others may be static and still. The emphasis can differ between styles of Chi Kung but essentially the goal is the same: to work with Chi to harness and focus our internal energy.

One particular style of Chi Kung often used in Tai Chi Chuan practice is Zhan Zhuang Chi Kung. It is a unique ancient Chinese exercise system based on the Taoist principles of harmony, simplicity and naturalness, and its aim is to cultivate, focus and balance the flow of Chi energy within the body, relaxing the mind, strengthening and improving health. It is used by many Tai Chi practitioners, and also as an independent exercise system, commonly practised by Chinese people in parks or gardens. Just like Tai Chi Chuan, it can be done by people of all ages, no matter what their lifestyle or state of fitness.

The Chinese words 'Zhan Zhuang' can be taken to mean 'standing like a stake or tree'. Zhan Zhuang Chi Kung consists of a set of standing postures that involves no obvious external movement. Some underestimate the simplicity of this exercise because of its static appearance. However, those who have had first-hand experience of Zhan Zhuang will acknowledge that, like Tai Chi Chuan, it is deceptively demanding physically and deeply absorbing mentally.

With consistent practice you can stimulate and concentrate Chi so that it can be used in different ways. Tai Chi Chuan is one method by which Chi can be applied. However, through Zhan Zhuang Chi Kung this energy can also be directly used for spiritual awareness and healing. Zhan Zhuang, and hence Chi, bring changes to both body and mind. Just as Tai Chi Chuan can be used as a mode of treatment for many illnesses, Zhan Zhuang and Chi cultivation can also be used to heal the sick. Numerous people with chronic conditions such as high blood pressure, heart conditions, asthma, weight problems, balance problems, etc. have found that regular practice has helped them, and improved their conditions. Moreover, in the hands of a Chi Kung Master, it is said that Chi can flow from one person to another and thereby a Master can heal other people – in much the same way as the Western concept of healing by the laying on of hands or spiritual healing.

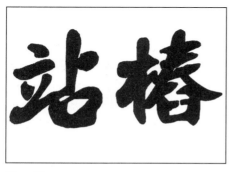

Zhan Zhuang

Push Hands (Tui Shou)

Tui Shou, which is literally translated as Push Hands, forms the third part of the traditional Tai Chi Chuan triad. Tui Shou is a fluid, rhythmical set of hand and body movements performed between two people together. It emphasizes the application of Chi, rather than its development and movement within the body. Tui Shou is based on the Tai Chi forms, drawing from many of their movements and postures. Hence, those principles and concepts found within the forms can be extended to Tui Shou. As such, there are many parallels that can be drawn between them. Both are fluid in action, and both focus on the movement of energy, so that they share the same stability of stance and solidity of structure. However, Tui Shou requires you to work in cooperation with someone else so that you can gain experience of putting Tai Chi principles into action – something that cannot be done by practising the forms alone. Tui Shou is applied Tai Chi Chuan.

Often teachers will teach Tui Shou only after you have learned the form for a period of time, and have familiarized yourself with many of the principles and concepts that lie behind Tai Chi Chuan. Once you have an understanding

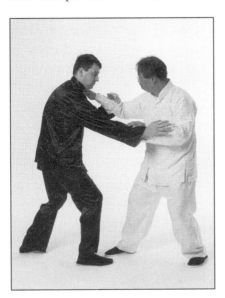

of these fundamentals, Tui Shou can then be taught to demonstrate how Tai Chi's principles can be applied. Tui Shou is primarily a dynamic exercise between two people who face each other. There are many types, which can range from a single-handed sequence of repeated movements to a full-length two-person set. Each type of Tui Shou has a particular use and function. Although little seen in public, Tui Shou is important, and forms a large part of Tai Chi practice.

Tui Shou demands interaction, cooperation and trust between the two students. It also requires a willingness to concede part of yourself to your partner in order to gain its full benefits. Tui Shou's most superficial aspect involves one partner constantly testing the other person's posture structure and stability by applying pressure in different directions. If you find yourself being pushed away by your partner, it shows a weakness in your own posture and represents a flaw in the application of the Tai Chi principles within that posture. Therefore, you can reflect upon the mistakes found by your partner, and correct them as necessary. Tui Shou is thus a process that encourages and reinforces the persistent correct practice of Tai Chi Chuan.

Through regular practice of Tui Shou, something quite extraordinary develops. Consistent correct practice allows the skin on the hands, arms and the rest of the body to become more sensitive and receptive to touch. With your heightened senses you become more aware of yourself and others. You develop sensitivity to your partner's forces and intentions during Tui Shou. Your reactions also speed up as you rely less on sight and more on touch to anticipate your partner's movements. You also slowly acquire the ability to project your energy directly through your partner, using it to push them away on contact. The Chinese believe that all these abilities and more are due to the development of energies (or 'geng') brought about by different methods of applying Chi. Thus Tui Shou's higher aspects involve the application of Chi through various methods in order to first recognize and then develop these energies.

Some common energies often associated with Tui Shou are as follows:

- Teng Geng (listening energy): the ability to feel the direction of push on contact
- Nien Geng (adhering energy): the ability to stick and keep in contact with your partner
- Far Geng (neutralizing energy): the ability to neutralize the force directed towards you by your partner
- Fa Geng (explosive energy): the ability to project your own Chi, and throw your partner away in any direction.

Master Ding demonstrating 'Fa Geng'

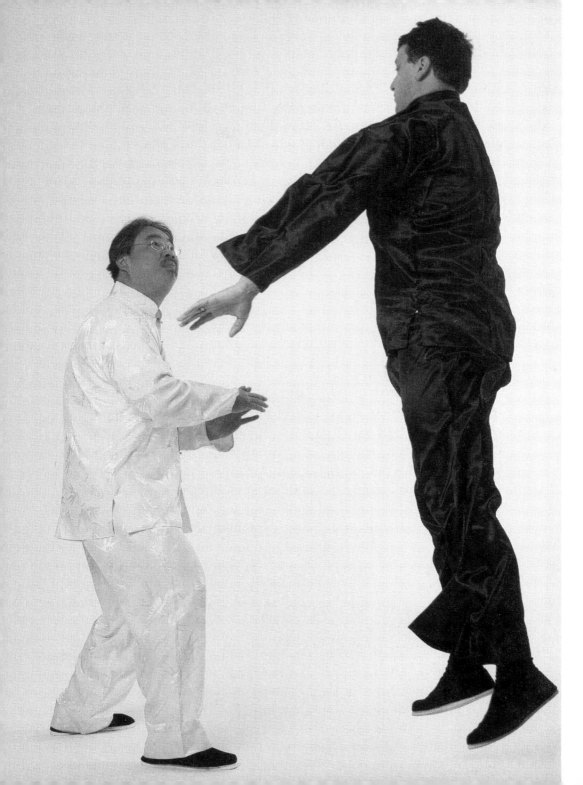

However, using these energies is not restricted to Tui Shou alone, but in fact has a much wider implication. Integrating the various forms of energies, or 'Geng Likk', creates a potent form of martial art that contains within it a powerful force that is also sensitive to the opponent. This is Tai Chi Chuan self-defence. Tui Shou, then, is a method that is multi-layered, whose essence is to develop the application of Chi so that ultimately it can be used for self-defence.

WHERE DO I START?

Traditional Tai Chi Chuan is a vast discipline that has many elements contained within it. In its full entirety the art is complex, taking time and commitment to refine and develop. To claim that this or any book could transmit the complete tradition would be a fallacy, and would do Tai Chi Chuan an injustice. The full art is simply too deep and too subtle. However, the beauty of Tai Chi Chuan is that to whatever depth you wish to take the art, and whatever level you aspire to, its core essence remains the same regardless of whether you are a beginner or advanced practitioner. Even with a small amount of practice you can still gain from Tai Chi Chuan's benefits.

To this end, *15-Minute Tai Chi* brings together those core essentials to give you an introduction to this fascinating art. It will teach you the fundamentals of Tai Chi Chuan to bring calm and tranquillity so that you can begin to cultivate the vital Chi energy. Thus, through regular practice you will not only become stronger and healthier in body but also in mind.

Tai Chi Chuan will change and settle you on many levels. Physically you will notice your balance improve, and your body strengthen and tone. Equally you will feel healthier and more revitalized from the inside. Tai Chi will not change the world around you, but it will change your outlook upon it. Whilst it may give you respite from the stresses and strains of modern-day living, the art is far deeper. It is not a way of simply avoiding the challenges and difficulties of life, but is a method which brings mental awareness and clarity of thought that will encourage you to live life more deeply, richly and truthfully.

15-Minute Tai Chi takes a concise and methodical approach to learning that allows you, even if you have little or no previous experience of Tai Chi Chuan, to explore and harvest its benefits, through carefully selected aspects of Traditional Tai Chi Chuan designed specifically to meet these needs. Furthermore, if you want to take the art further, it provides an introduction to Tai Chi's fundamental aspects. Each of the 10 routines in this book will take you on a journey that starts from Zhan Zhuang Chi Kung, through the Tai Chi form, and finally ends with settling breathing exercises. These sessions are adapted so that they are as easy to learn as they are safe and effective. Following in the Tai Chi Chuan tradition, they are open to all, and can be practised by everyone, irrespective of age, fitness or ability.

The three disciplines that you will learn in this book are:

John Ding Yeung San Chi Kung

The John Ding Yeung San Chi Kung is a set of eight postures based upon the Zhan Zhuang system. 'Yeung San' literally translated has the meaning 'cultivation of life'. Thus aptly, the name Yeung San Chi Kung represents a system whose essence is to harvest and develop the vital energy of life, Chi. Its method, similar to other types of Zhan Zhuang, involves standing in still postures that exhibit no obvious external movement. However, whilst standing in stillness may appear simple, the truth is that the Yeung San Chi Kung is deeply involving both physically and mentally.

As you begin to use these postures their stillness will gradually permeate you throughout, settling your mind and body so that you can become centred and focused. Your breathing should also be slowed and deepened. As each breath is taken, it is projected from the diaphragm and abdomen, and not from the chest. This effectively eliminates the use of the accessory breathing muscles within the chest, so that breathing is unforced, natural and relaxed. Indeed, in using Yeung San Chi Kung you should endeavour to relax and make the whole of your body free from tension. Once this is achieved, Chi will flow freely and will begin the cultivation process. Your mind too should be relaxed and cleared, as you use the intention of the

太
極
拳

mind, or 'Yi', to gather and focus the Chi at a point two inches below the navel, the Tan Tien – the body's central energy point.

Useful tips when practising Chi Kung

For complete beginners, start off by practising from 30 seconds to a minute on each posture. If you have problems with your knees, try not to bend them too low. Slowly increase the time to 5 or more minutes per posture. For more experienced and seasoned practitioners, when you find the posture too easy, it is a sign that you should lower your position by bending further at the knees.

Caution: Take care not to bend the knees too far, or beyond the toes in the early stages of practising Chi Kung, as there is danger of damage to the knees. Practise the Chi Kung at a comfortable level so that you will gradually strengthen your legs and knees. As they get stronger, you may decide to lower your stance slowly.

John Ding Tai Chi Chuan Form

In all the different styles of Tai Chi Chuan, the form is used as a tool to help you slowly bring together the natural harmony of the mind, body and spirit. The word 'natural' is important, as it requires the re-education of your mind, body and spirit so that Chi can once again flow freely and naturally. This process necessitates time, effort, perseverance and patience to achieve the ultimate state of naturalness. The essence of all Tai Chi Chuan forms is to achieve this by developing the 13 Tai Chi Chuan postures, which comprise the Ba Gua (or Eight Trigrams) and the principles of Wu Hang (or Five Elements).

Ba Gua is commonly referred to as the four sides and four corners of a square. The four sides are considered to be apparent and obvious within the form and consist of Pang (Ward Off), Lu (Roll Back), Ji (Press) and An (Push), whilst the four corners are unseen and disguised, and are composed of Cai (Pull Down), Lie (Split), Zhou (Elbow) and Kao (Shoulder). The principles of the Five Elements (Wu Hang) embody the concepts of Jin (advancing),

Tui (withdrawing), Gu (to be aware or attentive), Pan (gazing) and Ding (to be still).

Most traditional forms are complex and long, requiring both a large space and the luxury of time to learn and practice. The John Ding Form (JDF) is a simplified 20-step empty-handed form based on Traditional Yang Style Tai Chi Chuan that embraces the essence of the art – the 13 postures. It is also a form that is not only easy to learn but also requires less space to carry out. As such, it is ideal for the 15-minute Tai Chi programme. JDF has been put together for maximum holistic benefit. It is also based on the results of Tai Chi Chuan research and on over 30 years of my own martial arts and Tai Chi Chuan teaching experience for health, energetic and martial applications.

Embodying Tai Chi Chuan's essence and holistic nature, this form is suitable for men and women, young and old alike, whether strong or weak. Even with a small amount of practice, you will find beneficial effects to your health. For those who want to pursue Tai Chi Chuan training further, JDF will provide you with a good foundation and understanding to help you continue your training in the complete traditional system of Yang Style Tai Chi Chuan.

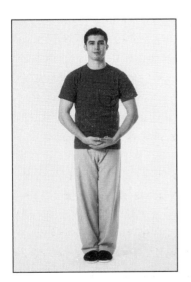

Settling Breathing Exercises

This Settling Breathing Exercise routine is usually carried out towards the end of any Tai Chi training session. The primary aim of this exercise is to re-establish the harmony of the mind, body and spirit by centring our mind and settling the Chi energy at our centre, i.e. the Tan Tien point, through the final standing meditative posture. Thus, while other parts of the session serve to cultivate, circulate and strengthen the Chi, it is through stillness and the quieting of the mind, body and spirit that we end each session.

As with Tai Chi Chuan, the Settling Breathing Exercise sequence also promotes the:

- circulation of Chi in our body by opening and unblocking the Chi meridians
- quietening of the mind and settling of Chi at the Tan Tien point
- gentle stretching and toning of the muscles
- relaxation of the mind and body
- development of natural and deep breathing
- maintenance of good balance.

PRACTICAL ISSUES

Every road has its twists and bumps, and the road to achieving the multitude of benefits that Tai Chi has to offer is no different. The Tai Chi journey can be fraught with simple problems that can waylay many students, and those of you who are in search of peace and relaxation through the art can instead be left dazed, as the senses are bombarded by the diversity of stimuli it brings.

Here are some of the most common questions students starting out on their study of Tai Chi ask. The answers will allow you to negotiate your way through some of the more usual problems novice students encounter, and will put you on a route that is as smooth and as trouble-free as possible.

How do I begin practising Tai Chi Chuan?

If you have not done Tai Chi Chuan before, the experience will probably be new and initially quite alien. However, in time you will become more familiar with the Tai Chi way of moving, and more accustomed to the effects of Chi flowing within the body. Always remember to approach Tai Chi in a relaxed way, and let your interest and involvement develop at its own natural pace. Try not to learn any new postures until you are fully confident with those that you have learnt before. Work at your own pace and bear in mind that not every-thing has to be learnt in the first session – quality is always better than quantity.

When can I practise 15-minute Tai Chi?

Tai Chi Chuan can be done at any time of the day or night. This gives you almost 24 hours from which to pick a quiet 15 minutes to go through these Tai Chi Chuan routines. Some people choose to practise in the early hours of the morning, when the world around them is at its quietest and the air is at its freshest. This not only is a great way to wake yourself up, but is also a brilliant way to energize your system before you start the day. If you are not a morning person, then Tai Chi can be performed at other times too. Some use it to refresh themselves and to regain focus during breaks after long hours in front of a computer or doing paperwork, whilst others, after a hard day's work, will practise these routines to revitalize themselves for the evening ahead. Tai Chi Chuan is flexible, and should you decide to a give it a little time each day, the rewards it brings are worth all the time and effort you put in.

Is 15 minutes enough and how often do I need to practise?

Fifteen minutes of Tai Chi a day is all that is needed to invigorate you from within and achieve many of the art's benefits. The key is to practise every day – even five minutes is better than none at all. This can be challenging, especially as many of us fail to give ourselves something as simple as 15 minutes of our own time each day. Whilst we may work late, service the car, pick up the children, mow the lawn and fix the house, too often we neglect our own needs, prioritizing others before ourselves. To take regular time out for ourselves is as important as giving our time to others. And using this time out to integrate short Tai Chi routines into our day-to-day lives will benefit all of us, in mind, body and spirit.

Make time for yourself by deciding on a realistic part of the day when you are able to put aside 15 minutes to practise the Tai Chi Chuan programme, and discipline yourself to adhere to the time you choose. Make any necessary arrangements to ensure that you won't be disturbed during these practice sessions; tell people what you are doing so that they know not to disturb you, and take the phone off the hook. Fifteen minutes in which you can be assured peace and quiet can be a haven, and creating this space will give you the peace of mind you need to relax and concentrate on your Tai Chi practice.

Once you have found the time to use these routines, you must also be consistent in your approach to practice. Regular daily 15-minute sessions are the key to success. There is little benefit in doing Tai Chi one day but then neglecting it the next. The more often you practise the more you are likely to benefit from it. Giving yourself realistic targets is one way in which you can develop a good habit. Try practising your 15-minute routine every day for a hundred days. This will not only give you a focus but will also pro-vide you with a method in which you can cultivate self-discipline. Sure, there will be some days when you really won't want to practise, but at the same time there will be other occasions when you feel 15 minutes simply isn't enough. Try to keep a balanced approach by sticking to the 15 minutes each day – any extra is a bonus. Positive habits are hard to develop, but once you begin to climb the hill and peer over the summit, you will begin to see and feel the attractions that Tai Chi has to offer and at that point you'll feel that it was all worth the effort.

Should I eat before practising?

Perhaps one of the only things that will restrict when you practise is the timing of when you eat. As a general rule, it is best not to practise for an hour after a full meal. During this time your digestive system is busily working, drawing a large supply of blood to the stomach. Practising Tai Chi in this instance will disrupt the digestive process as blood is drawn to other parts of the body. As a result this may give rise to feelings of nausea, stom-ach discomfort, dizziness and even fainting.

Similarly, practising when you are hungry is not a good idea either. The practice of Tai Chi Chuan will increase the activities of many of your physi-ological functions. This will increase the demands on you and your body, and fuel in the form of food must be at hand to supply these needs. Hunger is usually a symptom that fuel stores may already be low. To practise when you are hungry can therefore only lead to imbalance and illness, as fuel stores are unable to meet bodily demands.

Where should I practise?

Practising these 15-minute routines only requires a small amount of flat floor space. However, the bigger the space, the less claustrophobic you will feel, and the more aesthetically pleasant and comfortable it will be. Tai Chi Chuan can be practised both indoors and outdoors. Any indoor space used should be well ventilated and cool. The availability of mirrors in some training areas can be a blessing. Chinese masters often refer to the mirror as being 'the second teacher'. Looking into mirrors will heighten your awareness of each individual Tai Chi posture that you practise, and will enable you to adjust any incorrect body alignments to achieve the precision required of each posture. The use of mirrors can make practising Tai Chi postures much easier, and hence help you move forward that much more quickly.

If you decide to practise outdoors you should make sure that the wind isn't too strong, and that you dress appropriately for the temperature. Draughty, windy or cold conditions are said to cool the body too quickly and cause tension through the tightening of muscles. Direct sunlight should also be avoided, as this can cause our body systems to overheat and lose excess fluids through sweat. Parks, riversides and even our own gardens are usually ideal, especially in spring and autumn. But perhaps the most important factor of any venue you choose is that it should be quiet and free of disturbance or distractions, so that you can focus on the Tai Chi practice ahead.

What should I wear?

No special clothing is required for the practice of Tai Chi Chuan. Any loose-fitting clothing will be suitable as long as it will allow you to move with complete freedom. Simply dressing in tracksuit bottoms and a T-shirt are usually ideal for giving freedom of movement, even during the more expansive positions of the form.

Tai Chi Chuan, however, should be practised in light, thin-soled footwear or even barefoot. The Chinese slipper (or Kung Fu shoe) is perfect for practice. Usually made of black cloth, these shoes can come with a variety of soles – rope, rubber or plastic. Rope will rot if it gets damp, plastic will tend to slip on polished or wet surfaces, and rubber often will grip too well on the rough, so take your choice according to your normal practice surface. If you are unable to find this type of shoe then old-fashioned gym shoes or plimsoles are suitable, as are some dance or ballet shoes. Trainers can sometimes be heavy and with a high-raised sole can be cumbersome for sensitive floor contact as well as make twisting movements more awkward.

What kinds of physical feelings am I likely to experience when I start to practise?

You will be surprised at the range of sensations you will feel even with just 15 minutes of practice a day. Tai Chi Chuan will affect you on many levels and in ways that you would never expect. It will heighten the senses so that you will become more aware of each and every body component. Superficially, the stretching and toning process will allow you to unearth dormant muscles that you never knew existed. However, on a deeper level, it is through the cultivation and strengthening of Chi that you will discover a variety of strange yet wonderful sensations. Each of us will experience the movement of Chi in a slightly different way; here are just a few of the sensations that you may come across as you begin to practise Tai Chi Chuan.

Changes in body temperature: This is common in Tai Chi practice, and may vary from one extreme to the other. Whilst some may feel extremely hot, wiping beads of sweat from their brows, others may find parts of their bodies become cold and even slightly numb. All these sensations are

太
極
拳

normal and not only do they vary among us, but they also vary within us too. Some days you may feel warm and sweaty during practice, but other sessions may leave you feeling cool and fresh.

Sweating: This is a natural process that occurs in all of us, but it is sometimes exacerbated when we do Tai Chi. Sweating is a method to expel toxins from within us. It is also the main mechanism that helps to cool down our system after the generation of heat from exercise. Some people can experience large amounts of sweating during practice, and they can lose up to a litre of body fluid especially in hotter weather. But even if you don't sweat much, remember that you should always take enough clear fluids during practice to avoid dehydration. Water is usually best. Avoid coffee, tea and alcohol as they will cause dehydration rather than remedy it.

Also after any form of exercise, especially Tai Chi, try to let the body cool down naturally before having a shower or wash. Although you could feel hot, smelly and sticky after a routine, the sudden cooling down of the body system can be bad for your health, and you may end up doing more damage than good.

Shakes: Experiencing the shakes is perhaps the most common when we begin Tai Chi Chuan. They usually present themselves as fine shiver-like movements but can manifest as larger, almost flapping movements. Typically they start from the legs and move up the body. It is said that shaking is the result of the sinking of Chi energy to the Tan Tien point – an area two inches below the navel that acts as a reservoir of Chi. The body is said to be unable to cope with this sudden surge and concentration of energy at this point and hence reacts by shaking. However, over time the shakes can disappear as the body becomes accustomed to this movement of Chi.

Should the shakes persist, you could try the following:

1 Check your posture to ensure that you have carried it out correctly. You may be bending the knees too far and hence causing the Chi to flow too quickly and vigorously to the Tan Tien. Straightening the legs up slightly may help.

2 Use the intention of the mind or Yi to stabilize the Chi at the Tan Tien, stopping it from rising and causing the shakes.
3 Use the thumb and index finger of one hand to gently squeeze the last joint of the small finger of the other hand.
4 Raise the front part of the foot alternating from left to right to help disperse the Chi.

All these methods will generally help to stop the shakes while you practise. However, should they persist you may need to stop your practice for a few minutes to disperse the energy freely.

Tingling: Usually felt in the hands and fingers but can also be felt in other parts of your body too. Chi circulation is said to enhance and improve blood circulation. This will in turn open the pores of the skin, giving rise to tingling and sensations similar to pins and needles.

Numbness: You may feel this effect on different parts of the body; however, this will gradually fade and be replaced by a much more pleasant tingling sensation with continued practice.

Aches and pains: Almost all who begin Tai Chi Chuan will find that after a session or two, many of their muscles will ache and be mildly painful. Even those of you who practise other sports will not be immune to these effects. This is because the Tai Chi process slowly stretches, pulls and twists many of the muscles that were previously dormant. Aching muscles are simply a sign that they are gradually being awakened from their slumber. As you continue to practise, with time you will find that many of these aches and pains will disappear, and leave you with balance, poise and muscles that are toned and strengthened.

Many of these sensations are transient, and are a good sign that Chi is flowing freely within us. These feelings should not concern or distract you, but instead should encourage you that you are moving ahead in the right direction. If you allow these feelings to sidetrack you, you may find crossing this initial stage difficult. As you progress in training, so will the sensations you will feel. Tai Chi Chuan is dynamic and is a wonderful experience that will evolve with you the longer you continue with your practice.

Can illness, injury or disability stop me from practising Tai Chi Chuan?

Tai Chi Chuan can benefit all despite illness, injury or disability, and it is rare that its exercises do not improve or alleviate any problems or complaints. Whatever difficulties you may have, they need not restrict or compromise your practice of the art. Tai Chi Chuan is unique as its principles and concepts are of central significance to its health benefits. Its movements are a means to an end, and in many cases they can be adapted (with the help of an able Tai Chi instructor) to accommodate you and your needs. As long as you adhere to the principles you stand to gain as much as any other person. This is particularly true for those who have physical disabilities and are not able to practise Tai Chi in the conventional way. Tai Chi Chuan is about relating to the mind, body and spirit, and it is in their relationships with one another that we can *all* find ways of getting in tune with that inner experience, to harness and express Chi in a more natural way.

Is there any danger of injury?

Tai Chi is designed to be a safe and gentle activity for all to use. Its unique slow and graceful movements help to improve stability, balance and centredness. No extreme pressures and strains are applied to the joints or muscles during any of these exercises. Tai Chi Chuan will bring many strange feelings to your body that may include transient aches and pains through gentle stretching and toning. But these effects are far from injurious and are instead natural healthy signs that you are gradually achieving correct body alignment and improving posture through which Chi can flow freely.

Tai Chi and pregnancy

The holistic approach of Tai Chi Chuan makes it an ideal way of preparing expectant mothers for birth and motherhood. Regular practice of the slow, gentle and flowing movements of this ancient Chinese art helps bring together the natural balance and harmony of the mind, body and spirit – perfect when you are going through the dynamic changes of pregnancy.

- Mentally you will become more relaxed, calmer and self-confident
- Physically your body will become more centred, balanced, supple, stronger and flexible
- Spiritually you will develop inner stillness and peace

Within many Tai Chi classes there are always a handful of expectant mothers who practise right until the moment they give birth, because of the benefits that the art can bring. Not only can Tai Chi Chuan help to ensure a healthy pregnancy, but can also eradicate some common ailments such as backache, poor balance, fatigue and tiredness associated with pregnancy.

Note: If you are unsure about practising Tai Chi during pregnancy, always consult and seek advice from your doctor.

TAI CHI CHUAN – SOME GENERAL PRINCIPLES AND CONCEPTS

So far this book has emphasized the importance of the principles and concepts of Tai Chi Chuan. Outwardly we see the graceful forms that the art is most famous for. However, what we do not see are the thoughts, ideas and theories that lie behind the movement. It is these principles and concepts that guide us on how best to approach the art. They bridge the gap between the theoretical and the practical, and provide the fundamental elements that are needed for growth and development. Most importantly, though, it is from them that we derive all the benefits that the art has to offer. The principles and concepts are the core essence of Tai Chi Chuan. Without them Tai Chi would simply be aimless arm waving. Perhaps the fact that several books have been devoted solely to the art's principles and concepts serves to illustrate their importance. Whilst it is not the intention of this book to focus exclusively on this area, detailed below are some of the essential aspects that will help you to think of Tai Chi Chuan as something beyond simple body movements.

Breathing

Breathing is the most basic of all our bodily functions. It is the first and last thing we ever do. Breathing plays a large part in our general health and is closely linked to the way we think, feel and act. It can make us calmer and create emotional stability, or change in response to our physical and emotional needs. Indeed breathing drastically alters when we feel happy or sad, sing and dance or meet with threat and danger. But too often is it provoked and stimulated by the world around us, and we lose sight of our intrinsic and inborn method of breathing.

Through the practice of Tai Chi Chuan, we slowly relearn to breathe in a more natural and efficient manner. By remaining relaxed throughout your practice, without concentrating too much on your breathing, you will notice your breath reverts back to its more inborn and spontaneous form. Conversely too much focus on its control will instead lead the breath to be forced and unnatural, causing tension and disrupting the flow of Chi. Efficient breathing is more than just the re-education of the mechanics of inhalation and exhalation. It is equally important to understand that other Tai Chi Chuan principles have a huge bearing on breathing quality too. Good body alignment through understanding the relationships between the head, neck, back and chest is one of the principles that will provide an open, free-moving posture, and hence make your breathing as efficient as possible.

When you practise Tai Chi Chuan, breathe in and out normally through your nose, just as naturally as you are doing now as you read this book. With correct body alignment, breathing is made much easier, which in turn assists with the sinking of Chi to the Tan Tien point. Through regular practice, your breathing will gradually become coordinated with the Tai Chi Chuan movements. Eventually it will strengthen the diaphragm muscle and increase the volume of air capacity within your lungs, and at that point you will notice your breathing changes so that it not only becomes even but also deeper and longer.

Softness/relaxation (*Yau*)

It is not always possible to translate the true meaning of one Chinese word with one English word. Although the word 'Yau' is usually referred to as softness, it also contains within it the characteristics of pliability, flexibility, springiness and relaxation with structure and intent. When practising Tai Chi Chuan, softness, or more correctly Yau, should not be misunderstood to mean to be limp or collapsed. Instead it describes a defined structure that should be held and maintained with no tension and minimal physical force. In Tai Chi Chuan we all should endeavour to remain in Yau, a state that is not flaccid but is also far from using tensile muscular strength. It is similar to being in a swimming pool where the arms float with no effort.

Yau, and hence minimal physical strength, should be used in all parts of Tai Chi, be it in the forms, Chi Kung or Push Hands. Incorporating Yau within your practice will enable Chi to flow freely within you and gradually focus at the Tan Tien point. Once this concept is used correctly, your body paradoxically will feel more rooted, with the postures and movements becoming stronger and more stable. Relaxed and supple musculature enables Chi to flow through it, and the strength of your posture is derived from this energy and not from muscle. If tension or physical force is present then this will restrict and block the flow of Chi. Reverting to this physical force will mean that you are unable to harvest this intrinsic strength that is unique to the internal arts. This is a common mistake made by most beginners, and even by more experienced practitioners. Famous quotations in Tai Chi Chuan such as 'steel wrapped in cotton' perhaps help to describe the potent power of Chi.

Flow

The Tai Chi movements should be carried out in a smooth, even flow without any gap or pause. As one move finishes, the next begins, as if the form is in one continuous flow. It can be likened to reeling silk from a cocoon or emulating the gentle flow of water from a stream. If the form is hurried or with gaps and pauses, the flow will break and the Chi effectively will be unable to circulate efficiently. Practising Tai Chi Chuan in this controlled, unhurried, even and continuous flow helps to:

- gain focused mental and physical control in movement
- achieve complete balance
- strengthen and tone different parts of the body, i.e. muscles, tendons, ligaments and joints
- ensure the correct alignment of postures and movements – by doing Tai Chi Chuan slowly you are more likely to correct any bad postures and acquire good habits so that the flow of Chi can be maximized.

Consequently, practising Tai Chi Chuan movements with a continuous, even fluidity at a reasonably slow pace will allow many aspects and subtleties of the art to be maintained and nurtured in your training.

Intention of the mind (*Yi*)

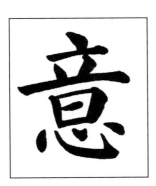

Yi can be translated to mean the idea or, more precisely, the intention of the idea. Whilst in Tai Chi Chuan intention is linked with the idea of outward projection, the art also insists that intention must be led by the mind as well. Hence within Tai Chi Chuan, Yi is taken to represent the intention of the mind. It is one of the most important and fundamental concepts that must be encompassed in all of your Tai Chi practice. Without the presence of Yi, movements are without focus and direction. Watch a cat stalk a bird or a mouse. The whole of the predator's intention is focused on one thing – to catch its prey. Its concentration is unwavering and its gaze fully engaged. Each movement is calculated, deliberate and economical. There is no wasted action.

Some misinterpret Yi as meaning 'to focus', but it is much more than that. It is a concept that binds together purpose, concentration and mental projection. It gives life to the movements of the forms. Movements and postures become purposeful – each having their own application and their own projection of energy. Awareness and good understanding of the postures give Tai Chi Chuan movements more meaning, and assist in your concentration and focus. But Yi is more; it must also contain the element of mental projection. Movements are projected beyond our hands using the mind. The Tai Chi classic writings emphasize the concept of 'Yi Dou Chi Dou' – when the intention of the mind arrives, Chi will also arrive and hence will flow and be projected. Thus, mental projection gives Chi the focus of a direction, in the form of an outward expression extending beyond our body.

For example, try pushing your partner. Ask him or her to put up a little physical resistance when you push. Do not attempt to push beyond the point of contact. In this instance, you will experience difficulty in pushing. Next, push again, but this time focus on pushing through and 10 feet beyond. With less effort on your part, your partner should be pushed away with what appears to be a much stronger force. Hence, when practising the form, Yi should always be present. Not only must we have purpose and concentration but we must also apply the use of mental projection out beyond our hands some distance.

Yin-Yang

The Yin-Yang theory has already been explained elsewhere in the context of health (see p.17). But the theory also extends to many other aspects of oriental culture. Often the Yin-Yang symbol is used to represent Tai Chi Chuan because its concepts play an integral part within the art. Tai Chi Chuan is intrinsically concerned with yin and yang, and there is a constant dynamic interplay between these two opposite forces in all aspects within our practice.

太
極
拳

The form in particular gives many examples of bringing the theory in practice. Throughout the form you will see that all the expanding, yang movements are followed by retracting, yin movements. Each flows seamlessly into the next, as yin flows into yang and back into yin in a never-ending cycle. Movements are also practised slowly (yin), yet at the same time must contain focused intent (yang). Our muscles are relaxed (yin), yet the structure of Tai Chi Chuan allows us to exhibit the inner strength of Chi (yang) – 'steel wrapped in cotton', as has been said.

Tai Chi Chuan has yin and yang everywhere within it. The entire philosophy of the art is based around it. But both theory and practice are equally important in Tai Chi Chuan. Endless theorizing and debate will yield little physical result. Likewise mere repetition of movement without input from the ideas contained within Tai Chi's principles and concepts will also reap little benefit. A Yin-Yang balance must be achieved between the two. Yin-Yang describes all things Tai Chi Chuan and beyond, and whilst the Yin-Yang symbol may look fairly simple it carries a much more profound meaning. Perhaps in much the same way that Tai Chi Chuan may look a simple exercise until you begin to do it!

Stances – rooting and weighting

Form practice dictates that the leg stances are no longer individual and instead become part of a collective of movements. Each complete stance must merge seamlessly into the next without hesitation or pause. Yet this fluidity must not come at the expense of strength, stability and rooting – the hallmark of a correct Tai Chi stance. Many practitioners make the mistake of over-emphasizing fluidity and neglect correct stance structure and weighting. Whilst this method may develop a sense of continuity what is lost is more fundamental – the ability to form a strong, stable and centred stance. Correct stances, and thus the development of rooting, not only provide you with stability within your movements and postures, but also form the solid platform from which you can project Chi.

The most common mistakes students make are that the stances are too narrow, too wide, too short or too close. As a general rule, the best way to start off is by using the following templates to help you get the correct stances with the correct weighting.

The square template stance

This can be applied in most of the stances when learning the Chi Kung or the Tai Chi Chuan forms. Start off by just standing with your feet parallel, facing forwards, with the heels shoulder-width apart. Visualize a square box with the sides being made up from the length of your shoulders' width. From this square you can make up most stances.

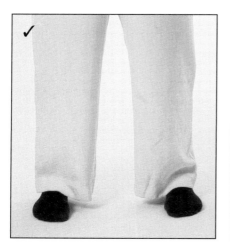
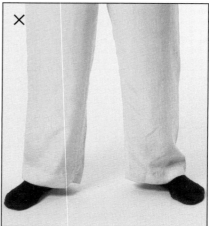

square

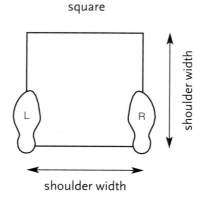

shoulder width

The rectangle template stance

This template is only applicable for people who are tall and who have longer legs. The same rules of the perfect square template apply except this time the two sides of the box become longer to accommodate the longer legs – hence forming a rectangle rather than a square. Note that the width of the rectangle is still the same – a shoulder-width apart. The length of your rectangle should be the optimal distance where you are able to bend the knees in a comfortable stance without feeling cramped or overstretching.

rectangle

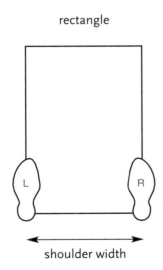

shoulder width

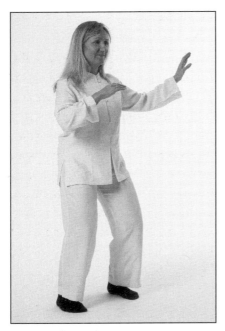

Horse Stance

Horse Stance (*Ma Bu*)

The Horse Stance is the basis of all Tai Chi footwork and resembles the riding horse position, hence the name. Use either the square or rectangle template format, i.e. standing with the feet parallel to each other and a shoulder-width apart. Then bend your knees, as you lower the body as if sitting on a stool. Keep the body relaxed and upright. An example of a Tai Chi Chuan posture using this stance is Cross Hands or commencing the form.

Bow Stance (*Kung Bu*)

Start off by using either the square template stance or, if you are tall, the rectangular template stance. With your heels at the bottom two corners of your square or rectangle, turn the right foot at a 45-degree angle. Step straight forward with the left foot, and place the heel at the corner of the top left corner of the square. Bend both knees, and shift the weight forward by bending the front knee more than the back one, so that the top half of your body moves forward. Try and adjust your knees so that 70 per cent of your weight is on the front leg and 30 per cent is on the back. Ensure that your hips are in line with the horizontal of the square, by turning your waist to the left and 'tucking in' the left Kua – the Kua represents the fold between the top of the thigh and the bottom of the abdomen. As you look down on your stance your left knee should be in line with your left toes while the right knee stays slightly bent and is rotated outward. You will feel some pressure on the left leg.

The common mistake with this position is to straighten the right knee, emulating the stances of external martial arts. Such a position causes the back leg to tense up and become rigid, thus when force is applied to the structure (as in testing) it is weak, unstable and un-rooted. Furthermore, in terms of self-defence a straightened back leg is vulnerable and can be easily broken when attacked.

This stance is suitable for everyone and is perfect for those with weakened knees. It is not only able to help heal them directly but is also able to strengthen and tone

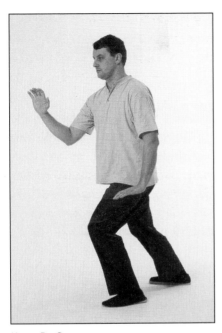

Kung Bu Stance

the muscles around the knee so that they can provide support and stability to the joint. Once your knees have become stronger, you should allow your front knee to bend forward further until the mid-point of the knee joint is in line with the front toes. Such a position makes the stance more stable and powerful and will also enable you to project Chi more effectively.

This stance is referred to as the Bow Stance, and is perhaps the most common stance within the Tai Chi Chuan form. Examples of Tai Chi Chuan postures using this stance are Brush Knee and Push, Step Forward and Punch, Ward Off and Single Whip.

Rear Bow Stance (*Hou Bu*)

In this stance, the feet are in the same position as the Bow Stance, with both knees bent. This time, however, the majority weighting is now on the back leg so that the back knee is bent more than the front: 70 per cent of your weight should be on your back leg and 30 per cent on the front. As you move backwards with the knees you should notice the top half of the body is moved backwards with the shift in weight. The back knee should be turning outwards away from the centre of the body. Indeed, turning the back knee inwards towards the centre of the body would collapse and weaken the lower structure as well as also block the Chi flow. Lastly the front knee should be slightly bent and not straightened as shown in the diagram below. An example of a Tai Chi Chuan posture using this stance is Lu (Roll Back).

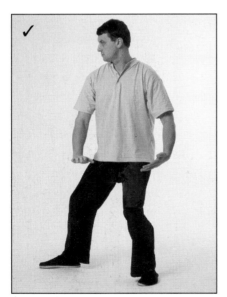
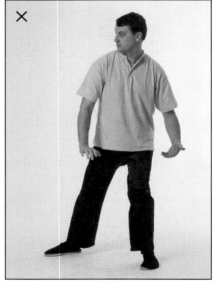

Incorrect posture:
Straightened right knee with body leaning too much to the left

Empty Stance (*Hoi Bu*)

In this stance the horizontal distance between the two heels is smaller and less than a shoulder-width. Here the square and rectangular templates above do not apply. Most of the weighting is on the rear leg with either the toes or the heel of the front foot resting lightly on the ground. The front knee should be slightly bent. For advanced students, the weighting should be fully committed on the rear leg, so that the front leg is empty, carrying no weighting – hence 'Empty Stance'. Again both knees are bent, with the back knee turned outwards away from the centre of the body. Examples of this stance in Tai Chi Chuan are White Crane Spread Wings, Lift Hands and Playing the Pipa.

太
極
拳

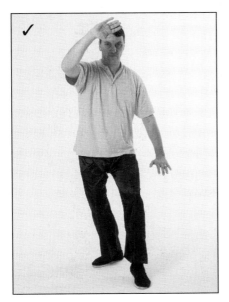 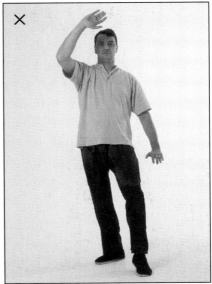

Incorrect posture:
Straightened right knee with the body leaning backwards

Body alignment

Correct body alignment is vital for the smooth flow of Chi within our body. It is particularly important in the following areas:

The head

Keep the neck straight by tucking the chin slightly inward, so that the back of the head is lifted and the neck remains vertical. Do not move the chin forward (a very common fault) as doing so causes the back of the neck to arch backwards, thus blocking the Chi flow, as shown below. Keeping a slight smile will help relax the facial muscles and reduce any tension. The eyes, being the opening to the external world, should also be opened and focusing ahead in the direction of the movement. You should keep your lips gently closed. As you do so the tip of the tongue will naturally touch the roof of the mouth, thus connecting to the circuit of the circular Chi flow. Breathing should always be done slowly and smoothly through the nose.

As we often crane our necks forward and hold our chins up unnaturally, this correct alignment may feel odd at first. But these subtle corrections to the alignment of the head allow the spirit to be lifted and Chi to travel to the crown of the head unhindered. This point is referred to by Great Grandmaster Yang Cheng Fu in one of his 10 important principles of Tai Chi Chuan. In Chinese it reads 'Xu Ling Ding Jin', which means 'Emptying the thoughts and raising the head as if the crown of the head is pressed up against the heaven'.

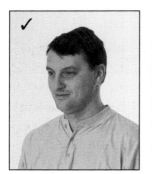 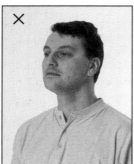

Incorrect posture:
Lifted chin which causes the neck to bend backwards

太
極
拳

The body

The emphasis on correct alignment here is to assist with the sinking of the Chi to the Tan Tien point and to enable efficient circulation of Chi through the body. The shoulder blades should be relaxed, allowing the shoulders to sink down. Lifting the shoulders causes the Chi to rise and prevents it from sinking to the Tan Tien point. We tend to carry a lot of tension in our shoulders, and you may find relaxing the shoulders difficult at first. Always check that your shoulders are relaxed when you practise. Incorrect positioning of the shoulders also affects the projection and circulation of Chi through the arms, as shown below. Relaxed shoulders help to weigh down the elbow. Weighing down the elbow lets the elbow be relaxed, drop downwards and hang loose within the arm structure. A raised elbow will cause the shoulder to lift, thus causing stagnation of Chi. This is referred to in another classic Tai Chi Chuan principle as 'Chen Lian Zhu Zhou', which means 'Sinking the shoulder and weighing down the elbow'.

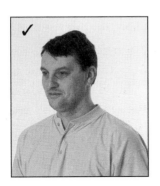 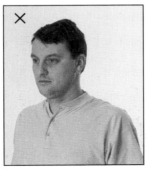

Incorrect posture:
The raised chest causes the shoulders to be lifted upwards

To assist with the sinking of Chi further, one should 'hollow' (or dip in) the chest at the base of the sternum (or solar plexus), which causes the back to rise naturally. The raised back will enable you to easily project the Chi through the spine as well as sink the Chi to the Tan Tien point. Conversely an expanded chest with a protruding sternum and the shoulders flung back causes tension, top-heaviness and lifts the heels. This will stop the Chi from sinking to the Tan Tien and will instead elevate it so that it becomes stranded at the top of chest, hence leaving you with a posture that is weak and unstable. This is another of the Tai Chi Chuan principles known as 'Han Xiong Ba Bei', or 'Hollowing the chest to raise the back'. In addition, the trunk and lower back should be maintained in an upright and straight position. It is very common to stick your tailbone out, which is bad for your back and general posture, as shown below. Instead, gently tucking the buttocks inwards causes the tailbone to move inwards and straightens your lower spine. Any backward bend of the spine will block the flow of Chi.

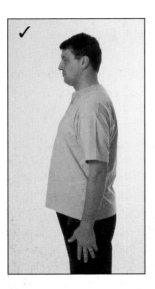
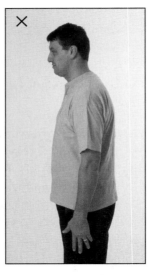

Incorrect posture:
The head and body are leaning forwards with slightly raised buttocks

Hand structure

Different hand positions in the Tai Chi Chuan form are used for different applications. The commonest is the open palm. In all open palm hand positions, the fingers should be relaxed, loose and brought together without any force or tension. The thumb should be relaxed and kept in the same plane as the fingers and palm. The most common fault observed with students is that the thumb is placed in front of the fingers, as shown below. A simple mistake in positioning such as this can cause the Chi flow along the Lung meridian to be hindered, making our whole posture weak and unstable.

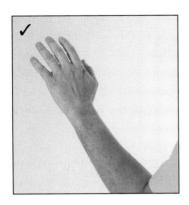
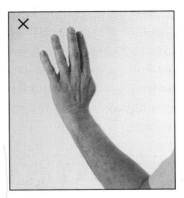

The next point to look at is the wrist. The back of the palm should not be bent backwards too much at the level of the wrist. Doing so will cause tension and impede the flow of Chi.

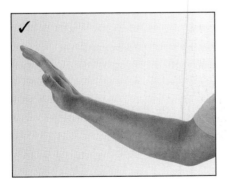
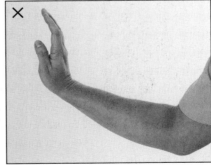

For the open palm application in the Aun or Push position, the wrist should be relaxed (see overleaf). The palms should face forwards but at the same time are also rotated slightly inwards so that the thumbs point backwards. By doing this Chi can be projected from the palms to meet at a point beyond you. If your palms are straight on and horizontal, the projected forces will be parallel and will hence never meet. This latter posture is therefore much more ineffective and weak. Testing with a partner will help validate this point.

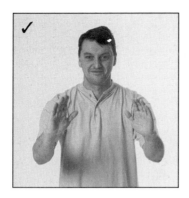 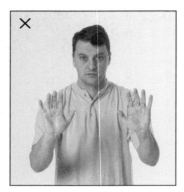

In Pang or Ward Off position, the back of the hand should be in alignment with the wrist and the forearm with the thumb pointing outwards. Here, the most common fault is allowing the left shoulder to be raised as shown below. Such faults disrupt or break the Chi flow, making the posture weak.

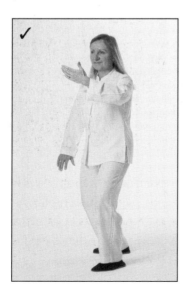 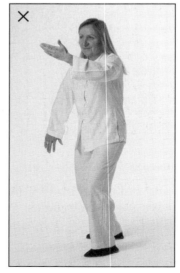

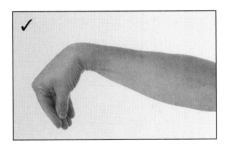 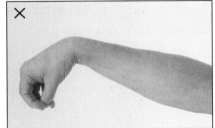

In Tan Pien or Single Whip posture, the left palm is in the Aun position while the right hand forms a hook. To form the hook, bring the thumb to touch both the index and middle finger while the remaining two fingers rest on the middle finger, creating a hook-like structure as you drop the palm downwards at the wrist. The dropped hand should be relaxed. The hook helps to loosen and increase the flexibility in the wrist joints.

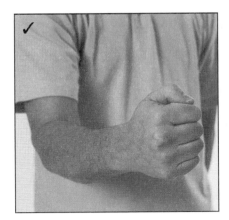 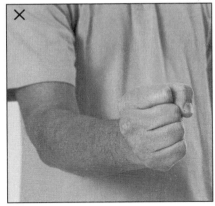

Fists are also used in Tai Chi Chuan form practices. Bringing the fingers together and folding them inwards, with the thumb resting on the index finger forms the fist. Keep your fingers loose and relaxed as if you were holding a small bird's egg. Any increase in pressure by clenching the fist too tight creates tension and thus blocks the flow of Chi. Again the back of the palm should be in line with the wrist and forearm.

The waist

The waist is an important part of Tai Chi Chuan postures. The Tai Chi Chuan classics state, 'The Chi is the wheel and waist is the axle.' This phrase stresses how important it is that all Tai Chi movements are initiated from the waist. Once the movement is initiated in this manner then Chi will flow – much like that of the relationship between the axle and the wheel. The waist should be loose and flexible, without tension. Only in this state will it enable the Chi to sink and gather in the legs to give a strong and stable base. Apart from the relaxed joints and muscles of the waist, another area of importance is the 'Kua'. This point is usually referred to as the fold at the top of the thigh and the bottom of the abdomen. The correct Kua positions enable you to sink more Chi to the legs, thus giving you more stability through a firmer base. Incorrect Kua positioning can hinder the flow of Chi to the legs and give rise to wasted Chi, which will result in poor rooting at the feet.

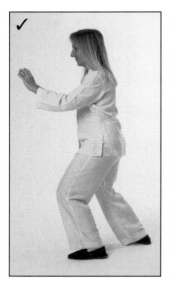 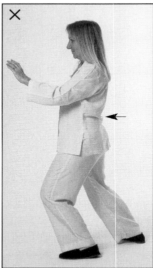

Incorrect posture: Arched back causes increased strain and tension on the spine as indicated

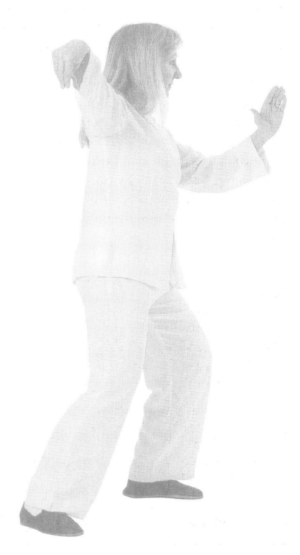

The Practice

PART THREE

Introduction

The 10 sessions of Tai Chi detailed here in 15-Minute Tai Chi have been specially designed to incorporate Chi Kung, Tai Chi Chuan and Settling Breathing Exercises to help you gain effective benefits through the practice of the ancient art of Tai Chi Chuan.

Each session is easy to learn and requires only limited space to practise, whether indoors or out. Through regular practice, you will be able to cultivate and harness the Chi for the maintenance of health, both of mind and body. Though the programme allows you to learn on your own, you will find it useful occasionally to practise with a partner, so that you can assess and monitor each other's progress.

Each of the 15-minute Tai Chi Chuan sessions is broken down into three sections:

1 John Ding Yeung San Chi Kung
2 John Ding Tai Chi Chuan Form
3 Settling Breathing Exercises

SESSION ONE

John Ding Yeung San Chi Kung

Posture 1: Wuji

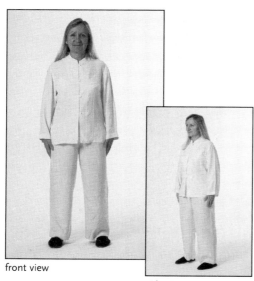

front view

side view

To begin:

1. Use the square template format, i.e. standing naturally with both feet parallel and shoulder-width apart.

2. The toes should be pointing forward and turned slightly inwards.

3. Ensure that the whole body, i.e. head, body and spine, is relaxed and correctly aligned.

4. The arms hanging down the side of the body should be relaxed and the fingers slightly separated, with the palms gently touching the thighs.

5. Your whole body should be slightly inclined forward by tucking in at the

hips with the knees a little bent and not locked.

6. Keep looking forward and slightly downward.

7. Breathe naturally through the nose and with the Yi (or intention of the mind) focused at the Tan Tien point, about two inches below the navel.

Stay in Wuji posture for at least two minutes and then relax. Shake the arms and legs and loosen up the body. Next proceed to the second part of this session.

John Ding Tai Chi Chuan Form

1. Hei Sai – Commencement

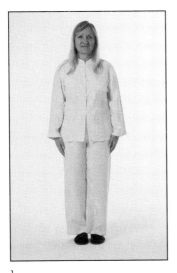

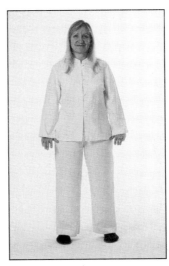

1.   2.

Preparation

1. Begin the movement with both feet together, legs straight but not locked. Keep the back straight and the shoulders down. The arms should hang down your sides with the palms of the hands touching your thighs.

2. Raise the elbows upwards and outwards, as the palms slide gently up the thighs. At the same time ensure that your shoulders are sinking downwards. Keep your arms rotated inwards with the elbows located at the side of the body. Next transfer all your weight to the left leg and move your right foot sideways, a shoulder-width apart from the left, keeping the feet parallel. Shift your weight to the middle, and make your hands trace an arc on your thighs, so that they move down just below the hips, to the side of the thighs, with the palms facing down.

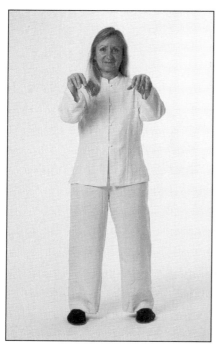

3.

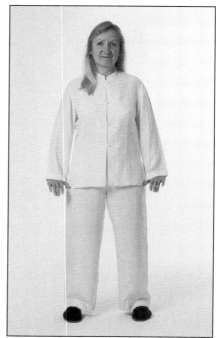

4.

Lift and Lower Hands

3. Slowly lift your hands forwards and up. As they move out, the wrists turn down. The hands should finish at shoulder height with the fingers hanging down, elbows bent slightly.

4. Next, the hands and arms move downwards and back to their original position. As they start to move down, turn your wrists up.

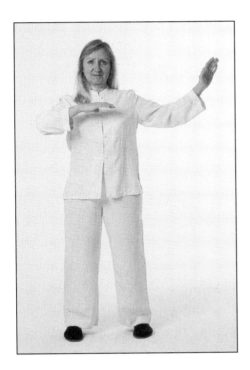

Tai Chi Circle Hands (Tai Gik Huen Sau)

Circle both arms anticlockwise in a semi-circle, starting from the right and then coming up and around to the left. The left hand should pass in front of the face, and extend out to the left at shoulder height with the elbow slightly bent. The right hand should finish up level with the centre of the chest. Make sure that you do not raise your shoulders.

2. Lan Chuek Mei: Jor Pang – Grasp the Bird's Tail: Left Single Ward Off

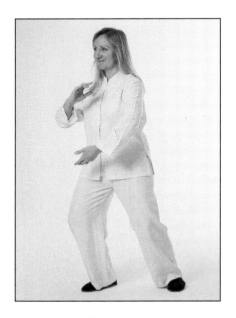

Hold the Ball (Hup Sau)

Bend the knees (Ma Bu or Horse Stance), and turn the right foot out 45 degrees, pivoting on the heel. Turn the hips slightly to the right, and let the weight move onto the right leg. The right leg is bent at the knee and you are squatting slightly. As you turn the hips to the right, both hands move across to the right-hand side of the body. The right hand ends up in a position with the palm facing down, at shoulder height, while the left hand moves underneath, and finishes with the palm turned upwards, as if you are holding a ball.

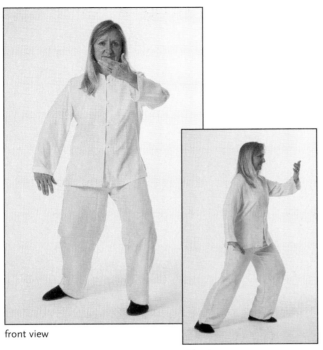

front view

side view

Left Ward Off (Pang)

Keeping your weight on the right leg, turn your hips to the left so that you face the front, square on. Step forward shoulder-width distance with the left foot, touching it down lightly with the heel first. As you move your weight forward on to your left leg to form the Left Kung Bu or Bow Stance, raise the left arm so that the forearm goes across the body. The left hand should finish level with your mouth, with the palm facing in.

Move your right hand down to your right side with the palm facing down.

Repeat the above Tai Chi Chuan movements over and over again for six to eight minutes until you are familiar with each posture. Ensure that you have incorporated all the Tai Chi principles described earlier within both the Chi Kung postures and JDF.

Settling Breathing Exercises

To conclude the first session of your 15-minute Tai Chi programme, the Settling Breathing Exercises will help you relax, settle down and also bring the mind, body and spirit together.

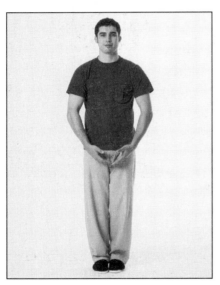

1.

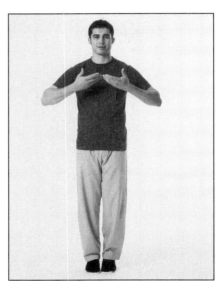

2.

1. Stand with both feet together, with the hands in front of the body, palms facing upwards.
2. Raise your heels so you are standing on tip-toe, and breathe in slowly as you bring your palms up to the chest area.
3. Turn your palms to face downwards and push downwards as you slowly breathe out and lower your heels (a and b). The raising and lowering of the heels should be in time with your breathing.

Repeat the breathing exercises slowly 10 times, maintaining a relaxed state.

4. Finish off in the 'meditative stance' by placing your palms one on top of the other, and resting them about two inches below the navel, at the Tan Tien point, facing up. The positioning of the palms is different for men and women. Women should place the left palm on top of the right, and men should place the right palm on top of the left. Gently half-close your eyes and breathe in and out slowly. Focus on the Tan Tien point and stay in this position for a few minutes.

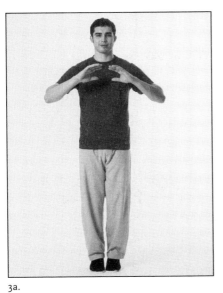

3a.

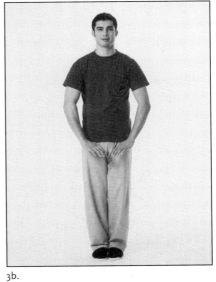

3b.

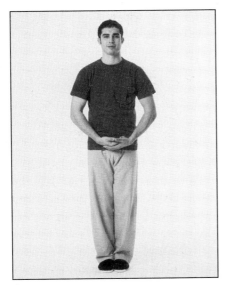

4.

This concludes the first session of the 15-minute Tai Chi programme.

SESSION TWO

John Ding Yeung San Chi Kung

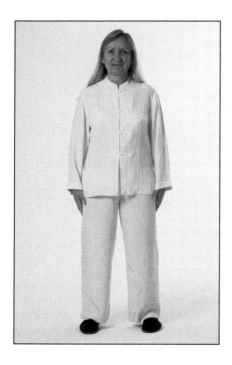

In this second session, begin with the Wuji position as practised in Session One (see page 68).

After standing for one minute, remain in the same position, and then follow the instructions below to carry out the second and the centring postures, each of which should be carried out for a minute.

Posture 2: Carrying the Ball

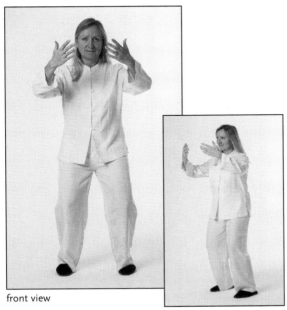

front view

side view

1. Bring both your arms upwards and outwards as if holding a beach ball (i.e. in a circular shape). Then slowly bend your knees as you sink your weight downwards to form the Ma Bu Horse Stance.

2. Your open palms should be at the level of your mouth. Both palms should be slightly rotated outwards and forwards by using the elbow as a pivot. Ensure that your wrist joints are not bent, as there should be no break in the line from the forearm to the back of the hand.

3. The fingers must be relaxed and slightly apart. Make sure that the thumbs are slightly extended and pointing upwards. Try to avoid bending the thumbs so that they point inwards, as this will cause blockage in the Chi flow of the Lung meridian.

4. The elbows should neither be pointing down vertically (which will close the armpits) nor be pointing out too far to the side (which can raise the shoulders), otherwise the energy may either be blocked or wasted. Instead the elbows should be placed in a position between these two extremes, making sure that the shoulders are relaxed and sunk downwards without closing the armpits.

5. Continue to keep your feet parallel and shoulder-width apart, with the toes pointing forwards and turned slightly inwards. The weight must be evenly distributed on both legs.

6. Keep your body relaxed with both the head and the trunk upright. Try to get your back as straight as possible by turning the your tailbone inwards and leaning very slightly forward.

7. Sink, relax and hollow the chest by dipping the breastbone inwards slightly, which indirectly causes the Chi to sink further to the Tan Tien.

8. Once again your eyes should be looking forward and gazing slightly downward.

9. Breathe naturally through the nose. Try to focus at the Tan Tien point. If you find difficulty in focusing at this point, just concentrate on your breathing – inhaling and exhaling.

Concluding Posture – Centring Posture

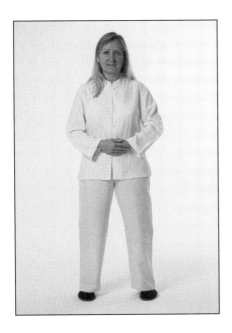

This is the concluding posture of the full eight-posture John Ding Yeung San Chi Kung set. It should be practised at the end of each Chi Kung session to help centre and settle the Chi further at the Tan Tien point.

Following on from the second posture, conclude your Chi Kung practice with the final posture of the set. Cup the right palm (or left palm if you are a woman) and gently bring it to rest at the Tan Tien point, about two inches below the navel. Rest your other palm on top of the first. Ensure that there is a hollow in the first palm. Keep the shoulders and arms relaxed. Then slowly straighten up the knees, but do not lock them. Half-close your eyes and maintain your mental focus or Yi at the Tan Tien point for the next minute.

Then shake the arms and legs and loosen up the body before going into the Tai Chi form.

John Ding Tai Chi Chuan Form

Practise the postures you have already learnt in Session One several times. Once you are happy and feel confident with these movements, move on to the following postures, which follow on directly from the previous session.

2. Lan Cheuk Mei – Grasp the Bird's Tail, continued

Right Double Ward Off (Siong Pang)

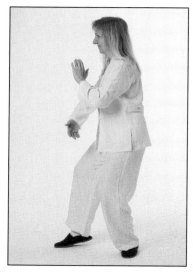

1.

1. From the previous Left Single Ward Off posture, turn your waist to the left, and move your right arm across to the left-hand side of the body. The right hand remains at hip level. Turn both the palms so that they face each other to form another 'Holding the Ball' posture. Then turn the hips fully to the right, so that the upper body faces the right-hand side. As you turn to the right, the weight shifts fully onto the left leg, and the right heel is lifted, so that the right foot can turn to the right, pivoting on the toes.

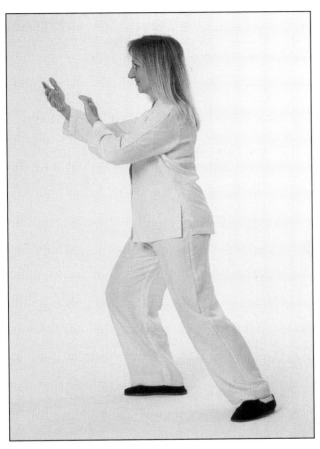

2.

2. Next, step out a shoulder-width distance with the right foot, first touching the ground with the heel. Following the centre of gravity, move forwards onto the right foot until it becomes a solid step, and turn the hips to the right (Right Kung Bu Bow Stance). At the same time, the right forearm comes upwards and wards off (pang) towards the right, with the right palm facing towards the body at nose height and the elbow slightly lower than the palm. The left hand pushes forward with the palm facing out, following the right palm, ending in a position that is slightly lower than the right hand.

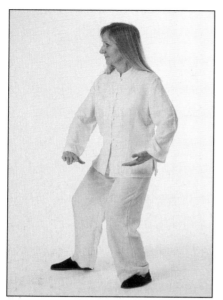

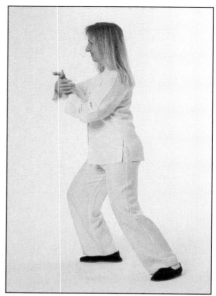

Roll Back (Lui)

Turn the right palm so that it faces downwards, and at the same time turn the left palm so that it faces upwards. The hands form a slanted T-shape – the left hand forming the vertical and the right hand forming the horizontal. Bring the weight back on to the left leg, and at the same time turn the hips to the left (Left Hou Bu, Rear Bow Stance). The hands keep the T-formation and follow the turning of the body to rest in a position beside your left thigh. Seventy per cent of your weight should be now transferred to your rear left leg. You should keep looking forward throughout this move.

Press (Jai)

The body turns slightly to the right and the right arm rotates out, causing the right palm to turn and face the body. The left arm rotates so that the left palm faces outwards. Place the left palm onto the right palm, with the left fingers pointing upwards. Turn the hips square, shift the weight forward (Right Kung Bu Stance), and push the hands out, keeping the right elbow slightly lower than the wrist. The press is more arc-shaped than a straight upward movement.

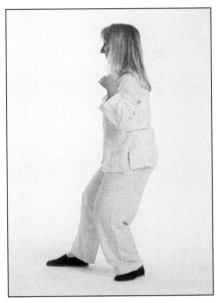

1.

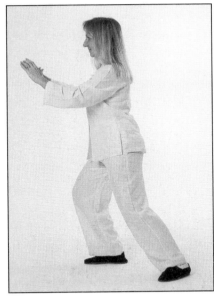

2.

Push (Aun)

1. Both arms push forward. The right arm rotates, causing the palm to face down. The left palm passes over the back of the right hand. The two palms then separate to a distance slightly narrower than shoulder width, with both palms facing downwards. The two elbows then gradually bend, and sink down, so that the hands are pulled back to rest in front of the shoulders. At the same time, the weight is gradually shifted to the rear left leg (Left Hou Bu).

2. Shift the weight forward on to the right leg and at the same time push forwards with the hands. As you push forward, the elbows sink down and your hands turn in slightly.

Practise the above Tai Chi Chuan movements for six to eight minutes until you are familiar with the postures. Ensure that you have incorporated all the Tai Chi principles described earlier within both the Chi Kung postures and the JDF.

Settling Breathing Exercise

Start off with the breathing exercise described in Session One (page 74) and repeat it six times. Then incorporate the next breathing sequence as described below.

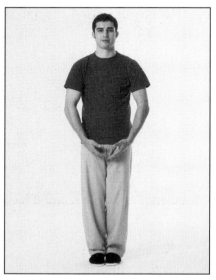

1a.

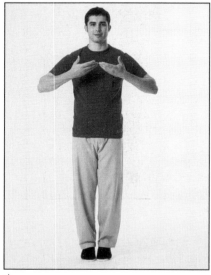

1b.

1. Complete the Session One breathing exercise and repeat six times.
2. Repeat the same movement again but this time, as soon as the palms reach the breastbone area, turn the palms out and extend the arms forward in front of the body.
3. Separate the arms and spread them horizontally to the side of the body as shown in diagram. Breathe in as you are carrying out this action.
4. Next, breathe out as you bring the arms back down to the front of the body. Keep repeating this exercise until you are familiar with the sequence. Then once you are happy, carry out the two breathing sequences you have learnt, consecutively, one after another, slowly and gently with correct body alignment. Repeat this six times.

Finish off in the meditative stance as described in Session One.

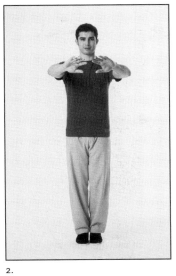

2.

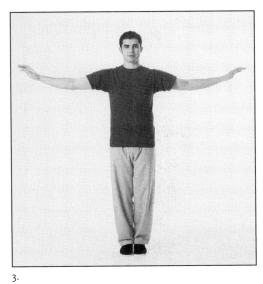

3.

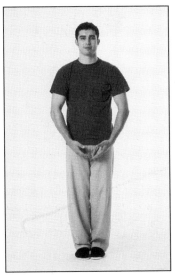

4.

Meditative Stance

SESSION THREE

John Ding Yeung San Chi Kung

Start the session by spending a minute in each of the Chi Kung postures you have learned. Begin first with 'Wuji' (page 68), and then move onto the 'Carrying the Ball' (page 77) posture. Follow these postures with the third Chi Kung posture laid out below.

Posture 3: Lowering the Ball

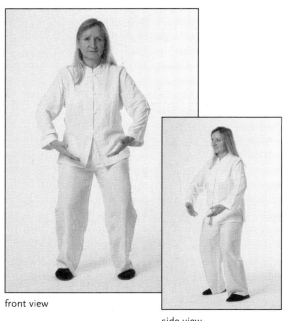

front view

side view

1. From the second posture, keeping the same position, lower both arms downwards slowly by using your elbows as pivots. Both forearms should slightly rotate outwards in the finished position, as shown above.

Be aware of the following points:

- Keep the fingers apart, with thumbs extended so that they point forward. Try not to curl the fingers inwards but keep them straight instead.

- Try not to bend the wrists inwards but instead try to make a continuous even line from the forearms to the back of the hands.

- Ensure that the armpits are slightly opened so that the arms are slightly away from the trunk.

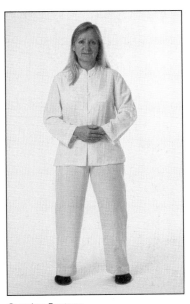

Centring Posture

2. Hold this posture for a further minute.

Conclude your Chi Kung session by returning to the Centring posture that you learned previously (page 79). Keep relaxed and maintain your Yi at the Tan Tien point.

John Ding Tai Chi Chuan Form

Begin by revising and repeating all the Tai Chi Chuan postures learnt from the previous sessions. Then start the new postures described below.

3. Jor Yau Toi Sau – Push Left and Right

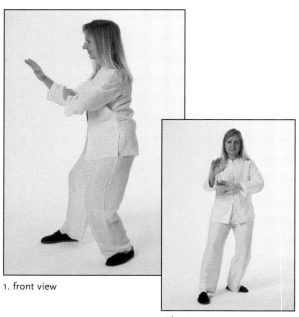

1. front view

side view

1. From the Push (Aun) posture shift the weight onto the back (left) leg. The left hand moves back to the inside of the right elbow so that the left arm is horizontal to the body with the palm facing the front and the thumb pointing down. The hips should still be square and the right leg remains bent (Left Hou Bo, Rear Bow Stance).

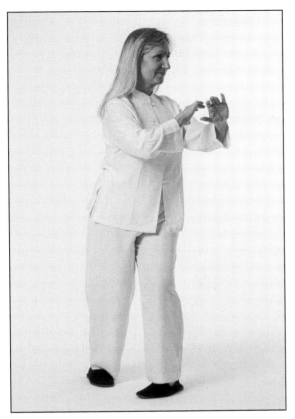

2.

2. Turn the hips to the left and turn the right foot in, using the heel as a pivot. The weight should remain on the left leg. As the hips turn, the hands follow the body and as the turn completes they push out to the left with the right hand finishing just inside the left elbow.

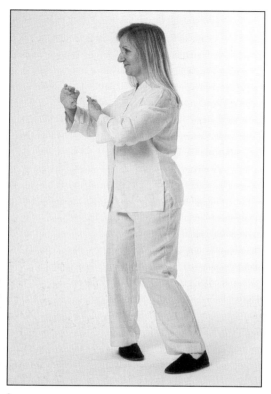

3.

3. Shift the weight onto the right leg, and bring both arms back so that they are in front of the chest at shoulder level.

 Turn the hip to the right and push both hands out to the right side with the left hand finishing just inside the right elbow.

4. Tan Bien – Single Whip

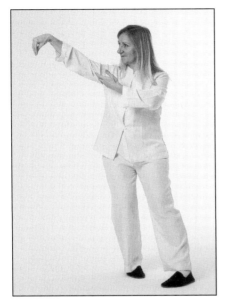

1.

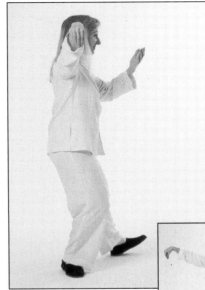

2. front view

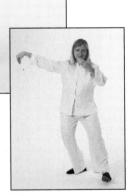

side view

1. Turn the hip to the left, keeping the weight on the right leg. As you do so the right arm moves across to the left, passing the face. Turn the right wrist downwards bringing the fingers together, so that the index and middle finger touch the thumb. Turn the hips back to the right, and extend the right arm outwards to the right side, in a hook like fashion. The left forearm then rotates outwards so that the palm faces you.

2. Sink the weight onto the right leg and turn your hips to the left so that your body directly faces the left hand side. The left leg follows the turning of the hip and steps out a shoulder-width distance round to the left. Touch the ground with the left heel, but keep the weight on the right leg. The left hand should move with the body, so that it is continues to be in front of the chest with the palm facing in.

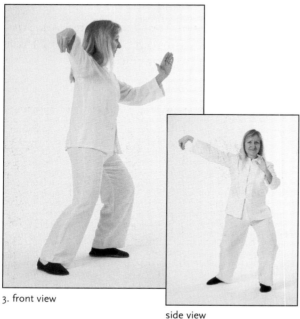

3. front view

side view

3. Turn the left hand so that the palm now faces outwards. Then gradually transfer the weight to the left leg (Left Kung Bu, or Bow Stance). As you do so, push forwards with the left hand and, at the same time, extend the right hooked arm backwards.

Practise the above Tai Chi Chuan movements for six to eight minutes until you are familiar with the postures. Ensure that you have incorporated all the Tai Chi principles described earlier within both the Chi Kung postures and Tai Chi Chuan form.

Settling Breathing Exercise

Begin by using the two sets of breathing exercises learnt previously. Practise them consecutively, one after another, and repeat the exercises six times. Once you have done this, incorporate the next and final breathing sequence described below.

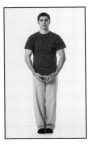 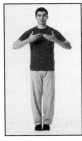 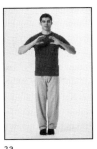 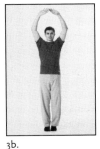 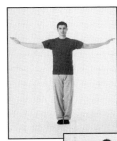

1. 2. 3a. 3b. 4.

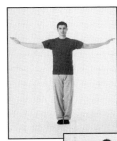

Meditative Stance

1. Practise the two sets of breathing exercises, and repeat six times.

2. On the next movement, as the palms reach the breastbone area turn the palms out and extend the arms.

3. Once again initiate the beginning move to the sternum area. Then, turn the palms up and push the arms upwards gently as if pushing up towards the sky. Remember to relax and breathe in as you extend your arms upwards.

4. Keeping the arms extended, use the shoulders as a pivot to bring the arms down slowly in an arc along the side of the body until they meet at a resting point in front of the body.

Repeat the sequence several times until you are familiar with the new exercise. Then carry out all three breathing sequences consecutively, one after another, slowly and gently with correct body alignment, another six times. Finish off in the meditative stance as described in Session One.

SESSION FOUR

John Ding Yeung San Chi Kung

Begin with the three Chi Kung postures that you have learnt previously. Each of the postures should be practised for one minute before moving onto the next. To link the third posture to the fourth, gently clench your hands and bring them to the waist, ensuring that the elbows do not go behind the body. From this position, bring the hands up to eye level with the palms facing outwards.

Posture 4: Pushing Outwards

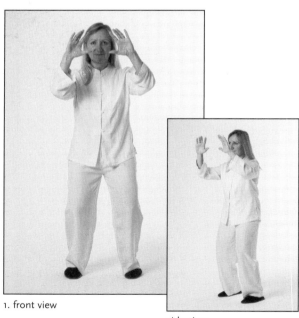

1. front view

side view

1. The hands should be level and placed in front of the forehead. Try to ensure that the hands are neither too far in front of you, overstretching the arms, nor too close to the forehead, closing the armpits. The thumbs should point slightly backwards and should be placed at a level just slightly above the nose.

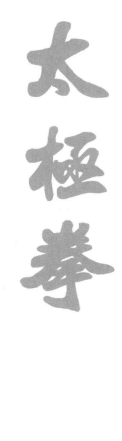

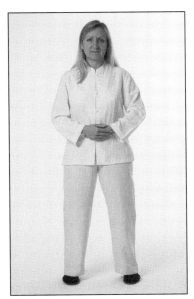

Centring Posture

2. Keep the backs of the hands in line with the forearms by making sure that you do not bend your wrists (which would effectively cause a blockage of Chi energy at the wrist joint).

3. The fingers and thumbs should be relaxed and opened. Try not to over-stretch the fingers. Doing so could cause excess tension that will indirectly block the flow of Chi.

4. The rest of the body positions remain as they were described in Posture 2. Hold this posture for a minute.

Once again, conclude the Chi Kung session with the final Centring posture.

John Ding Tai Chi Chuan Form

Begin by revising and repeating all the Tai Chi Chuan postures learnt from previous lessons. Then begin the postures described below, which carry on directly from those learnt previously.

5. Chou Di Chui – Fist Under Elbow

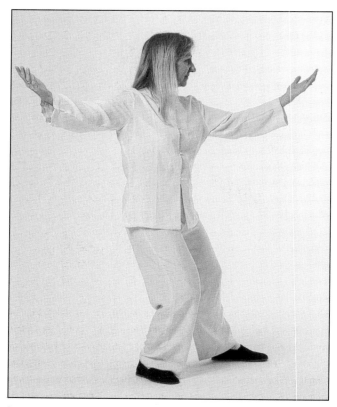

1.

1. Turn and project both your arms outwards with palms facing upwards as you turn your hips 45 degrees while shifting your weight to your right back leg.

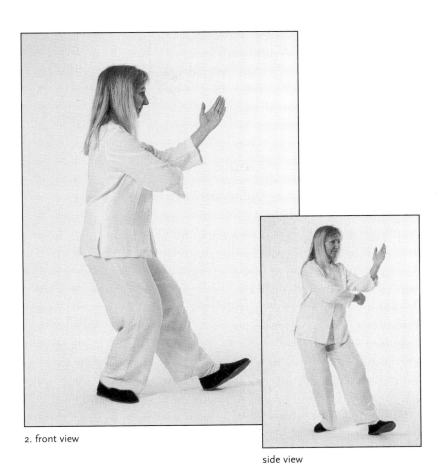

2. front view

side view

2. Lift the left leg, and gently place the left heel on the ground in front of you, in a position where the horizontal distance between the two heels is less than a shoulder-width apart (Right Hoi Bu or Empty Stance). Next, keeping the weight on the back leg, turn the hips to the left. As you do so, bring the left hand back so that it stays in front of the shoulder but at the same time allows the elbow to drop down further. The left palm should be facing the right side. Then as the hips continue to turn, the right hook forms a fist and moves to tuck under the left elbow, with the right arm going across the body.

6. Dou Nien Hou – Back-stepping Monkey

Back-stepping Monkey Right (Yau Dou Nien Hou)

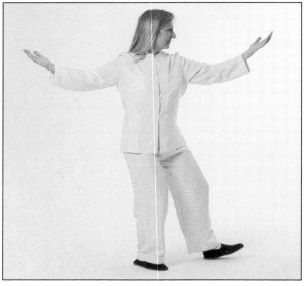

1.

1. Maintaining the previous stance, rotate the hips to the right. As you do so, you will find that the upper body will also turn to the right-hand side. While the body turns, the two arms move simultaneously. The left arm extends slightly forward with the palm facing up at the level of the shoulder. The right fist changes to an open hand, and the arm swings horizontally across to the right side, and ends up in an extended position behind the body, as shown in the photo. As the right arm swings across, it also rotates so that the right palm gradually faces upwards. Keep the shoulders relaxed, both hands at ear level, and at all times keep looking forward.

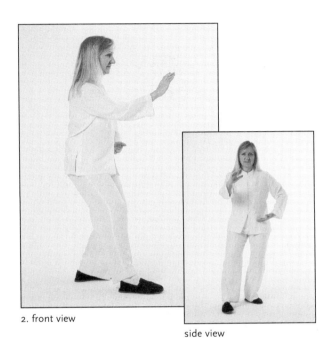

2. front view

side view

2. Bend the right elbow, bringing the right palm, facing down, beside the right ear. Then move the left leg back a step, touching the heel to the ground. Make sure that the back left foot is turned out 45 degrees, and that the two heels are slightly less than a shoulder-width apart. Then shift your weight back on to the left leg (Left Hoi Bu, Empty Stance). As you shift the weight back several things happen at the same time. First your hips move so that they now face the front square on. The right foot also turns to face the front, using the heel as a pivot. As you do this, the right hand pushes forward past the side of the right ear so that the arm extends forward with the palm facing out, at shoulder height. The left arm comes to rest on top of the left hip, with the palm facing up and the fingers pointing towards the body.

Back-stepping Monkey Left (Jor Dou Nien Hou)

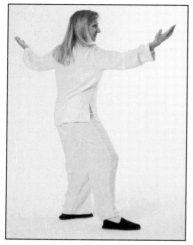

3.

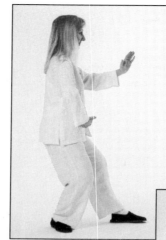

4. front view

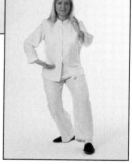

side view

3. Repeat steps 1 and 2 but this time on the left-hand side as this will mean that, with your weight now on the left leg, the hips turn to the left, with the right arm extending slightly forward and the left arm moving back in an arc that will allow it to end up behind the body.

4. The step back is taken with the right leg, and you will end up with the right hand at the waist and the left hand pushing forward level to the shoulder, using Right Hoi Bu Stance.

Back-stepping Monkey Right (Yau Dou Nien Hou)

Repeat the same move as in steps 1 and 2 above, stepping back on the left leg again.

Practise the above Tai Chi Chuan movements for six to eight minutes until you are familiar with the postures. Ensure that you have incorporated all the Tai Chi principles described earlier within both the Chi Kung postures and Tai Chi Chuan form.

Settling Breathing Exercises

Repeat the previous three different breathing exercises, consecutively, one after another, (page 93) and repeat the sequence 12 times. Finish off in the meditative stance.

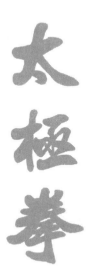

SESSION FIVE

John Ding Yeung San Chi Kung

Begin with the four Chi Kung postures that you have already learnt. Each of the postures should be practised for one minute before moving onto the next. The fifth posture directly follows on from the last posture you have learnt.

Posture 5: Pushing Downwards

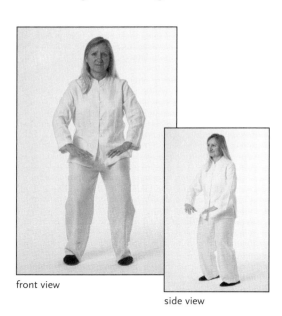

front view

side view

Lower the arms down to the level of the hips. The arms should still be circular with both sides of the palms pushing slightly down and out. Keep the fingers relaxed and slightly apart. The thumbs should be facing towards the hips and should not be allowed to point downwards. Keep the shoulders relaxed and the Yi focused at the Tan Tien. There should be no change in the position of your legs and feet. Hold the posture for a minute.

Once again conclude the Chi Kung section with the final Centring posture.

John Ding Tai Chi Chuan Form

Begin by revising and repeating all the Tai Chi Chuan postures learnt in the previous sessions. Only when you are confident with these movements should you then commence to learn the new postures described below.

7. Yau Che Fey Sai – Right Diagonal Flying

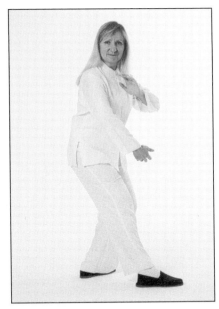

1.

1. Keep your weight on the left leg and turn the hips to the left. As you do so the right hand comes down across the body, so that the right hand rests at the left hip, with the palm facing up. The left hand comes up with the palm facing down as if 'Holding the Ball' (Hup Sau).

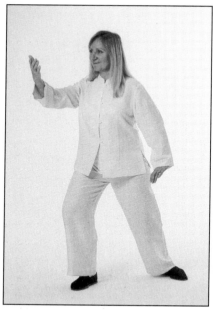

2.

2. With your weight resting over the left leg, the body turns to the right. At the same time the right foot takes a step out and moves around about 135 degrees toward the right rear. First touch the ground with the heel, then gradually shift your weight to the right leg and plant all of your weight solidly in the foot by bending the right knee. Then turn the hips to the right. As the upper body follows the movements of the hip to the right, the right arm should move upwards and outwards to the right side of the body, with the palm facing up. The right hand ends up in a position at eye level. At the same time the left palm faces downwards and pulls down in an arc to rest beside the left hip.

8. Tei Sau – Lift Hands

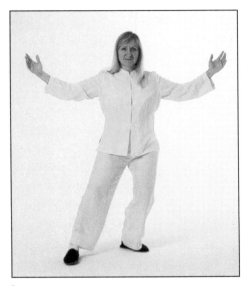

1.

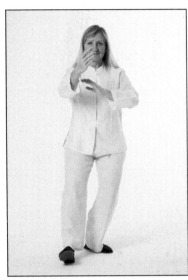

2.

1. Shift the weight to your left leg and extend both arms upwards and outwards to the sides. The hands should be at ear level with the palms facing to the front. The hips face the front, and the right knee should be bent.
2. Lift the right foot and bring it in line with the left heel. Ensure that the right heel touches the ground with the toes

lifted up to form a Left Empty Stance (Left Hoi Bu). Bring in the hands to form 'lift hands' – the left hand is brought in at chest height with palm facing right, and then the right hand with the palm facing left is brought in and rests at nose height. Both hands are almost in line, in front of the chest.

9. Yau Pang – Right Ward Off

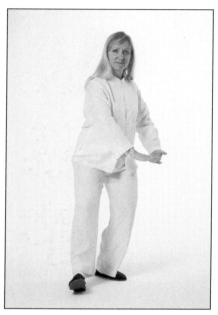

1.

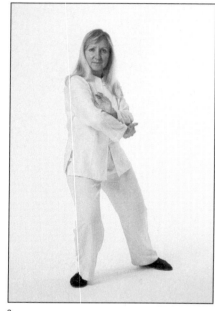

2.

1. Turn both hands so that the palm of the left hand faces upwards whilst that of the right faces downwards. Both hands, again, form a T-shape on its side.

   Bring the weight back on to the left leg and at the same time, turn the hips to the left. The hands keep the T-formation and follow the turning of the body to rest beside the left thigh. Your weight should be fully over your left leg (Left Hoi Bu). Try to keep looking forward during this move.

2. Turn the palms in the opposite direction so that the palm of the left hand faces downwards whilst the right faces upwards. Lift the right foot and place the heel to the right, away from the centre of the body so that it rests a shoulder-width apart from the left foot.

   As you gradually transfer your weight onto your right foot, push forward in the same direction with the right elbow. The left hand is then brought up and rests lightly on the inside of the right elbow.

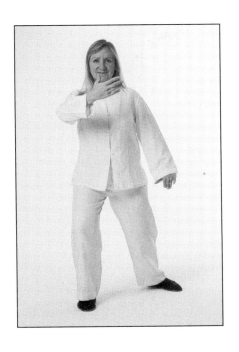

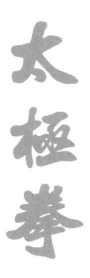

3. Turn your upper body to the right so that it faces forward. As you turn the hip the right hand is raised to the level of the face with the palm facing in. The right arm ends up in a position across the body to form Right Ward Off. The left hand slips back down to the left hip with the palm facing down. Your weight should be 70 per cent on the right leg, the hips are square and your back is upright (Right Kung Bu or Bow Stance).

Practise the above Tai Chi Chuan movements for six to eight minutes until you are familiar with the postures. Ensure that you have incorporated all the Tai Chi principles described earlier in both the Chi Kung postures and Tai Chi Chuan form.

Settling Breathing Exercises

Repeat the complete breathing exercise cycle 12 times and finish off in the meditative stance.

SESSION SIX

John Ding Yeung San Chi Kung

Begin with the five Chi Kung postures that you have learnt previously. Each of the postures should be practised for one minute before moving onto the next. To link the fifth posture to the sixth posture, gently clench the hands and bring them to the waist, ensuring that the elbows do not go behind the body. From this position, bring the hands to chest height.

Posture 6: Holding the Ball

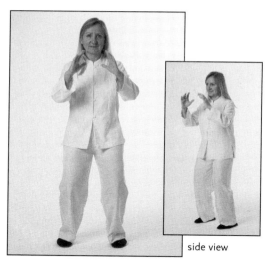

side view

front view

The palms should face outwards in a position that is almost like holding one side of a beach ball. Let the thumbs point back and both arms extend forward, about a foot in front of the chest. The elbows should neither be pointing down vertically (which will close the armpits) nor be pointing out to the side too far (which can raise the shoulders), otherwise the energy may either be blocked or wasted. Remember also to hollow the chest.

Once again conclude the Chi Kung session with the final Centring posture.

John Ding Tai Chi Chuan Form

Begin by revising and repeating all the Tai Chi Chuan postures learnt in the previous sessions. Once you are happy with the movements, follow the new postures described below.

10. Bak Hock Leung Che – White Crane Spreads Wings

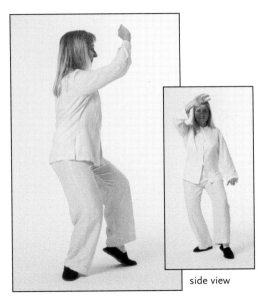

side view

front view

From Ward Off, lift the left foot and bring it forward slightly, placing only the toes lightly on the ground. Keeping the weight on the right leg, turn the hips fully to the left, so that the upper body now faces the left hand side. As you turn the hips, the left foot also turns to face the left, by using the toes as the pivot. The right arm turns upwards and outwards to the left, ending up in a position in front of the forehead, with the palm facing out. The left hand, with palm facing downward, rests beside the left thigh. All the weight is now on the right leg with the heel of the left foot raised (Left Hoi Bu Stance).

11. Jor Lou Sut Aou Bo – Left Brush Knee and Push

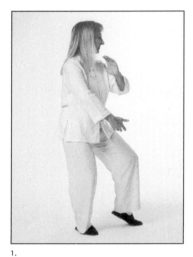

1.

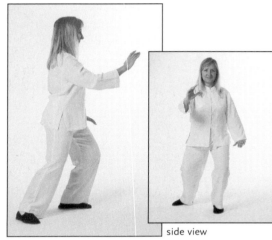

2. front view

side view

1. The right arm rotates down in front of the body to the level of the lower abdomen so that the palm faces up. Keeping the weight on the right leg, turn the hips to the right, and bring the left hand up (with the palm facing down) to form the 'Holding the Ball' position.

2. As you continue to turn the hip, the lower right arm extends out behind the body, to end up in a position where the right palm is facing upwards at ear level.

The right arm then bends at the elbow to bring the right palm facing down next to the right ear. The fingers should be pointing forwards. Step out a shoulder-width distance with your left foot, touching the ground gently with the left heel. As you gradually shift 70 per cent of your weight to the left leg, turn the hips to the left (Left Kung Bu or Bow Stance). The left hand brushes past the left knee with the left palm facing down, and the right arm pushes forward with the palm facing out.

12. Yeh Ma Fun Tsung – Parting the Horse's Mane

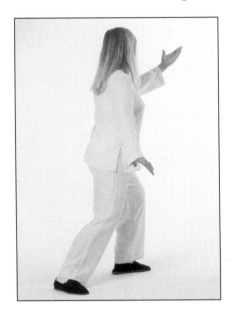

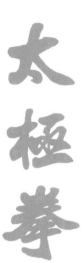

Keeping the weight on the front, left leg, turn the left foot 45 degrees outwards using the heel as a pivot. At the same time turn the hips to the left and bring the left arm round upwards and outwards to the left, so that it ends up in a position with the palm facing up at eye level. As you do this, the right arm pulls down in an arc to the right so that the right hand ends up in position away from the body at thigh level with the palm facing down.

Practise the above Tai Chi Chuan movements for six to eight minutes until you are familiar with the postures. Ensure that you have incorporated all the Tai Chi principles described earlier in both the Chi Kung postures and Tai Chi Chuan form.

Settling Breathing Exercises

Repeat the complete breathing exercise cycle 12 times and finish off in the meditative stance.

SESSION SEVEN

John Ding Yeung San Chi Kung

Begin with the six Chi Kung postures that you have learnt previously. Each of the postures should be practised for one minute before moving onto the next. The next posture follows on directly from the previous posture and is described below.

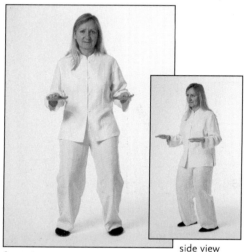

front view   side view

Posture 7: Resting the Arms

Lower the arms until they rest in a horizontal position at the side of the body – almost as if sitting in an armchair. The upper arms should vertical in a position directly next to the chest. The elbow joints are bent almost to 90 degrees, where the forearms protrude forwards and are level to the ground with the palms facing down. Keep the shoulders relaxed with a slight gap under the armpits. Ensure that the fingers are slightly opened without allowing the thumbs to drop – they should remain in line with the rest of the hand.

Conclude the Chi Kung section of your practice with the Centring posture. You have now learnt the complete John Ding Yeung San Chi Kung set.

John Ding Tai Chi Chuan Form

Begin your form by revising and repeating all the Tai Chi Chuan postures learnt from previous lessons. Then begin the new postures described below.

13. Yau Teng Geuk – Kick with the Right Leg

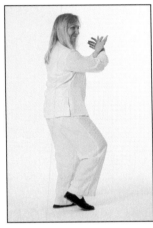
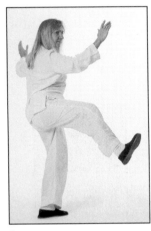

1.　　　　　　　　　　2.

1. Keeping 70 per cent of your weight on the left leg, turn the hip further to the left. As you do so, bring the right forearm across the body so that it ends up in a position crossing in front of the left arm. Note that in the movement of the right arm across the body, the palm gradually turns to face you. Now with both palms facing you, shift all of your weight onto the left leg, and bring the right foot forward so that it rests near the left.

2. Straighten (but do not lock) the left knee so that the body rises. Then separate your arms by lifting them upwards and outwards to the side. You should end up in a position with palms facing outwards at ear level. The right arm should point in front, 45 degrees to the right, whilst the left arm should point backwards, 45 degrees to the left.

Gently kick out with the heel of your right foot. The kick should be in the same direction as the right arm. If you cannot kick high, kick to the height at which you are comfortable. Once you have kicked, keep the right thigh elevated so that it is horizontal, but bring the foot down by bending at the knee, as shown above.

14. Jor Teng Geuk – Kick with the Left Leg

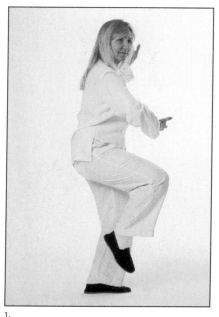

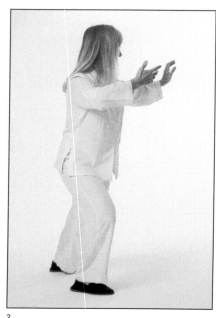

1.

2.

1. Bend the left knee, and then turn your hips slightly to the left. As you do so, roll the right hand down so that the palm faces up, as if diverting a punch. The left arm remains in the same position.

2. The right foot takes a step diagonally to the right with the heel touching the ground first. Gradually shift your body weight onto the right leg. As you do so, the hips turn to the right, and the right arm moves out and upwards to pro-

tect the face, with the palm facing in – almost like Right Ward Off (see p.81). The left arm then comes forward in front of the body in an almost horizontal anticlockwise arc in front of the chest, and pushes out to the left side. Although the body faces the right, look towards the left – the intended direction of the next kick.

3. Keeping the weight on the right leg, bring the left arm across the body so that it ends up in a position crossing in

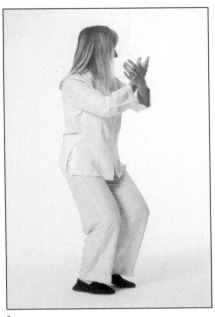

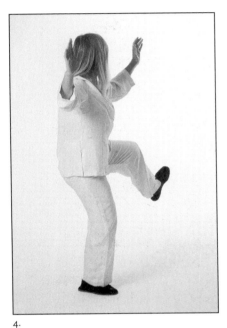

3.

4.

front of the right arm. As you bring the left arm across to the right, the palm gradually turns to face you. Now with both palms facing you again, shift all the weighting from the left leg to the right, and bring the left foot in to rest near the right foot.

4. Straighten (but do not lock) the right knee this time, so that the body rises. Then separate your arms by lifting them upwards and outwards to the side. You should end up in a position with palms facing outwards at ear level. The left arm should point in front, 45 degrees to the left, whilst the right arm should point backwards, 45 degrees to the right.

Gently kick out with the heel of your left foot. The kick should be in the same direction as the left arm. Once you have kicked, keep the left thigh elevated so that it is horizontal, but bring the foot down by bending at the knee.

15. Jor Lou Sut Aou Bo – Left Brush Knee and Push

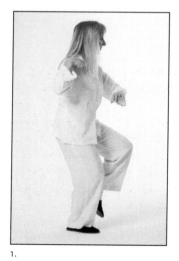

1.

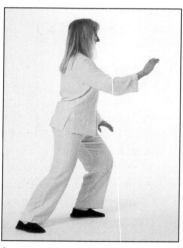

2.

1. Bend the right knee, so that the body sinks downwards slightly. Turn the hips slightly to the right, and at the same time, bend the left elbow to bring the left arm back to a position where the palm is in front of the chest, facing down. As you do this, the right arm bends at the elbow to bring the right palm facing down next to the right ear so that the fingers point forward.

2. Step out with your left foot so that it is a shoulder-width distance from your right, touching the ground gently with the left heel. As you gradually shift 70 per cent of your weight onto the left leg, turn the hips to the left (Left Kung Bu, Bow Stance). The left hand brushes past the left knee with the left palm facing down, and the right arm pushes forward with the palm facing out.

Practise the above Tai Chi Chuan movements for six to eight minutes until you are familiar with the postures. Ensure that you have incorporated all the Tai Chi principles described earlier in both the Chi Kung postures and Tai Chi Chuan form.

Settling Breathing Exercises

Repeat the complete breathing exercise cycle 12 times and finish off in the meditative stance.

SESSION EIGHT

John Ding Yeung San Chi Kung

Having learnt all the individual postures of the John Ding Yeung San Chi Kung set, you are now in a position to practise the complete sequence of eight Chi Kung postures from beginning to end. Start with the Wuji, and work through each of the postures in order. Practise each position for a minute and then, at the end of each minute, try to change smoothly and seamlessly into the next. The total time you should spend on Chi Kung should be around eight minutes. Try to discipline yourself to stick to this time period, and ensure that you are incorporating the Tai Chi principles and concepts at all times. If you are unhappy with any postures, check and correct them by referring to the text. You may find that checking your posture in a mirror can help too.

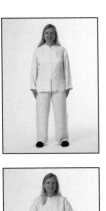 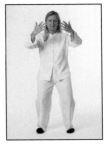 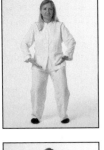 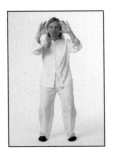

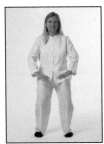 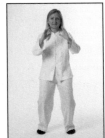 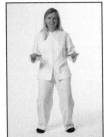 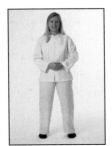

John Ding Tai Chi Chuan Form

Begin your form by revising and repeating all the Tai Chi Chuan postures learnt from previous lessons. Then begin the new postures described below.

16. Pi San Chui – Deflect, Parry and Push

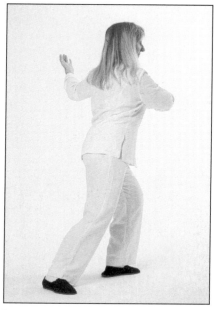

1.

1. Keeping the weight on the left leg, turn the left foot out 45 degrees, pivoting on the heel. At the same time turn the hip to the left. As the body turns, the left hand turns so that the palm faces up next to the knee, and the right hand makes a fist. The arms then move simultaneously. The right arm moves in an arc, first coming down and across the body close to the left knee and then ends up in a position near the left shoulder. The left arm extends out behind the left side of the body to end up in a position where the left palm is facing upwards at ear level.

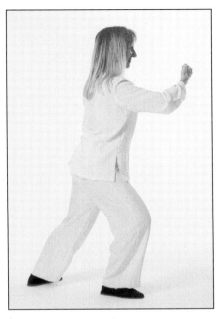

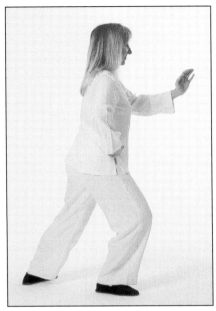

2.

3.

2. Step forwards with the right foot a shoulder-width distance, touching the ground gently with the right heel. In this posture, although you should be looking straight ahead, the right foot does not point directly forward, but instead is turned 45 degrees away from the centre of the body to the right. Gradually shift 70 per cent of your weight onto the right leg. As you do so, punch forward with the

back of the right fist, and bend the left arm at the elbow to bring the left palm facing down next to the left ear.

3. Then continue the right back-fisted punch downwards so that it arcs down to the right hip. At the same time, the left arm pushes forward with the palm facing out.

Your hips should be square on to the front, with 70 per cent of your weight on the right front leg.

17. Sheung Bo Boon Lan Chui – Step Forward, Parry and Punch

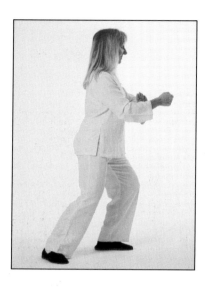

1. Turn the hip to the right, and as you do so, push to the right with your left palm.
2. Shift all the weight to the right leg and then bring in the left foot to rest near the right. Next, step out a shoulder-width distance with your left foot, touching the ground gently with the left heel. Gradually shift 70 per cent of your weight onto the left leg (Left Kung Bu), and punch forward with the right fist.

The left palm rests on the inside of the right forearm.

Practise the above Tai Chi Chuan movements several times until you are familiar with the postures. Ensure that you have incorporated all the Tai Chi principles described earlier in both the Chi Kung postures and Tai Chi Chuan form.

Settling Breathing Exercise

Repeat the complete breathing exercise cycle 12 times and finish off in the meditative stance.

SESSION NINE

John Ding Yeung San Chi Kung

Practise the complete sequence of eight Chi Kung postures from beginning to end, allowing one minute for each position.

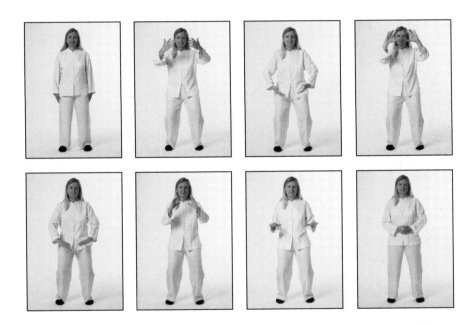

John Ding Tai Chi Chuan Form

Begin by revising and repeating all the Tai Chi Chuan postures learnt from previous lessons. Next commence the new postures described below.

18. Yue Fung Che Bie – Apparent Seal Off

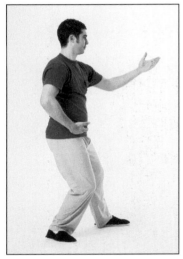

1.

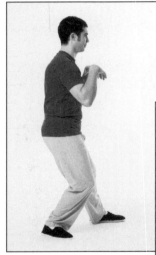

2.

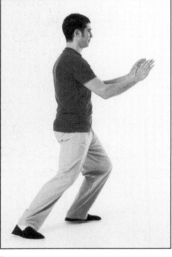

3.

1. Move the left arm under the right, so that the back of the left hand is in contact with the right elbow. Turn both palms facing upwards. Gradually shift 70 per cent of your weight back onto the right leg (Right Hou Bu, Rear Bow Stance). At the same time, slide the right arm back over the left forearm so that the right palm ends up beside the right hip with the palm facing up.

The left arm extends forward so that the left hand is level to the left shoulder.

2. Turn the hips square and bring both hands directly in front of the shoulders with the palms facing down.

3. Transfer 70 per cent of your weight to the left foot as you push forward (Left Kung Bu), with both the arms in the Aun, Push posture.

19. Sup Zi Sau – Crossing Hands

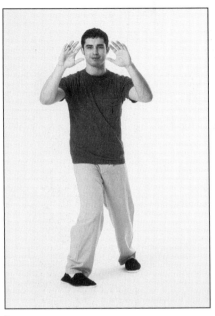

1.

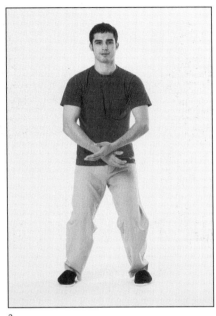

2.

1. Turn the hips fully to the right, and at the same time shift the weight to the right foot, so that the upper body turns 90 degrees in a clockwise direction. As you do this, the left foot also turns 90 degrees clockwise, pivoting on the heel. The arms follow the movement of the body and rotate to the right too. As you turn move your arms slightly upwards and out.

2. Shift the weight back fully to the left leg and bring the right foot back so that it is parallel with left foot. The feet now should be shoulder-width apart in Ma Bu, Horse Stance. The palms push slightly outwards and the arms swing in an arc, down in front of the body to form 'cross hands' at the level of the Tan Tien, two inches below the navel. Both palms face up with the left hand on top of the right.

20. Hup Tai Gik Sai – Conclusion

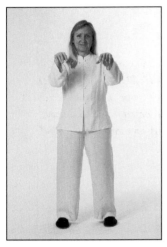

1.

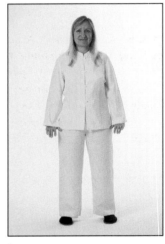

2.

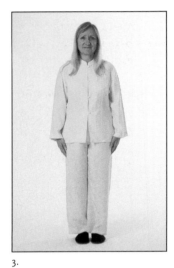

3.

1. Uncross your hands and drop the arms to your sides, with the palms facing up. Raise the arms to shoulder height, and at the same time straighten both the legs. Turn the arms so that the palms face down.

2. Then pull the arms down and back so that the hands come to rest beside the thighs with palms facing down.

3. Turn the wrists so that the palms touch the sides of the thighs and then bring the feet together by stepping in with the right foot.

Keep the mind, body and spirit relaxed and calm by staying in this meditative posture for a minute.

Bow forward slightly in respect for the founder of the ancient art of Tai Chi Chuan.

This concludes the 20-step John Ding Tai Chi Chuan Form.

Settling Breathing Exercise

Repeat the complete breathing exercise cycle 12 times and finish off in the meditative stance.

SESSION TEN

In this last session of the 15-minute Tai Chi programme you will be able to complete each of the sections within 15 minutes.

- John Ding Yeung San Chi Kung:
  8 minutes
- John Ding Tai Chi Chuan Form:
  4–5 minutes
- Settling Breathing Exercises:
  2–3 minutes

Having completed the 15-Minute Tai Chi programme, there is still a lot of work to be done to fine-tune your postures. Only through consistent practice will your movements bring about harmony of the mind, body and spirit.

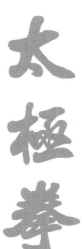

Note: If you are unsure of any particular posture or movements, read the notes again and repeat the sequence a number of times until you become familiar with it.

POSTURE LISTING

John Ding Yeung San Chi Kung

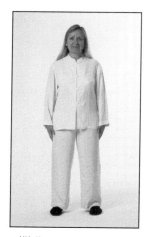

1. Wuji

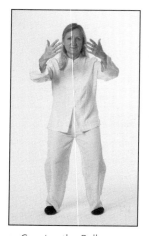

2. Carrying the Ball

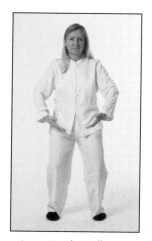

3. Lowering the Ball

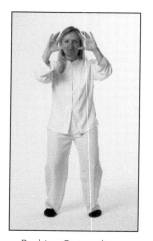

4. Pushing Outwards

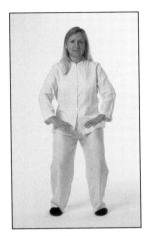

5. Pushing Downwards

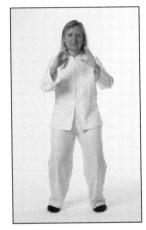

6. Holding the Ball

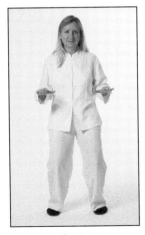

7. Resting the Arms

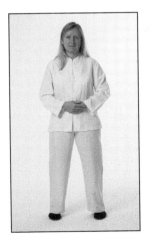

8. Centring

John Ding Tai Chi Chuan Form

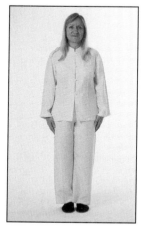

1.1. Hei Sai – Commencement, Preparation

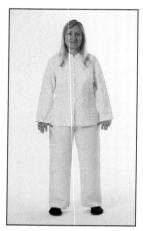

1.2. Preparation

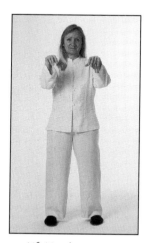

1.3. Lift Hands

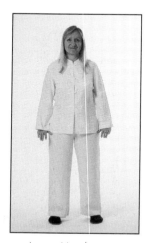

1.4. Lower Hands

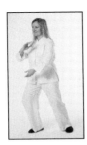

Link Posture

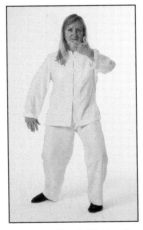

2.1. Lan Cheuk Mei Jor Pang – Grasp the Bird's Tail: Left Single Ward Off

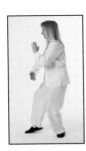

Link Posture

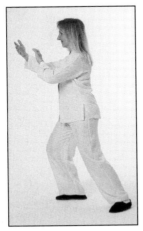

2.2. Right Double Ward Off (Siong Pang)

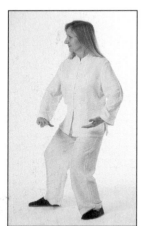

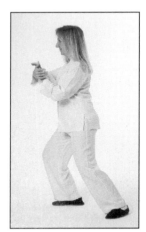

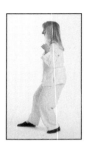

2.3. Roll Back (Lui)   2.4. Press (Jai)   Link Posture

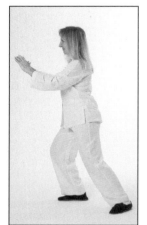

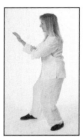

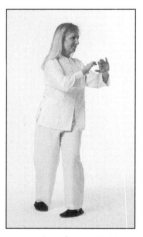

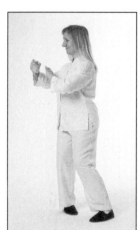

2.5. Push (Aun)   Link Posture   3a. Push Left and Right   3b.
                                   (Jor Yau Toi Sau)

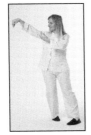

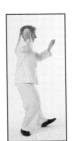

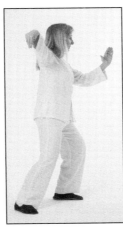

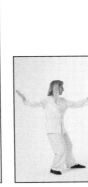

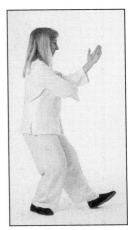

Link Posture   Link Posture   4. Single Whip (Tan Bien)   Link Posture   5. Fist Under Elbow
(Chou Di Chui)

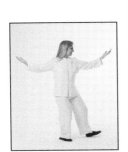

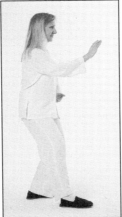

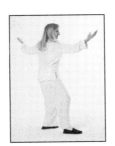

Link Posture   6.1. Back-stepping   Link Posture
Monkey Right
(Yau Dou Nien Hou)

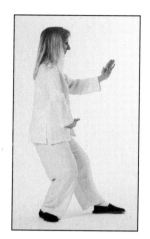

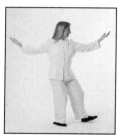

6.2. Back-stepping
Monkey Left
(Jor Dou Nien Hou)

Link Posture

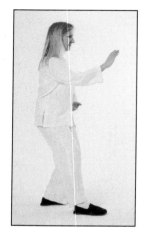

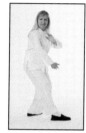

6.3. Back-stepping
Monkey Right
(Yau Dou Nien Hou)

Link Posture

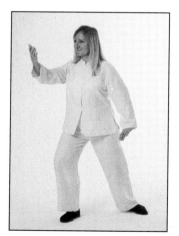

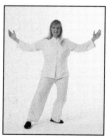

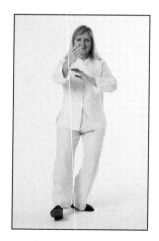

7. Right Diagonal Flying (Yau
Che Fey Sai)

Link Posture

8. Lift Hands (Tei Sau)

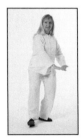

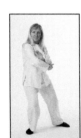

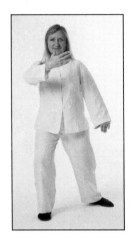

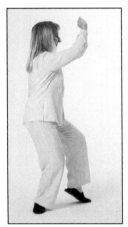

Link Posture

Link Posture

9. Right Ward Off
(Yau Pang)

10. White Crane Spread
Wings (Bak Hock Leung Che)

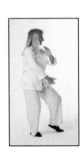

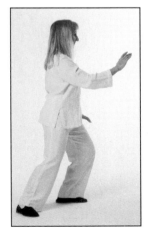

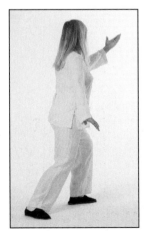

Link Posture

11. Left Brush Knee and
Push (Jor Lou Sut Aou Bo)

12. Parting the Horse's Mane
(Yeh Ma Fun Tsung)

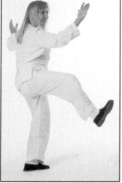
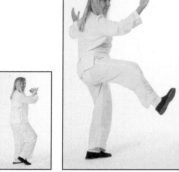
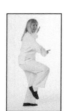
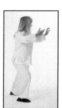
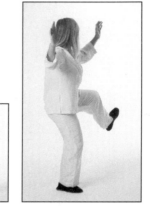

Link Posture   13. Kick with the Right   Link Posture   Link Posture   Link Posture   14. Kick with the Left
               Leg (Yau Teng Geuk)   Leg (Jor Teng Geuk)

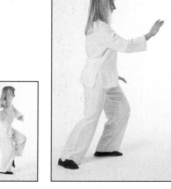
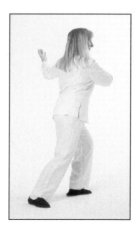
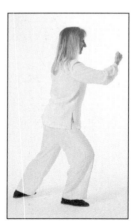

Link Posture   15. Left Brush Knee and   16a. Deflect, Parry and   16b.
               Push (Jor Lou Sut Aou   Push (Pi San Chui)
               Bo)

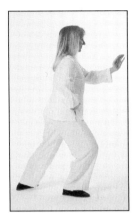

16c.

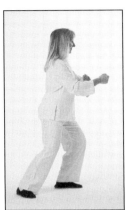

17. Step Forward, Parry and Punch (Sheung Bo Boon Lan Chui)

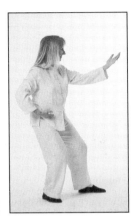

18. Apparent Seal Off (Yue Fung Che Bie)

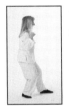

Link Posture

Link Posture

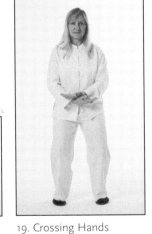

Link Posture

19. Crossing Hands (Sup Zi Sau)

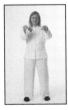

Link Posture

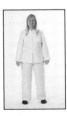

Link Posture

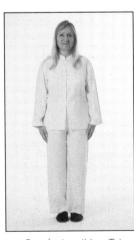

20. Conclusion (Hup Tai Gik Sai)

Settling Breathing Exercises

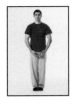 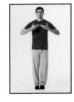 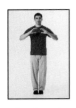 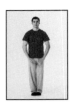

1. Bring the hands to chest level and down again

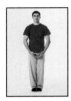 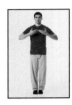 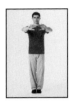 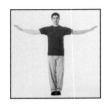

2. Bring the hands to chest level, push forward and out and down again

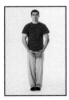 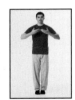 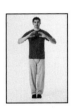 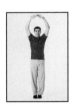 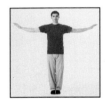 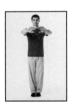

3. Bring the hands to chest level, push up, round and down again.

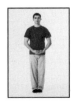

Meditative stance.

Tai Chi Chuan in Daily Life

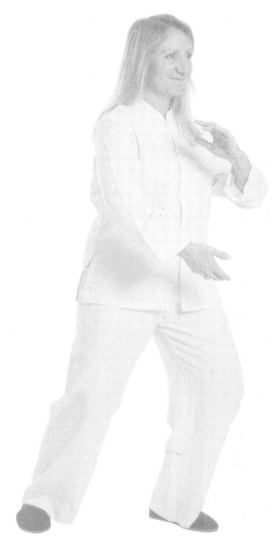

PART FOUR

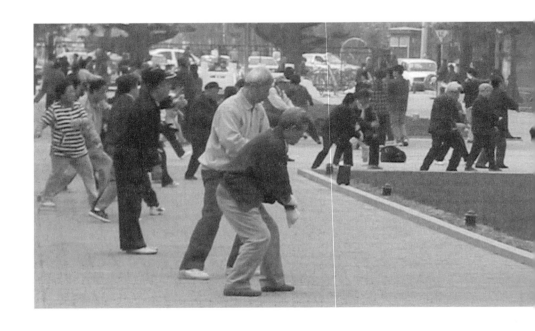

Introduction

Tai Chi's potential extends far beyond the 15-minute haven of undisturbed and quiet space that your practice session provides. Look further and you will soon see with time that Tai Chi Chuan is more than just simply plucking an isolated 15 minutes of time out of each day, but is something that can be integrated in all aspects of our daily life.

Each of the 15-minute sessions seeks to refresh and invigorate you by re-establishing an open, balanced and continuous flow of Chi. This will reverse blockages in your life force that are caused by the pressures of day-to-day life. But as you continue with your practice and become more acquainted with the art, what you will realize is that Tai Chi principles can be brought into almost every aspect of your daily life. Tai Chi Chuan should not be perceived as an

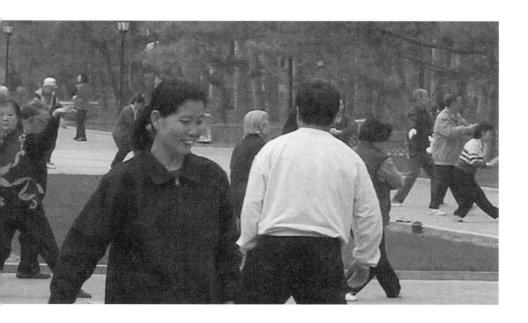

abstract exercise that you make time for to relieve the physical strains and the mental stresses of your life. It should eventually become integrated throughout your day so that the free, even and unblocked circulation of energy can be maintained, providing continuous benefits to you.

The crossover of Tai Chi Chuan into our everyday lives can occur on many levels. It will balance, inform and enrich your life experience by developing both mental and physical attributes. In all activities of your daily living, whether you are at home or at work, sitting, standing or walking, you will find that many of the Tai Chi principles can be applied. Not only does Tai Chi act to relax and energize you, it also serves to teach you ways in which you can use your energies most effectively. When you are ill, Tai Chi does not only help to relieve symptoms but can also help to improve many diseases, and speed recovery. It will provide you with more emotional stability and strength too. As our minds are increasingly preoccupied with the stresses of modern society, Tai Chi Chuan provides the perfect antidote, by creating the mental space that will bring relaxation, concentration and clarity of thought.

Tai Chi Chuan permeates through to you and your everyday life with infinite diversity. It creates a positive influence on the way you think, the way you move and, most importantly, the way you feel. Take Tai Chi Chuan one step at a time and you will find that many of its principles will naturally diffuse into your daily life. There is no need to deliberately impose or force the transition. Indeed, this would be abrupt and unnatural, yielding tension rather than holistic benefit. With a correct and consistent attitude to practice comes a greater understanding and awareness of your body and mind, and it is this that is reflected back into your day-to-day life.

Tai Chi Chuan is a deeply personal journey that blends itself differently with each of its practitioners. It is also a journey in which the intimacy between the art and its practitioner is forever changing. Some will experience its effect immediately; others will initially experience the art in subtler, and even obscure, ways before later discovering more of the fruits it has to bear. We are all unique and so too is our interaction with Tai Chi Chuan. What follows are just some of the countless ways in which the art can be applied in life. Tai Chi Chuan is a route that is your own, and through its process you will discover your own ways in which the art will best change you.

TAI CHI CHUAN IN EVERYDAY LIFE

There are countless moments throughout the day in which the principles of Tai Chi can be applied. As you become more familiar with the art's postures and movements, you will begin to gain an ability to apply them to situations you encounter each day. The process of merging Tai Chi Chuan principles into the everyday things that you do amplifies the benefit the art brings. It will encourage mental and physical relaxation so that tension can be released as and when it becomes apparent. Blockages in the energy system caused by incorrect body alignment and tension are also effectively removed. This in turn allows the Chi to circulate more freely within the body to leave you feeling refreshed and focused.

Bringing Tai Chi Chuan into the physical aspect of our lives enhances our activities with suppleness, poise and fluidity. You will become more centred, balanced and stable. Coupled with the ability to develop flexibility and coordination, this means that the art is ideal for those who seek to improve mobility. But a greater awareness of your body will also lead to a greater understanding of how simple everyday movements can be used more efficiently. The principles of Tai Chi will enable you to use less effort to achieve the same results, by conserving your energies and using movements more effectively. This will mean that you economize on your effort and feel less tired at the end of a long day. Even basic things like opening tight lids and turning taps can be done with efficiency and ease.

Here we take a look at just a few examples of where and how Tai Chi Chuan principles can be encompassed into the activities of daily life.

Posture

Posture is vital to everything that we do. We stand in a particular way to do the ironing; we sit in a particular way to work at a desk. But the way in which we sit, stand or walk can have a huge effect on the circulation of Chi, and therefore on our physical and mental well-being. A posture that is tense and rigid, with poor body alignment, will block the flow of energy within us and disrupt the balance of Chi. The practice of Tai Chi Chuan enables us to become aware of these shortcomings, and then gives us an excellent method by which we can seek to improve our posture.

Whether you are sitting at a desk or at home in front of the television, or whether you are standing in a queue at the bus stop, there are always ways in which you can ensure that the Tai Chi principles are applied. Part Two of this book, The Basics, and in particular the section that deals with the general principles and concepts on pp.46–64, is the ideal reference from which you can begin to understand how the Tai Chi principles can directly correlate with the postures and movements you use every day. Read the section again, but this time extend your thoughts beyond applying the principles to Tai Chi Chuan, and think about the ways in which they may be integrated into the real-life activities you do. With a little mental projection, you will begin to appreciate that not only are there thousands of examples of how and where the principles can be incorporated, but that many of the core principles can be universally applicable to the day-to-day postures we adopt. In any normal posture that you assume, try to be especially aware of the following common core principles:

- Be sensitive and aware of the physical tension that you may hold
- Relax and be soft throughout the body to release tension
- Breathe naturally through the nose
- Drop your chin slightly downwards to straighten and release tension from the neck
- Straighten your spine
- Sink the shoulders down
- Avoid over-expanding the chest and being top-heavy
- Slightly hollow the chest
- Be centred and let the energy settle at the Tan Tien.

When you are sitting at your desk try also to bear in mind the following:

太
極
拳

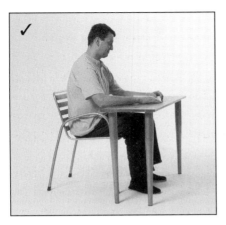 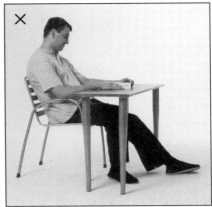

- Try not to slouch
- Keep the armpits slightly open
- Do not lean against the back of the chair to prop up your upper body; adjust your back yourself so that it remains upright and straight
- Adjust the height of the chair so that your feet rest comfortably on the ground
- Avoid crossing your legs
- If you rest your arms on the desk or on the armrests of the chair, be aware that this may raise your shoulders. Sink the shoulders so that you remain relaxed. Dropping the elbows can help to sink the shoulders further.

When you stand, think about these principles:

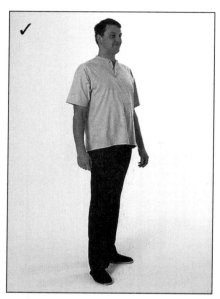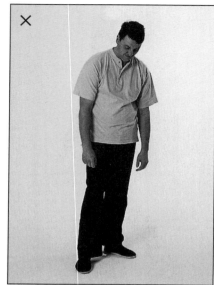

- Keep the arms relaxed and loose by the side of the body
- Allow the elbows to be slightly open away from the body
- Loosen the waist
- Avoid forcibly locking the knees; allowing them the freedom to move, and bending them ever so slightly, can avoid excess tension
- Distribute your weight evenly between both feet. Alternatively, if you want to exercise while you stand and cultivate the energy further, transfer your weight to one leg. Bend the weight-bearing knee slightly further so that a Chi Kung posture is adopted. When the weight bearing leg tires, transfer your weight to the other leg, so that both sides can be exercised. You can use use this method to practise Chi Kung discreetly while you are queuing or waiting at a bus stop – nobody need know that you are practising Tai Chi Chuan.

When you walk:

太
極
拳

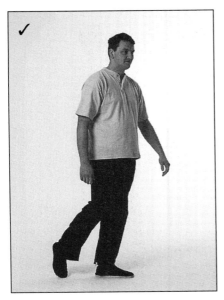

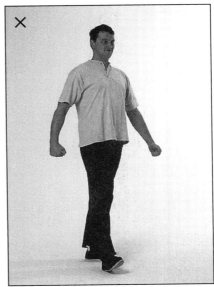

- Let your body be coordinated, so that its movements are synchronized
- Walk with an even momentum and let the movement flow while you walk
- Look ahead and be aware of your surroundings
- Relax the chest and let the energy settle to the Tan Tien to help you stay grounded and centred as you walk.

Although the ideas and concepts may seem easy in theory, it is much more difficult to put them into practice in your everyday life. It is a transition that will ask you to address and change the habits you have absorbed over a lifetime, and certainly this is not a task that can be done overnight. To allow the principles to consistently cross over to your everyday postures requires thought and the mental appreciation of their possible applications. You will also have to practise Tai Chi Chuan regularly to enable you to experience and understand the principles in the physical form. However, over time, you will find that Tai Chi Chuan naturally infuses into your life.

Household tasks

Even in the everyday cleaning tasks that we do around the house, the Tai Chi principles can be used to good effect. Chores such as washing up, ironing, dusting and cleaning the floor are often done using too much force and physical effort, quickly leaving you feeling tired, worn out and with a backache. Tai Chi Chuan can help you conserve your energies by re-educating your body to move in a more efficient manner.

Actions that are forced and deliberate will use excess muscular strength that is simply not needed. Tai Chi teaches us early on to relax and be supple. Constantly being mindful of relaxing your movements as you perform each task will mean that you will be able to use far less physical strength, yet at the same time achieve the same end result. In Tai Chi Chuan, strength and power come from an understanding of using coordinated whole body movements. Therefore instead of using individual body components to do tasks, you can economize on your efforts and conserve your energies.

Take one simple example – mopping the floor. Not only do we usually grip the mop too tightly, we also tend to rely only on the muscles and movements of the arms to carry out the mopping actions. All this creates a lot of tension, especially in the arms, neck and back, making the work physically exhausting and even causing aches and pains. Instead try to hold the handle of the mop less tightly, using the minimal amount of physical strength that you can to maintain control of the mop. Also try to involve more of your body movements in your mopping action. Rely less on the movements of your arms and instead use the rotation of the hips to achieve the same action. You will effectively use less effort, and will feel less tired once you have finished.

Shopping

Many of the simple things we take for granted in our everyday lives can be more involved than we think and can take their toll on our energy reserves. When we are out shopping, for example, there are plenty of instances where the Tai Chi principles can be incorporated.

When carrying your shopping basket or bag, remember not to hold the handle too tightly or hunch your back. Sink the carrying shoulder down and keep it relaxed, so that the arm hangs freely almost like a pendulum. This will effectively reduce tension and strain on the muscles of the arm, shoulders, neck and spine.

When pushing a supermarket trolley, rest your hands on the handle of the trolley and push it forward from the waist by shifting the weight forward from the back to the front leg. Too often many of us fail to use our body movements in this way, and instead use only the arms to push forward.

Lifting heavy shopping bags or any other heavy object are tasks that we all do, but it is too often something that we get wrong. Bending forwards over an object to lift it uses only the muscles of the back and pelvis to create the upward movement of lifting. As you can imagine, this creates immense pressures on your lower back and spine that can ultimately lead to pain or injury. Instead, any sort of heavy lifting should endeavour to use whole-body movements so that it can be done as safely and as efficiently as possible. Relax your arms, shoulders and upper body and let the body weight sink into the legs. Try not to bend over the object you pick up, but instead squat next to it, ensuring that your back is straight and relaxed. Take a good solid grasp of the object, holding it near to your body. In one smooth action slowly stand up. By doing this you are using the entire body to lift the weight. The upper body holds the object whilst your legs propel you upward, minimizing the risk of injury to your back.

Sport and leisure

In any physical activity we do the rate at which we tire is much to do with how relaxed and coordinated we are. If you use your body in a more relaxed manner – particularly coordinating your upper and lower body movements effectively, you will be able to use your energy much more efficiently, and increase your stamina. Conversely being physically tense, or getting angry and frustrated (which also makes the body tense), uses a lot of your energy reserves very quickly. Sport requires a focused effort and can either depress or excite both the participant and the audience. It is, in essence, an activity in which your physical and mental reserves are used to the fullest extent. Using your energies effectively is therefore the key to sporting success.

In sport, competition means that we often get tense under pressure. Trying too hard to win can cause tension and waste valuable mental and physical energy. Tai Chi Chuan is the ideal method to help you to stay relaxed and coordinated so that your energy is used most effectively. Just like Tai Chi Chuan, to improve in any sport requires a very precise understanding of the physical activities and movements involved. Repeated practice, coupled with this understanding, will mean that movements change from being mechanical to something that is second nature.

Follow some of the basic Tai Chi principles shown below and you will find that your games, especially those that involve striking a ball, will be more relaxed and hence that much more fluid:

- Relax the upper body
- Relax and loosen the waist so that movements originate from here
- Sink the weight down into the lower body or legs
- Sink the shoulders

- Coordinate the upper and lower body in a smooth effortless manner. In this way your body will provide you with continuously controlled and smooth power: ideal when hitting a ball.

Apart from the physical changes that can be made, your mental state and game play is critical to success. To be successful at sport you need to be clear what you are trying to achieve with the action you are doing. Providing yourself with a clear intention, or Yi, is thus vital.

Finally, it is easy to get into a routine playing sport and not to notice when and what you or your opponents are doing. Lacking sensitivity to others, in life as well as in sport, means that you will not notice what people around you are doing and how they are achieving their results. Developing sensitivity to others and your environment will help you to control situations better to achieve the results you want.

TAI CHI CHUAN IN ILLNESS

Tai Chi Chuan can be used directly as an effective therapy against disease by strengthening the internal energy within us. Using the postures of Zhan Zhuang Chi Kung and practising the movements of the Tai Chi form will allow you to remove blockages in the energy system that exist in illness. This serves to maximize the circulation of Chi, so that it can permeate freely throughout the body. Allowing our energy to flow freely will curb many disease processes and enhance your ability to heal. Simply practising the 15-minute routines in Part Three can often help us effectively alleviate or cure many illnesses, allowing us to be healthy in both body and mind.

Although Tai Chi Chuan is largely an exercise system that depends upon the movement of the body, the Tai Chi process can be used no matter how debilitating the illness. Adapting and using specific elements of the Tai Chi Chuan system, in particular Zhan Zhuang Chi Kung, will mean that we can use Tai Chi Chuan despite the most severe of illnesses. Often standing in still Chi Kung postures alone can prove to be an effective method to cultivate your internal energy to provide relief from illness. Research has also shown that simply visualizing exercises in detail will often bring many of the benefits of the exercise itself. Thinking about our golf swing or our tennis forehand action alone helps to improve that shot, if you pay attention to the specific sequence of events involved. In the same way, mentally rehearsing Tai Chi Chuan when we are too weak physically to do the form can often bring about many of the art's benefits, and improve our health to a large degree.

Thus Tai Chi Chuan can be used directly to treat illnesses throughout all their phases. When you feel at your worst or at your weakest, you can practise Zhan Zhuang Chi Kung alone, and just mentally rehearse your Tai Chi form. However, once the worst has passed and when you feel more able, you can gradually resume the full 15-minute practice. Tai Chi can be used regardless of your physical limitations and the degree of illness. By carefully and systematically adapting the Tai Chi Chuan method to your own physical capabilities you can ensure that the art works as best as it can to help you on the road to recovery.

Whilst Eastern medicine will prescribe Tai Chi Chuan as a stand-alone treatment, the method can also be used side-by-side with other therapies. It works well in combination with Traditional Chinese Medical practices, but can work equally as well to complement more Western approaches to health care. Surgery is an effective and at times a very necessary form of treatment. But it is also invasive and damaging to surrounding tissues, which means that the journey to full recovery is often one that is long and protracted. Tai Chi Chuan can often help in the recovery stages after surgery. Its ability to improve and enhance healing is ideal for post-operative recuperation. Using the Tai Chi process from day one after surgery, in the graduated process explained above, can help to increase the speed of your recovery.

The concept of illness, though, does not simply equate to disease. In fact, it is a much more complex state that is the result of an interaction between the disease process and our beliefs about it. Illness takes into account the ways in which symptoms may be differentially perceived, eval-

太
極
拳

uated and acted upon by each of us. It is as much about how we feel about ourselves as about the pathology of disease. Integrating Tai Chi Chuan into ill health gives us a method by which we can deal with illness at its root level. It can directly be used as a therapy to combat disease, and can also address mental attitudes towards our current state of health.

When you are ill or worried, make sure that you allow time for yourself. Illness is not only a sign that your physical self needs maintenance, but can also indicate that the mind and spirit need attention too. When you are ill allow yourself to use Chi Kung meditation and the Tai Chi form to provide you with the mental space you need. Let the mind lead the body (just like when you practise Tai Chi Chuan), so that you can take charge and improve your state if you are unwell. Use your intention, and direct your thoughts and attention to the problem or disease. In this way show yourself consideration and give your illness the respect it deserves. This will help you come to terms with the ailment, and maybe even understand the illness and why you have it. Indeed, acknowledging and paying respect to the illness may in itself change your attitudes towards it, and change the symptoms that you experience.

Focus the mind and think about your intentions and outcome. If you are ill, think about all that the illness means to you, and the effect it has upon you. Ask yourself these questions: What do you really want? What is your intention? How important is it to get better? In what ways does being ill serve you? What do you want instead of being ill? When you are clear about your intentions, you can bring focus to your actions – lack of Yi, or intention, means that your energies and your thoughts will wander aimlessly of their own volition. This can be good, but far better to harness those thoughts if you have an unsatisfactory situation, like an illness, that you want to resolve.

Tai Chi Chuan and our well-being, both mentally and physically, go hand in hand. Whilst the art will undoubtedly benefit those of us who are ill, it has wider implications for our health. Chinese physicians believe that taking steps to keep your energy system balanced and healthy will prevent illness in the first place. Hence the use of Tai Chi Chuan in health goes beyond the treatment of illness and also takes a role in disease prevention.

Take a simple analogy. If you drive your car hard all the time and neglect its regular maintenance, it will start giving you trouble and will deteriorate quickly. Keep neglecting it and it will break down and force you to attend to it. Pushing a system beyond its limits and neglecting proper maintenance invites deterioration and breakdown. Just like machines, human systems have limits and breaking points and in the same way they too require regular maintenance. If you are under pressure, push yourself too hard and neglect the proper maintenance on yourself, you will also deteriorate and eventually break down. Eventually your body will force you to stop and take notice by manifesting its neglect as illness.

Rather than finding a solution after a problem or illness has already set in, it is far better to regularly maintain and overhaul your system when you are well so that you stay healthy instead. Prevention is always better than cure, and using Tai Chi Chuan as a preventative measure, as well as a curative one, will provide you with the ideal strategy to maintain good health. Regularly practising the art and adapting it into daily life will maintain the free flow of Chi within us. It will strengthen us internally, boost our immune systems and increase out stamina, which will all enable us to lead lives as healthy and disease free as possible.

Going beyond the physical, Tai Chi will create quiet mental space in which you can reflect. It will allow you to enhance your awareness, gain focus and give you the ability to be centred and mindful of your aims and intentions. The calming influence the art has tames the immediacy of our knee-jerk reactions and instead encourages us to give ourselves the time in which we can observe ourselves, the environment and those around us, so that we respond with appropriate sensitivity and compassion to events.

Ultimately Tai Chi Chuan is a system that takes a holistic approach to our well-being and, regardless of whether you are in good health or not, the art can help all who follow its method.

TAI CHI CHUAN AND STRESS

Stress is an unavoidable consequence of life. However, contrary to popular belief, stress, or more precisely the stressors around us, are not necessarily harmful. As a positive influence, they can help compel us to action. They provide us with the means to realize our true potential so that we can express our talents and energies fully. Stress can result in a new awareness and give us fresh perspective, adding excitement and diversity to our lives. We all thrive under a certain amount of pressure, and increased stress can result in increased productivity and satisfaction – up to a point.

Stress, though, also has a strong negative influence. It can cause exhaustion and illness, both physical and mental. Emotionally, it can bring about feelings of anger, depression, rejection and unhappiness. Often stress can manifest itself physically and can affect any of the systems within our body. It can present itself as gastrointestinal disturbances, like abdominal upset or peptic ulcers. It can also affect our cardiovascular system, bringing high blood pressure and an increased risk of coronary heart disease and stroke. Neurologically too, it can manifest itself as headaches and insomnia. Indeed stress's negative effects have become more apparent with the hustle and bustle of today's society. Recent studies have shown that between 75 and 90 per cent of all visits to primary health care centres are due to stress-related problems, and as a result our economies have lost billions through the high level of sickness. *Time* magazine refers to stress as 'our leading health problem'. Negative stress has a marked effect on our lives causing physical, emotional and behavioural disorders, affecting our health, vitality and peace of mind as well as our professional lives and personal relationships.

Stress then is an entity that must be kept in balance, like yin and yang. Stress is not only about the external factors in our environment that are put upon us but our own individual ability to deal with stressors we encounter too. What may be stressful and distressing to one person may bring enjoyment and pleasure to another. There is no one level of stress that is optimal for everyone. We are all individuals with unique abilities and requirements and as such our intentions should not be to banish stress completely, but to find our own ideal level of stress, which will motivate but not overwhelm us.

Too much stress may be a negative experience that is the result of a substantial imbalance between life's demands and our capability to fulfil those demands. Too little stress and life becomes dull and tedious. In the same way, too little tension and stress on the strings of the Chinese instrument, the Pipa, will produce a muffled and dull tone; too much and the string will shrill and break. However, just the right amount of stress produces the perfect note. Stress, like anything else in life, must be kept in harmony and in balance.

The Western model of stress

Through human evolution and natural selection mankind developed critical life-saving responses that allowed our ancestors to deal with physical challenges and stresses. This response, known as the sympathetic drive (or more commonly as the flight or fight response), prepares our body for defensive action. The nervous system, in particular the sympathetic nervous system, increases in activity, as adrenaline, cortisol and other stress-related hormones are released. As a result our senses are sharpened, the pulse is quickened, the breathing is deepened and our muscles become tense, ready for any threatening situation that lies ahead.

But the stresses that are encountered in the modern world are not the occasional encounter with a wild beast or fight with another person, but rather a host of emotional challenges. Common events like being stuck in traffic jams and arguments with your boss or customers, which occur several times a day, result in the same, prehistoric flight or flight responses. These pre-programmed biological remnants of our former selves serve much less purpose in modern society and instead are potentially damaging, even fatal. Short-lived or infrequent episodes of stress pose little risk. However modern-day stresses tend to be persistent and insidious in nature, and with stressful situations going on unresolved (often further compounded by other stressors), the body is kept in a constant state of alert. This chronic activation of the stress hormones increases the wear on our biological system and, with the ability of the body to repair and defend itself compromised, the risk of disease and injury escalates. The short-term relentless pressures of stress ultimately have medium- to long-term consequences on our health and well-being.

The Traditional Chinese model of stress

Traditional Chinese Medicine takes a very different approach to our health than the Western model, and hence views stress in an alternative light. This system of medicine is not one based upon biochemistry or pathology but instead it is the concepts of balance and harmony that hold central significance. Yin and yang, the Five Elements, the Six Pathogenic Factors and the Seven Emotions are all Chinese medical theories that involve balance and, according to Eastern medical practice, it is excess or deficiency – imbalance – that causes illness. Furthermore, good health requires the vital energy we call Chi to flow smoothly through 14 major channels or meridians in the body. Observing imbalances as they arise allows us to address them before they develop into more serious illnesses or pathologies. The regular practice of Tai Chi Chuan is a method that works on balancing our whole system to prevent disease from arising. In Chinese medicine this includes the physical, emotional and mind/spirit dimensions. Stress is no different, and must be kept in balance in the same way. Here we take a look at how Wu Xing, or the Five Elements, can be applied to stress.

Wu Xing – the Five Elements

In oriental medicine our energetic system, and therefore our health, is mirrored in the environment in which we live. Mankind is just one manifestation of myriad expressions of energy (Chi), and follows the same universal laws of yin and yang and the consequent movement of energy.

One model for explaining the movement of Chi is that of Wu Xing or the Five Elements. 'Wu' means five, and the most common English translation for 'Xing' is elements. But 'elements' fails to convey the vital concept of movement. 'Phases' is a word that perhaps comes closer to 'Xing'. In fact Xing is even more than phases, and describes a constantly moving dynamic of energy, where each of the elements/phases is continually nourishing and controlling others in the cycle to maintain balance. The Five Elements in oriental thinking are Fire, Earth, Metal, Water and Wood. Each one represents an aspect of the environment in which we live, the functioning of the body, mind and Shen (spirit), and a direction and movement of energy. In fact, there are countless things in and around us that correspond to each of the elements/phases, such as the internal organs of the body, seasons, colours, tastes and sounds.

For the purposes of health and our well-being, each element corresponds to specific organs, with each organ/element association serving diagnostically to clarify symptoms from a specific disharmony or imbalance. For instance, Fire is the most yang of the Elements, the peak of energetic activity, represented in the seasons as summer and in time as midday. In health, Fire's associated organ is the heart. Here we do not only mean the physical organ, but also the energetic, Chi functions designated as 'Heart'. Any person with a typical Fire (Heart) imbalance might be slightly over-emotional, ungrounded and over-excitable. They may well speak quickly, and have difficulty in maintaining relationships and in knowing what is appropriate. If this is allowed to develop unchecked, it could ultimately lead to further health problems related to circulation, palpitations, insomnia or hypertension, which are all areas energetically associated with disharmonious Heart Chi at various levels.

In a state of health and balance, each Element nourishes or gives rise to the next one in what is known as the Sheng or Generating Cycle. This is sometimes also referred to as the 'mother/child' relationship. For example Fire (Heart) is the mother, giving rise to and nourishing its child, Earth (Spleen). This continues through to each element as shown by the direction of the arrows in the diagram opposite.

Each element is equally kept in check and controls another in the Controlling or Ke Cycle in order to maintain a harmonious balance amongst the five elements. As the second diagram opposite indicates, Fire controls Metal, Metal controls Wood, Wood controls Earth, Earth controls Water, and Water controls Fire.

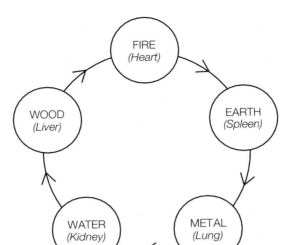

Take, for instance, the still and grounded yin quality of the Water (Kidney) Element. It controls the more yang tendency of the Fire (Heart) Element from rising up, expanding and becoming over-active.

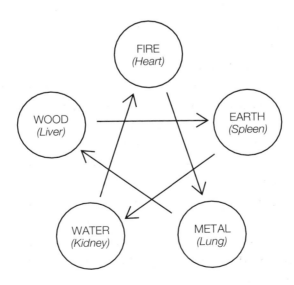

Putting these two dynamics together, it can be seen that disharmony in any one element has a potential implication for the whole cycle. Commonly, though, each of us has a constitutional weakness or a tendency to under- or over-express one or more of these elements.

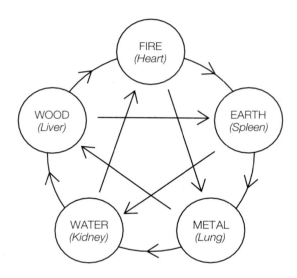

Wu Xing and stress

We all respond differently to stress. Some people thrive on responding to demands and being constantly stimulated. Provided they have the ability to switch off afterwards, the system can then return to a state of balance. However, for people with high-stress jobs, or who find it hard to relax, or whose constitutions respond poorly to stress, there can be a variety of difficulties with maintaining health. Inappropriate stress commonly affects the Wood and Water Elements in the cycle. The Wood Element is responsible for the free flow of Chi within the system, providing energy to us when and where it is needed, giving the body and the mind the flexibility to move and change as necessary. Under stress this function becomes blocked, creating aches, pains, tension in the body, irritability, inappropriate anger and frustration, and any other symptoms on p. 161.

Bearing the above cycles in mind, we can see that the disruption of the Wood (Liver) Element alone will have direct implications on other Elements.

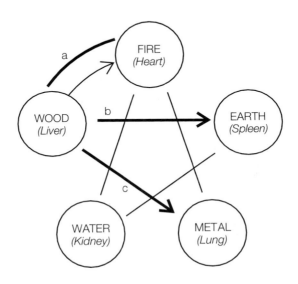

WOOD/FIRE

The Wood (Liver) Element fails to nourish and generate Fire (Heart) in times of stress. A typical symptom pattern here would be timidity, lack of courage, indecision, palpitations and insomnia.

WOOD/EARTH

Stress constrains the Wood (Liver) Element, causing Chi to stagnate. As a result it spills over and over-controls Earth (Spleen), giving rise to symptoms such as upper abdominal pain, feelings of distension, irritability, loose stools, poor appetite or other digestive problems.

WOOD/METAL

Instead of being controlled by Metal (Lungs), the Wood imbalance creates a backlash of energy, which could affect the Metal (Lung) element in the following ways: cough, asthma, feelings of distension in the chest and in the abdomen. This reverse of the controlling Ke cycle is pathological, and is commonly known as the Insulting Cycle.

WOOD/WATER

The Water (Kidney) energy fails to nourish the Wood, giving rise to tiredness, indecision, stress from having to make decisions; dry skin, hair, nails, eyes; amenorrhoea, headaches, etc.

Excess or deficiency

Imbalances can be caused by an Element having too strong an influence on the cycle or because it is weakened in some way (for example, by not being nourished by its mother Element in the cycle).

So, looking at the list opposite of some examples of signs and symptoms, we can see that in the Wood Element, an excess of Chi could build up, typical of that induced by excess stress. The person would feel as though they were bursting with energy that was stuck inside them. Then as the yang energy suddenly releases upwards, like a dam bursting through, it could give rise to angry outbursts, heat in the face or head, emotional instability, headaches, eye problems or even a stroke. This would be the Chi rising from an excess yang condition.

However, the yang can also rise as a result of there being insufficient yin energy to stabilize it. This would manifest as a more deficient condition and the signs and symptoms would be less severe, with an underlying feeling of fatigue and weakness, rather than the bursting, need-to-work-it-off feeling of the excess.

Benefits of Tai Chi

The following tables show some examples of signs and symptoms that could be generated by excessive stress and how that would manifest in each

太
极
拳

Element. Bear in mind that, because of the interaction of the Phases, more than one Element is often implicated.

The effects of the regular practice of basic Tai Chi principles in helping to promote the healthy functioning of each of the Phases are also explained.

Element/Phase	Examples of related signs/symptoms	
	Physical	*Psychological*
WOOD (Liver/Gall Bladder)	stiffness, rigidity of muscles/sinews	stress
	aches, pains that come and go	inability to make decisions, having too much choice
	abdominal pain	mood swings
	tight neck or shoulders	inability to plan
	lack of flexibility in sinews	feelings of being stuck
	poor eyesight, dry eyes	over-controlling or lack of control
	digestive problems due to fat intolerance	inappropriate anger
	problems with sexual functioning	frustration, resentment
	tiredness, unable to motivate	inflexibility of thought
	migraine, headaches	no sense of direction
	premenstrual syndrome	feeling unable to cope
	hip problems	

Tai Chi practice can encourage the regulation of the Wood energy by:

- Developing flexibility of mind and body
- Allowing the continuous flowing movements to move Chi to prevent stagnation in body and mind
- Allowing blood to nourish the whole system, particularly the sinews and eyes
- Sinking shoulders to reduce tension
- Developing focus for the intention
- Regulating the storage and distribution of blood.

Element/Phase	Examples of related signs/symptoms	
	Physical	*Psychological*
FIRE (Heart/Small Intestine/ Percardium/Triple Heater)	tightness/pain in the chest palpitations angina insomnia dream-disturbed sleep circulatory problems speech impediments hypertension	emotional constriction in chest depression over-excitability mania/hysteria over-emotional relationship problems long-term memory problems

Tai Chi practice can encourage the regulation of the Fire energy by:

- Calming the mind
- Increasing blood circulation
- Grounding the emotions in the centre
- Integrating the spiritual into the physical
- Freeing up physical/emotional constriction in the chest (sinking the chest).

Element/Phase	Examples of related signs/symptoms	
	Physical	*Psychological*
EARTH (Spleen/ Stomach)	digestive problems over/underweight eating disorders weak muscles/limbs fluid retention poor/voracious appetite anaemia varicose veins prolapse diabetes, hypoglycaemia tiredness menstrual problems	feelings of unmet need lack of fulfilment over-thinking need for support over-anxious over-supportive of others poor or over-active intellect feeling ungrounded

Tai Chi practice can encourage the regulation of the Earth energy by:

- Teaching to feel support from the Earth
- Grounding
- Training the intention/intellect
- Relaxing the mind
- Energizing by facilitating the absorption and transformation of food and drink into Food Chi
- Giving feelings of self-sufficiency
- Improving energetic balance to restore optimum weight
- Allowing the 'don't think, just do it!' approach
- Strengthening the limbs
- Encouraging two-way flow of Chi (up/down, Yin/Yang).

Element/Phase	Examples of related signs/symptoms	
	Physical	*Psychological*
METAL (Lung/ Large Intestine)	distension/tightness in chest constricted breathing respiratory problems weak immune system nose, sinus, throat problems lack of vitality coughing skin problems tiredness (from poor breathing/elimination) bowel problems	depression unable to let go of grief no/excessive boundaries isolation/detachment inability to let go melancholy holding on to old ideas fear of the new defensiveness lack of vitality

Tai Chi practice can encourage the regulation of the Metal energy by:

- Developing vitality
- Regulating the breath and opening the chest
- Sinking the chest – harnesses the Air Chi in the Tan Tien
- Opening the upper back
- Developing the quality of letting go
- Energizing, by maximizing use of Air Chi through breathing into the Centre or Tan Tien
- Cultivating Chi, strengthening defensive/immune system
- Relaxing the lower abdomen to facilitate the function of the large intestine.

Element/ Phase	Examples of related signs/symptoms	
	Physical	*Psychological*
WATER (Kidney/ Bladder)	low energy reserves	inappropriate feelings of fear
	lower back ache	poor will-power
	knee/ankle problems	timidity
	oedema below the waist	lack of endurance
	feelings or fear of cold	short-term memory problems
	urinary problems	lack of courage/ determination
	reproductive problems	inability to switch off
	nervous system disorders	driven to point of exhaustion
	weak constitutional strength	
	hormonal/endocrine problems	
	ear/hearing problems	
	asthma	
	early signs of ageing	
	no connection with lower part of the body	

Tai Chi practice can encourage the regulation of the Water energy by:

- Developing the Tan Tien — restores energy, revitalizes, strengthens lower back
- Opening and strengthening the spine
- Freeing up lower torso, hips and legs
- Strengthening the parasympathetic nervous system (PNS) — induces rest and recovery at a deep level
- Nourishing Jing/Essence (energetic reserves)
- Strengthening the will
- Developing confidence
- Using weight-bearing exercise to strengthen the skeletal structure/ bones
- Counteracting the effects of ageing (by nourishing the Tan Tien)
- Counteracting the effects of stress (by developing the PNS via stillness).

BRINGING TAI CHI CHUAN INTO YOUR LIFE

Tai Chi Chuan is ultimately an art that brings changes. Far from only being an isolated exercise, it crosses all boundaries to touch all aspects of our lives. The examples in this section alone have highlighted three large areas in which Tai Chi Chuan can affect us. But the art has infinite diversity. It can influence you physically, emotionally, cognitively and spiritually. Practise Tai Chi Chuan correctly and you will see these changes infuse your everyday life. Don't just take it from me though. There are millions of people who practice Tai Chi Chuan for its multitude of benefits and effects. Certainly many of my own students have seen the positive consequences the art can bring. And as such I leave the final words to one of my instructors, Sara:

Tai Chi has had many and varied effects in my everyday life. Some have been obvious straight away: feeling happier, sleeping better, being less stressed; other effects have been more subtle and sometimes come in the form of insights. I will be practising the form one day or even going about my daily business and suddenly I will understand something a fellow student or instructor was trying to tell me months before. I no longer shout at other drivers who cut me up or engage in conflict with others at work and home. It seems so unnecessary and a waste of good energy. On the health front, I am no longer asthmatic, nor do I suffer from the range of respiratory problems that I suffered from periodically in my life. Emotionally, I am much happier – in my experience daily practice of Tai Chi eradicates depression, restores energy and helps one to see everything in a positive light. It has enabled me to establish healthy boundaries in all areas of my life and brought me greatly enhanced and loving relationships. In my experience, Tai Chi brings with it a gentle energy which comforts, sustains and informs our life experience.

I have used the principles of Tai Chi at work on many occasions to resolve conflict situations. I've found that by not meeting force with force, it is impossible for people to fight with you. Staying centred and grounded prevents one becoming angry or upset by another person and enables one to view problems from many different perspectives. When the energy is sunk or grounded it is impossible to feel anxious about anything. Many people experience stress, anxiety and other negative emotions because their energy is being carried in the chest area, or all their energy is in their head, which is cut off from the rest of the body in the person's body-mind. This is why Tai Chi is so good as a reliever of stress. It brings the person's energy back into their body and to their centre. I have experimented with many students looking at problems in their lives with their energies in different locations of the body. When students sink their energy to their centres the problem does not go away but somehow the problem changes – it appears less overwhelming, solutions seem to come to mind that could help the situation, they see it from a more objective point of view – sometimes it simply does not seem like a problem any more.

Tai Chi is both sudden and subtle in its effects. Everyone can benefit from the first lesson. For some people it will be as simple as going home after a class and getting the best night's sleep they've had in a long time; for others it is recovery from serious illness. Its deepest effects may not be realized for many years, however. I am constantly amazed at the insights that come with regular practice of Tai Chi. The greater appreciation of the flow of life, understanding of energy and how to go with the flow rather than trying to battle against it have all saved me so much wasted time and energy.

Tai Chi has sustained me through so many difficult and trying times; it has enabled me to deal calmly with difficult people and situations, and it has helped me to develop discipline and integrity in my character. Tai Chi trains the body, mind and spirit to work in harmony and, when all these elements are aligned, the power is incredible. I wouldn't say I'm there yet – in Tai Chi you never reach the destination, there is always something else to learn – but my focus is much improved. I feel I have gained wisdom about what is most important to me in my life and how to draw that to myself.

For me it is the spiritual development that takes place in Tai Chi which is the most beautiful. It is perhaps the least written about because it is so difficult to put into words. I know how I have changed myself and see also how my students change as they come to lessons. Many have reported that they are less concerned about things that used to annoy or worry them. They stop attracting uncomfortable situations to themselves, they no longer become angry when someone tries to push their buttons, they feel more compassion and comradeship with the people around them. I see their faces change, becoming softer and laughing more, as well as their bodies becoming healthier and more flexible. Many change their job or start out on a new road – they discover what is really important to them in their lives and feel confident enough to strike out and get it. It really is a joy to experience.

I never thought that I would have the confidence to get up in front of a room of people and teach, but now it seems like the easiest and most enjoyable thing to do. I am deeply thankful to my Sifu and all the instructors and students at the Academy for the positive effect that their teachings have had on my life.

Appendix

LOOKING BEYOND: FINDING THE RIGHT TEACHER AND CLASS FOR YOU

15-Minute Tai Chi serves a purpose. It was specially designed to provide readers with the opportunity to gain a balanced introduction to the art's theoretical and practical aspects, and begin a journey that would allow the benefits of Tai Chi to spill over into everyday life. Having now completed the 15-minute programme, and having begun to experience its unique rewards first hand, the natural next step, should you wish to take the art further, is to start a class that offers the traditional system. Books can facilitate the art's practice or provide an introduction to Tai Chi, but no text can replace the tangible experience of a real class and the tailored instruction and guidance from a reputable and knowledgeable teacher.

However, finding a suitable class with the right teacher can be a difficult and frustrating exercise. The variety of styles and approaches, the misconceptions of what the art involves, and the quality of teaching itself are just a few of the factors that can deter the would-be beginner. In the days when Tai Chi Chuan was only taught to a select few, these and other difficulties were to be expected. Obstacles were placed in the path of these students, to test their character and determination, ensuring that only the most dedicated survived.

Today, however, attitudes are different. The benefits of Tai Chi are available to all, and whilst the higher levels of training remain open only to those who are fully committed, teachers will welcome anyone who has a genuine interest in the art. There are classes in all parts of the country, in leisure centres, adult education colleges, church halls, or even full-time Tai

Chi schools. However, not all Tai Chi classes are the same. They can vary considerably, depending upon the knowledge and experience of the instructor, who the instructor was taught by, the emphasis of the class, the size of the class, and so on. With so many factors to consider, choosing a Tai Chi class that is right for you is a decision that should be carefully thought out. To help you, here are some of the main points you should bear in mind.

Know yourself and know Tai Chi

Perhaps one of the first things you can do is to try and find out as much as you can about Tai Chi Chuan. The contents of this book will provide you with a balanced insight into the art, which will also serve well as a guide to what a genuine Tai Chi class may offer. But there are also plenty of other sources of information. Libraries and bookshops should contain books on the art, as will more specialist outlets like martial-arts stores, health-food shops or a local Chinatown. The Internet also offers a wealth of information on the art too. Whilst there is no guarantee that the information you gather is representative of the true art, it will give you an overall picture of the Tai Chi Chuan that is on offer in your area.

People practise Tai Chi for different reasons, and there are a multitude of classes to cater for these different needs. Finding out as much you can about the art, and then deciding what you want from it, can save time and make the choice of a class that much easier. If you want to learn the art solely for its health benefits or for spiritual discipline, then a class that emphasizes those aspects may be more suited to you. However, if your requirements are wider or even a little blurred, then a class with a traditional approach can usually offer the complete Tai Chi Chuan system and provide the ideal way in which you can consolidate and enhance what you have already learnt.

Different Tai Chi styles

There are three main styles of Traditional Tai Chi Chuan: Chen, Yang and Wu. These names relate to the original family names of the founding masters, and are seen as being separate and distinct styles, which can make the beginner's choice difficult. However, they all have the same origin, and their general principles should remain the same regardless of the style. These principles should focus on a holistic perspective, i.e. mind, body and spirit, that encompasses the:

- Harnessing of Chi – achieved through various Chi Kung systems
- Circulation of Chi – through correct practising of the Tai Chi Chuan form
- Application of Chi – by using the Chi for health, self-healing, healing others and self-defence.

Quality of instruction

Standards vary from school to school. Large schools and organizations will issue their own certificates and qualifications to instructors. However, this by no means ensures quality instruction. The quality of teachers can vary a lot depending on their knowledge and experience. There are even teachers professing to teach Tai Chi who are not actually teaching Tai Chi at all! So finding a knowledgeable and experienced teacher/master can be difficult, although not impossible.

No genuine teacher/master will mind telling you from whom they have learnt Tai Chi Chuan, and from what lineage their particular style of Tai Chi Chuan comes. The lineage of the teacher/master often gives authenticity to the style of Tai Chi Chuan taught. To be part of the official lineage, the teacher has to be an accepted disciple of a master from the existing branch of the family tree lineage. Your teacher should be as near to the trunk or centre line of the family tree as possible, ideally a disciple, so that the instruction you get is from an authentic source. However, you should be aware that many teachers put themselves on official lineages without having first been accepted as disciples. Students may have to change teacher/master, sometimes a number of times, until they finally meet the right master. This is fate or 'Yuen Fan' in Chinese. Be prepared to travel if you want top-level instruction in Tai Chi Chuan. Quality tuition saves time, effort and energy.

Also, beware of those who have learnt Tai Chi Chuan for only a short time or those who teach several different styles of martial arts. The art is complex, and is not a skill that can be mastered within a few months or years. There is a saying that only after practising it for 10 years do you really begin to take the first step into the realm of the true art of Tai Chi Chuan.

The school

Observe a Tai Chi class in session. Most teachers will not mind you observing them conducting a class. Some of them even have open sessions to introduce potential newcomers to Tai Chi Chuan. Ask yourself the following questions when you are there (remember that 'gut feeling' is important):

- What is the general atmosphere like while the class is in session?
- Will the environment be comfortable and conducive for growth?
- Are the students having fun and at ease with their teacher/master?
- What is the relationship between the students and the teacher/master?
- Are students being taught how to test their postures properly?
- Are the movements smooth, flowing and relaxed?
- Is there evidence of the Tai Chi principles?

Take the opportunity to chat with the students when they are having a rest during the session and find out how long they have been in the class, the benefits they feel, their perception of the teacher/master and any other questions that you may have. Generally in a good Tai Chi Chuan school, even though there may often be a high drop-out rate among beginners, you will find that teachers/instructors as well as students have been training with their master for a very long time.

Remember that at first you may be taught by instructors rather than by the master himself, until you reach a higher level. To this day, the higher aspects of Tai Chi Chuan are still a guarded secret and handed down only to a few selected disciples who have shown patience, dedication, commitment, sincerity and trustworthiness.

Students must show these characteristics before the master is prepared to share in-depth knowledge and experience of Tai Chi Chuan, a process that can take time.

Schools often offer group or individual sessions. There are advantages of both types of lesson. In group classes, there is the opportunity of working with people who are at different levels. It is important that students treat each other with respect, friendliness and consideration. In pair work, they should try and help each other in whatever exercises they do. Tai Chi Chuan should be non-competitive. The idea is to 'invest in loss' and let go of one's ego and of a 'winner takes all' mentality. The latter causes one to tense and resort to the use of physical strength, which leads to the blockage of Chi flow. The power derived from Chi energy takes time to nurture and requires complete softness and relaxation. Individual private sessions, though they may be more expensive, mean that learning is quicker, and is tailored to the student's specific needs.

■ ■ ■

Learning authentic Tai Chi Chuan is not easy. It needs lots of dedication, perseverance and regular practice under the constant guidance of a knowledgeable master to achieve a high level. Without such guidance, your progress can be very slow or even negligible. Tai Chi is a very subtle art, in which detail is vital. It must be taught properly, otherwise its essence will be lost, and precious time will be wasted. Like the saying in the Tai Chi classics, 'Miss by an inch, miss by a thousand miles.' However, if you invest the time and effort needed to learn Tai Chi, you will be rewarded many times over.

Further Reading

The following articles provide a selection of the scientific studies that have been carried out as to the benefits of the practice of Tai Chi.

Channer, KS, Barrow, D, Barrow, R, Osborne, M and Ives, G (1996), 'Changes in haemo-dynamic parameters following Tai Chi Chuan and aerobic exercise in patients recovering from acute myocardial infarction'. *Postgrad Med J* 72(848): 349–51.

Henderson, NK, White, CP and Eisman, JA (1998), 'The roles of exercise and fall risk reduction in the prevention of osteoporosis'. *Endocrinol Metab Clin North Am* 27(2): 369–87. Review.

Hong, Y, Li, JX and Robinson, PD (2000), 'Balance control, flexibility, and cardiorespiratory fitness among older Tai Chi practitioners'. *Br J Sports Med* 4(1): 29–34.

Jin, P (1989), 'Changes in heart rate, noradrenaline, cortisol and mood during Tai Chi'. *J Psychosom Res* 33(2): 197–206.

Jin, P (1992), 'Efficacy of Tai Chi, brisk walking, meditation, and reading in reducing mental and emotional stress'. *J Psychosom Res* 36(4): 361–70.

Lan, C, Chen, SY, Lai, JS and Wong, MK (1999), 'The effect of Tai Chi on cardiorespiratory function in patients with coronary artery bypass surgery'. *Med Sci Sports Exerc* 31(5): 634–8.

Li, JX, Hong, Y and Chan, KM (2001), 'Tai Chi: physiological characteristics and beneficial effects on health'. *Br J Sports Med* 35(3): 148–56. Review.

Qin, L, Au, S, Choy, W, Leung, P, Neff, M, Lee, K, Lau, M, Woo, J and Chan, K (2002), 'Regular Tai Chi Chuan exercise may retard bone loss in postmenopausal women: A case-control study'. *Arch Phys Med Rehabil* 83(10): 1355–9.

Shapira, MY, Chelouche, M, Yanai, R, Kaner, C and Szold, A (2001), 'Tai Chi Chuan practice as a tool for rehabilitation of severe head trauma: 3 case reports'. *Arch Phys Med Rehabil* 82(9): 1283–5.

Wang, JS, Lan, C, Chen, SY and Wong, MK (2002), 'Tai Chi Chuan training is associated with enhanced endothelium-dependent dilation in skin vasculature of healthy older men'. *J Am Geriatr Soc* 50(6): 1024–30.

Wolf, SL, Sattin, RW, O'Grady, M, Freret, N, Ricci, L, Greenspan, AI, Xu, T and Kutner, M (2001), 'A study design to investigate the effect of intense Tai Chi in reducing falls among older adults transitioning to frailty'. *Control Clin Trials* 22(6): 689–704.

Wu, G (2002), 'Evaluation of the effectiveness of Tai Chi for improving balance and preventing falls in the older population – a review'. *J Am Geriatr Soc* 50(4): 746–54. Review.

About the Authors

Master John Ding
Sixth Generation Lineage
Yang Style Tai Chi Chuan

John Ding, BA (Hons), DMS began his study of martial arts at an early age under various Shaolin Kung Fu masters, before devoting himself entirely to the internal system of Tai Chi Chuan. He is one of the few people to have studied under all three formal disciples of the late Grandmaster Yang Sau Chung of the Yang family. On 1 January 1998, John Ding, founder of the John Ding International Academy of Tai Chi Chuan, based in London, was accepted as the first disciple of Grandmaster Ip Tai Tak.

Master Ding is also the publisher and editor-in-chief of *Tai Chi and Alternative Health* magazine, one of the leading international Tai Chi magazines.

■ ■ ■

Doctor Alan Ding
Seventh Generation Lineage
Yang Style Tai Chi Chuan

Dr Alan Ding, MBBS began his study of Tai Chi Chuan at the early age of five under his father, Master John Ding. During his Tai Chi Chuan training, he has also studied under Master Chu Gin Soon (Second Disciple of Grandmaster Yang Sau Chung), who teaches in Boston, USA.

In his pursuit of excellence in Yang Style Tai Chi Chuan, Alan Ding still continues his studies with his father and Grandmaster Ip Tai Tak.

He is a doctor in the UK's National Health Service, as well as an accomplished Yang Style Tai Chi Chuan practitioner and Chief Instructor of the John Ding International Academy of Tai Chi Chuan.

Other Tai Chi Resources by the Same Authors

15-Minute Tai Chi Chuan Video
Strong Body, Still Mind
By Master John Ding with Dr Alan Ding
Price: £20.00
Running time approximately 45–55 minutes

This video is an excellent accompaniment to *15-Minute Tai Chi*. It is a good source of reference and also provides a very useful visual aid to learning the step-by-step specially designed 10-session training programme as described in the book. A valuable and informative video for beginners and other levels of Tai Chi practitioners. The complete holistic workout for body, mind and spirit. (DVD also available.)

Yang 200 Video
An insight into Tai Chi Chuan
By Master John Ding
Price: £20.00
Running time approximately 50 minutes

The video provides a fascinating insight into the ancient Chinese art of Tai Chi Chuan and provides quality demonstrations with commentaries explaining the different aspects of Tai Chi Chuan. This video will be of interest to people from all walks of life and all levels of Tai Chi practitioners or external martial-arts practitioners. Highly recommended.

Traditional Yang Style Tai Chi Chuan Video
Complete long form in easy to follow stages
By Master John Ding
Price: £27 per tape or £74 for all three
Running time approximately 45–55 minutes each

This best-selling set of three videos looks at the Traditional Yang Style Tai Chi Chuan form as demonstrated by Master Ding with the assistance of his students. As well as showing each posture, it also shows you how to test the postures out with a partner to ensure they are correct. The commentary explains how each move is carried out as well as identifying the major points to watch for.

- Volume 1 covers the Principles and Part 1 of the form
- Volume 2 covers Part 2 of the form
- Volume 3 covers Part 3 of the form and some basic self-defence applications

Tai Chi Chuan Self-Defence Applications Volume 1 Video
A real insight and understanding of Tai Chi Chuan for self-defence
By Master John Ding
Price: £27.00
Running time approximately 55 minutes

The tape covers some basic principles and concepts of Tai Chi and its applications. All techniques are shown step-by-step and then at normal speed to appreciate the power of Tai Chi Chuan. Essential for all who are interested in gaining an insight into the martial aspects of this internal art.

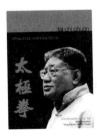

Tai Chi Chuan Revelations
Principles & Concepts
By Grandmaster Ip Tai Tak,
Translated by Master John Ding
Price: special limited hardback edition with Grandmaster Ip's signature: £55
Paperback: £29.99

In his first book, Grandmaster Ip, Fifth Generation Yang Style Tai Chi Chuan, First Disciple of Great Grandmaster Yang Sau Chung of the Yang Family Tai Chi Chuan and one of the leading authorities on the Traditional Yang Family Tai Chi Chuan, shares his deep insight and understanding of the Tai Chi classics, including some original interpretations and concepts not found in other Tai Chi texts and some rare pictures of Grandmaster Ip and Great Grandmaster Yang Sau Chung. Without a good understanding of Tai Chi principles and concepts students will never attain a high level in the art. This book contains a wealth of knowledge, which will assist both beginners and advanced practitioners seeking to improve and gain deeper understanding in the principles and concepts of Tai Chi Chuan. This rare and informative book on Tai Chi Chuan is a must for practitioners of all styles of Tai Chi.

Tai Chi and Alternative Health Magazine
Edited and published since 1994 by Master John Ding
Price: £3.00 (UK only, exclusive of postage and packaging)

Every quarterly issue features in-depth articles on all aspects of Tai Chi Chuan – its history, theory and martial application as well as interviews with leading Tai Chi Masters. The magazine also features the theory and practice of Alternative Health Therapies – Shiatsu, Acupuncture, Aromatherapy, etc., plus articles on Chinese philosophy, Taoism, Zen Buddhism, reviews and news. *TCAH* is essential reading for those with an interest in Internal Arts, Alternative Therapies and the philosophies that shape them. To subscribe, contact the address below.

To order any of the above item/s please send a cheque or sterling bank draft (for all overseas orders) payable to TCAH to:

TCAH
P.O. Box 6404
London E18 1EX
United Kingdom

Please ensure that you add the following amount for postage and packaging:
UK only: £2.50 for the first item and £1 for each subsequent item.
Europe: add 30 per cent of the total cost of order.
Rest of the world: add 60 per cent of the total cost of order.

For more information, visit our website: www.taichiwl.demon.co.uk
or email: tcah@taichiwl.demon.co.uk

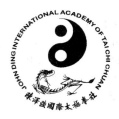

The John Ding International Academy of Tai Chi Chuan

Founder: Master John Ding,
6th Generation of Yang Style Tai Chi Chuan

Chief Instructor: Dr Alan Ding,
7th Generation of Yang Style Tai Chi Chuan

The Academy was established in 1994 in London, United Kingdom to promote the practice of Traditional Yang Style Tai Chi Chuan. Since then it has expanded internationally with numerous branches established worldwide.

The Academy provides tradition, authenticity, depth and excellence of training in all aspects of the Traditional Yang Style Tai Chi Chuan for all levels through its international branches. In addition, we now also provide courses in 15-minute Tai Chi and stress management.

The Academy welcomes Tai Chi instructors or practitioners with at least 4 years of Tai Chi Chuan experience in Yang Style Tai Chi Chuan wishing to train as qualified instructors of the JDIATCC and to receive high quality training in the traditional approach.

Master Ding and Dr Alan Ding are available for workshops for club members in any areas or countries, covering all aspects of Yang Style Tai Chi Chuan.

To find out more about the John Ding International Academy of Tai Chi Chuan and its branches, or for nearest classes in your area, please email us at: jdiatcc@taichiwl.demon.co.uk or visit our website: www.taichiwl.demon.co.uk

Index

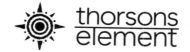

Praise for *Mail Obsession*

'Almost every page contains at least one thing
that you'll be itching to startle your friends with'
Reader's Digest

'Turns up trivia at every stop'
BBC Radio 4

'Awesome – full of amazing facts'
The QI Elves

'I didn't know post could be so interesting'
The One Show

'Fascinating'
Daily Mail

Mark Mason is a lover of trivia, the 'little facts that slip down the back of life's sofa'. Before becoming a writer, he sold Christmas cards at Harrods, played guitar in a blues band, and made radio programmes for the BBC. His previous books include *The Importance of Being Trivial*, *Walk the Lines* and *Move Along, Please*.

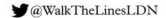@WalkTheLinesLDN

www.theimportanceofbeingtrivial.com

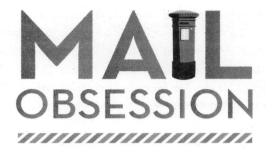

OBSESSION

//////////////////////////

A Journey Round Britain
By Postcode

MARK MASON

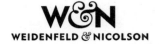

WEIDENFELD & NICOLSON

A W&N PAPERBACK

First published in Great Britain in 2015
This paperback edition published in 2016
by Weidenfeld & Nicolson,
an imprint of The Orion Publishing Group Ltd
Carmelite House, 50 Victoria Embankment
London, EC4Y 0DZ

An Hachette UK Company

1 3 5 7 9 10 8 6 4 2

A CIP catalogue record for this book is
available from the British Library.

ISBN: 978 1 780 22833 4

Typeset at The Spartan Press Ltd,
Lymington, Hants

Printed and bound by CPI Group (UK) Ltd,
Croydon, CR0 4YY

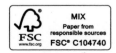

www.orionbooks.co.uk

CONTENTS

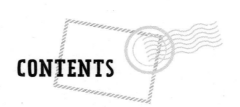

INTRODUCTION

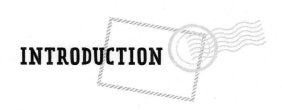

I sometimes wonder if the great Victorian administrators knew what they'd started. The men (it *would* have been men in those days) who first laid out Britain's railway system, and created ways of classifying the trains that ran on it. The men who met in a London pub to form the Football Association, codifying the game's rules and establishing a league. The men, in particular, who decided that the country's postal system needed formalising, and started putting letters and numbers at the end of our addresses.

The reason I wonder about them is nothing to do with what the administrators were trying to achieve. It's what they *accidentally* achieved that fascinates me. One man's list, you see, is another man's challenge. The Victorians who covered Britain with a rail network also, without meaning to, set in train (I'm sorry) the process by which lots of people (again, mostly male) ended up trying to 'spot' every locomotive in the book. The league started by the FA has now grown to four leagues, containing 92 teams – which means that there is something called 'The 92 Club', a group of fans who have visited all those team's grounds to watch matches. Whenever a new team is promoted, or an existing one moves stadium, members have to watch a game there to maintain their record.

But it's the postcodes that have really got me thinking. A century and a half after Sir Rowland Hill first split London into ten districts, the UK now has 124 postcode areas. Wherever you live in this green and occasionally pleasant land, your home falls into one of those areas. A letter, or more probably two letters, features at the end of your address, followed by some numbers and some other letters, all of them combining to aid Sir Rowland's successors in bringing you bank statements, birthday cards, TV licences and the other necessities of modern life. This is what the administrators were trying to achieve. What they have accidentally achieved is to provide me with the perfect method of conquering Britain. Because I have decided to collect at least one fact – one piece of historical, geographical or cultural trivia – from every one of those 124 postcode areas.

I've been looking for a 'completist' way of discovering my home country ever since finishing a Land's End to John O'Groats trip. That was great fun, and made me see Britain in several new lights, but it was just one line across the country. The route – dictated by local bus services, that being my chosen means of transport – was just one route. In Leeds, say, I could have chosen to head north-east towards York, instead of (as I actually did) north-west towards Ilkley and the Lake District. From Glasgow I could have travelled up the west coast of Scotland rather than the east. Plus, of course, there were whole areas of Britain which, given the nature of a roughly straight line between Land's End and John O'Groats, were never going to be on the itinerary at all. Kent, for instance – no way I'd be enjoying England's only one-syllable county on that trip. Wales remained unsampled. As did Northern Ireland, that being not just over the water but outside Britain full stop. It isn't outside the postcode system, though, which is a United Kingdom one. If you want to get that kingdom done, you can't choose a more exhaustive method than its postcodes. As soon as I saw the list of those

124 areas the challenge formed in my mind: I had to do the AB to ZE of my home country.[1]

The project holds several attractions. Firstly, the joy of exploration inherent in any journey. Much of the research will be done on the road. Which roads, though, and which bits of the country will they lead me to? Maybe my BN (Brighton) fact will concern Beachy Head, where the worn patch of grass from which people jump to their deaths is known locally as the Launch Pad? Perhaps LL (Llandudno) will be Plas Newydd, the country seat of the Marquess of Anglesey, where you can see the wooden leg used by the 1st Marquess after his real one was blown off at the Battle of Waterloo? ('By God, sir, I've lost my leg!' he cried, to which the Duke of Wellington replied, 'By God, sir, so you have!') Could EH be Edinburgh itself, where the Bay City Rollers chose their name by throwing a dart at a map of the USA and hitting Bay City, Michigan? Who knows? The only certainty is that lessons lie in wait.

Talking of maps, I'm not far behind Les and the boys in an appreciation of the inspiration cartography can provide. Crossing off the postcodes as I achieve them will be another of the project's joys. The irony occurs to me that it's only by splitting something up that you can unify it. My way of unifying it, anyway, the way that entails learning about every part of it so you can claim 'ownership'. Without those parts being segregated, you could learn a fact, *any* single fact about the UK and claim you knew the country. But once you've partitioned it into 124 chunks, you have to learn something about every one of them. Only then can you say you know the country – but that knowledge is so much more comprehensive.

[1] Aberdeen and the Shetland Islands. The latter are ZE because until 1975 the Shetlands were known as Zetland. Did the change happen after Sean Connery voiced a marketing campaign?

Something else the map triggers is wordplay. All but eight of the 124 codes are double-lettered ones. I find myself wondering if B.B. King ever visited Blackburn, if the residents of Hemel Hempstead eat much HP Sauce, if people in Preston are especially keen on proportional representation, or indeed on public relations. I even realise, with childish delight, that by splitting the word 'postcode' into 'PO', 'ST', 'CO' and 'DE' you can reference Portsmouth, Stoke-on-Trent, Colchester and Derby. The delight is even more childish because one of those postcodes is my own. Not that I was very happy about this at first. Having moved from London to a village in Suffolk, I was disappointed to learn that my postcode began 'CO'. Why should I be tarred with the brush of Essex? I'd never worn white stilettos in my life.

Although I've warmed to the neighbouring county in the ten years since, that episode was still a sign of the role postcodes play in our lives. You'd think they would have withered away as emails replaced letters, but no, a different form of technology has made them more relevant than ever: the satnav. Millions of people type postcodes into one every week. Then there's that phrase 'postcode lottery', complained about whenever different councils provide different levels of service, though it always seems to me the people doing the complaining were the same people calling for more decisions to be taken at a local level in the first place. There are also the insurance implications. Residents of SE2 have campaigned for a change to the Bexleyheath code so they won't have to pay London premiums. Conversely, an Ilford businessman wants E19 instead of IG so he can claim his business *is* in London.[2] People in Windsor

[2] E19 has never been used. E20 used to be reserved for Walford in *EastEnders*. The soap now shares it with the real-life Olympic Park in Stratford.

and Maidenhead, meanwhile, dislike their SL code because it comes from common-sounding Slough: they're calling for the invention of 'WM' instead. Although as to most of us those letters say 'West Midlands' you have to conclude they haven't really thought that one through.

Once you add in the media's use of postcodes (for instance the story a few years ago that Tesco now had a store in every one[3]), you realise they're going to be part of our national life for a long time yet. They were certainly iconic in my childhood: the only way to get in touch with your favourite TV programme, magazine or fan club was by post, so postcodes were burned into your subconscious. The times Tony Blackburn's voice crackled across the Radio 1 airwaves, for instance, telling us to send our letters to W1A 4WW. I was particularly excited one year when the Post Office gave the BBC their own special code for the seminal 'Shot of the Championship' competition at the World Snooker in Sheffield: S14 7UP. For the non-snooker fans among you, 147 is the game's highest possible break. Although given that the competition's popularity merited its own postcode, as a non-snooker fan you would have found the early 1980s a rather lonely time.

It wasn't always thus. For well over a century the postal authorities struggled to get people using their postcodes. That first London scheme was set up by Sir Rowland Hill in 1857. He split the capital into N, NE, E, SE, S, SW, W and NW, adding the two 'middle' areas of EC and WC (East and West Central). A decade later Anthony Trollope, not content with being a successful novelist (don't you hate these industrious Victorian types?) used his position at the Post Office to get rid of NE and S, leaving London with only the eight codes, poor thing. The 1930s saw postcodes introduced in larger towns

---

[3] The last area to hold out was HG (Harrogate).

and cities across the land. Some of them entered popular lingo – for instance by the 1940s many people, Ringo Starr among them, were saying that they lived in 'Liverpool 8'. But by and large people were too lazy to comply. Perhaps this isn't surprising, given the campaign slogan deployed to encourage them: 'For speed and certainty always use a postal district number on your letters and notepaper.' Hardly 'go to work on an egg', is it?

Some sticks remained in the mud until the 1970s. Michael Palin's diary for 16 February 1971 records his resentment not at the new decimal coins introduced that day, but a fear that postcodes 'will one day replace towns with numbers – and after towns streets, and after streets . . . ?' He also bemoans the loss of letters from phone numbers. Exchanges often had witty names, such as FREmantle (373) for Earl's Court, because lots of Australians lived there. Well, Michael, if it's wit you're after, postcodes offer it in spades. Father Christmas is SAN TA1. Sheffield Wednesday are S6 1SW, while across the city their rivals United glory in S2 4SU.[4] The part of HM Revenue and Customs which deals with VAT is at BX5 5AT, V being the Roman numeral for 5. Over in Cardiff, Lloyds Bank are CF99 1BH, the letters standing for 'black horse'. Said symbol, ironically, dating from the days before addresses existed at all, never mind had postcodes in them: businesses were identified not by street numbers but by symbols outside their premises. The black horse was the symbol of the goldsmith whose firm evolved into the modern Lloyds. I'm looking forward to investigating the system's arcane secrets. Zeroes are high rather than low, apparently (in other words they're only used after 1 to 9 have been exhausted). To avoid confusion with numbers

---

[4] More humour from those who name Sheffield's streets: a road housing the base for a police helicopter has been christened Letsby Avenue.

the final two letters in a postcode are never taken from the list CIKMOV, which sounds for all the world like an organisation in a John le Carré novel.

Beyond all this, though, what I'm really looking forward to is poking into every one of the UK's 124 nooks and crannies, discovering the country's past and its present, the quirks of its history and the humour of its residents. In Lincolnshire, for instance, the road sign at the turning for a couple of tiny villages says 'To Mavis Enderby and Old Bolingbroke', and underneath someone has written '...the gift of a son'. Where will the project take me? To Woking, the town that found fame in a Jam song as the one called Malice? Or Woking*ham*, home to the Transport Research Laboratory, the body which settles such issues as the maximum time you can spend waiting at a pedestrian crossing (two minutes)? Could Kilmarnock be on the agenda, the birthplace of Johnnie Walker with his square bottles (so more could be fitted into the same space) and angled labels (so the whisky's name could be larger)?[5] Perhaps the itinerary will include Merthyr Mawr in Wales, whose sand dunes were used for the location filming in *Lawrence of Arabia*? So many facts from our nation's past could flit into the torch beam of my research. WHSmith was started by someone called H. W. Smith. (It was his son William Herbert who really built the business up.) When newspaper crosswords became popular in the early twentieth century staff at Dulwich library blacked out the empty squares to prevent people being distracted from the news. The BBC chose Beethoven's Fifth as the call sign for its Second World War 'V for Victory' campaign because the 'der-der-der-DER' opening is Morse code for V. Surely it says an awful lot about Britain that in fighting a German dictator we used the work of a German composer.

[5] The angle in question being 24 degrees.

And so, as Blur might put it, the story begins. I have to assemble a history of the United Kingdom containing at least one fact from each of its 124 postcode areas. It's time to lose myself in some mail obsession.

1
LIFE NEAR THE FAST LANE

Perhaps it's because my research starts in the run-up to Christmas, but pretty soon I come to see Britain as nothing less than one huge advent calendar. Instead of 22 windows hiding chocolates, it has 124 windows hiding trivia. If information had the same calorific value as chocolate, I would soon be incapable of leaving the house.

The image of an advent calendar coincides with my first investment of the project: a postcode map of Britain. This is obtained (as just about any map in the world can be) from Stanfords, whose presence in London's Covent Garden gives them the postcode a friend of Evelyn Waugh's always called 'West Central' because 'WC' had 'indelicate associations'. The map shows each area's geographical boundaries, and these look like 124 advent windows. The fact they're all different shapes and sizes merely adds to their charm. The only wall space big enough for the 4 foot by 3 foot sheet is in my young son's bedroom, but this is fine: it's never too early to introduce children to maps. The bits of Blu-Tack round the edge don't provide enough support, so extra anchoring comes from blobs underneath WR (Worcester) and KY (Kirkcaldy).

In one or two cases the trivia doesn't exactly come tumbling out of the advent calendar: it's more a case of poking around in the dark recesses, desperately hoping that something's there. Kirkcaldy itself, for instance, yields only the fact that when St Andrews golf course was first established in 1552 it also functioned as a rabbit farm. This is moderately interesting – and a return to the policy would certainly make the Open Championship more entertaining – but it's not grade A trivia. It does lead to the additional info that golf was banned in Scotland by James II because it distracted men from training for the wars against England – but even this isn't the standard we're aiming to set. There's also stuff that *is* top-drawer but doesn't relate to a particular postcode area. Like the fact that in 2012 'John' fell out of the top 100 names given to boys in England and Wales. (How can this be true?) Or the fact that that defining phrase of Britishness 'stiff upper lip' isn't British at all: it was first recorded in the Boston newspaper the *Massachusetts Spy* in 1815.

When a postcode does deliver, though, *boy* does it deliver. The Northampton (NN) window is positively quaking as it struggles to hold back the trivia behind it. There's Borough Hill in Daventry, from where the BBC's World Service (then called the Empire Service) used to be broadcast. The announcement 'Daventry calling' was the reason the literal pronunciation became the accepted one – before that people had said 'Daintree'.[1] There's Corby, which although it didn't invent the trouser press (that was done in Windsor by someone *called* Corby), has a crater on Mars named after it. This is in tribute to a conversation between the Apollo 11 crew and mission control, who relayed Neil and Buzz and Mike items of world news to help them feel bonded to their home planet. 'In Corby,' went one story, 'an Irishman named John Coil won the World's Porridge Eating Championship by consuming 23 bowls of instant oatmeal in ten minutes.' Another NN representative is Margaret Bondfield, who, not content with being MP for

---

[1] The same hill, at around the same time (1935), also saw the first demonstration of radar. Signals were bounced off a Heyford bomber flying overhead, allowing its position to be estimated.

Northampton, also became (in 1929) the first ever female member of the British Cabinet. Then there's the yard-long lock of hair preserved in a Wellingborough church, taken from an ancient queen in the era when long hair was a status symbol (which is why the Romans, when they first invaded a country, made everyone cut theirs off as a sign of defeat) ... the start, in Kilsby, of the A361, cherished by seasoned pub-quizzers as the longest three-digit road in Britain ... and (sticking with the motoring theme) the country's first ever arrest following a car chase. Sergeant Hector Macleod was our man behind the wheel in 1899, when he caught and flagged down a Benz car driven by a wanted criminal. The heady speed of 15 miles per hour was reached, though my favourite detail is the crime for which the man was wanted: selling counterfeit circus tickets.

Much of the material I unearth comes, like Macleod and his screaming tyres, from the Victorian era. Whenever you read about this period you come away with the feeling that Britain crammed more achievement, adventure and all-round derring-do into those 64 years than we've managed in the rest of our history put together. Yes, I know there were children up chimneys and all that, but for sheer energy the last two-thirds of the nineteenth century just can't be beaten. It's the inventions that always get you: there were so *many* of the things. The average Victorian couldn't turn around without inventing a revolutionary new industrial process or the cure for a fatal disease. Things had been going this way for a while – take Joseph Bramah, for instance, the Yorkshireman who died a couple of decades before Victoria took the throne, though not before he'd given us the hydraulic press, the beer pump, an improved design for the toilet, a type of lock he challenged anyone to pick (the challenge went unmet for 67 years, until well after Bramah's death, and even then it took the successful man 51 hours to do it), and a machine for printing banknotes with consecutive serial numbers. Once the new queen was in place, though, things really took off. Take Hiram Maxim. He's most famous as the inventor of the machine gun, but he also held patents on a mousetrap, a set of hair curlers and an automatic fire-sprinkler that didn't just douse the flames, it alerted the nearest fire station, too. One of Maxim's other brainwaves was a steam inhaler for bronchitis sufferers called the Pipe of Peace. People criticised him for pandering to 'quackery'. Maxim replied: 'It will be seen that it is a very creditable thing to invent a killing machine, and nothing less than a disgrace to invent an apparatus to prevent human suffering.'

But the award for the greatest concentration of inventive talent per square yard surely goes to the Nottingham pitch that played host to a game of football in January 1891. This event, which makes a strong early claim to be my NG fact, is recorded as the first ever game to use goal nets. They were the recent creation of John Alexander Brodie, a civil engineer from Liverpool. Despite being responsible for the Mersey Tunnel and the initial planning of New Delhi, Brodie said the goal net was the invention of which he remained most proud. What I really love about the story is that it's an example of how your assumptions can be challenged. The reason nets were needed is simple: to stop people having to run miles to retrieve the ball, right? Wrong. It was actually because there had been frequent arguments about whether the ball had passed inside or outside the post. Brodie invented the net as an easy way of settling the issue – if the ball ended up in the net it was a goal, if not it wasn't.[2] Therefore when the Everton striker Fred Geary scored

---

[2] On the 'miles to get the ball back' question: Geoff Hurst has admitted that his third goal in the 1966 World Cup final wasn't an attempted shot at all – he was trying to leather the ball way over the crossbar so a few more seconds would be wasted at the end of extra time.

for the North against the South, he became the first player ever to hit the back of the net. The reason for the 'greatest concentration' title, meanwhile, is that the match referee that day was Sam Widdowson – inventor of the shin-pad.

For my own postcode (CO) I'm tempted to use one of the facts I already know. We do a nice line in nursery rhymes round here – the original Humpty Dumpty was a Royalist cannon during the Civil War, shot down by Parliamentary troops from the wall protecting Colchester ('all the King's horses and all the King's men, couldn't put Humpty together again'), while the village of Lavenham gave us 'Twinkle Twinkle Little Star'. Jane Taylor, who lived there with her sister, wrote the words in 1806 (several years after Mozart had provided the music).[3] I think about Taylor a lot these days – a couple of years ago the local council starting turning off my village's street lights at midnight, a decision prompted by budget cuts but which has had the delightful effect of making the night sky even brighter than it was before. Gazing up at the galaxy, I always relish the mind-blowing fact that the light from any star further than 200-odd light years away (in other words, lots of them) is older than 'Twinkle Twinkle' itself: it left the star before Taylor wrote the words.

Despite knowing these facts, however, it really doesn't seem in the spirit of things to use them for CO. This project is all about discovery, the joy of the new, the unencountered. What's particularly thrilling is learning a fresh detail about a story I *thought* I knew. The Jack Russell terrier, for instance. I knew it was named after the man who first bred it, and I'm pretty sure I knew he was a clergyman, the Reverend John Russell

---

[3] A local friend went to school with someone who lived in Taylor's house in the 1980s. She got very fed up with American tourists taking photos of her bedroom window.

of Swimbridge in Devon. What I didn't know is why he bred them. And so we arrive at the project's first fact:

EX (Exeter): The Jack Russell was bred with a predominantly white coat so that, unlike darker terriers, it could be easily distinguished from the fox during a hunt.

Russell bought his first terrier, Trump, from a milkman in 1819, during his last year at Oxford University. Though a man breeding his best friend to have particular physical characteristics was nothing new: the bulldog's backward-sloping nose was engineered for bull-baiting (so it could breathe without letting go of the larger beast). This may not sit very well with twenty-first-century sensibilities, but at least we Brits only design our dogs to attack other animals. The Dobermann hails from Germany, where it was bred by the tax collector Karl Dobermann to accompany him on his rounds.

After this the facts mount up with pleasing regularity. As so often in life the best stuff comes along when you're not actually looking for it. Watching a TV quiz show I learn that:

WV (Wolverhampton): Wolverhampton Wanderers have the longest name (22 letters) of any football team in the top four English divisions.

Reading an article about the referendum on Scottish independence, I discover that:

EH (Edinburgh): The shade of blue in the Scottish flag is slightly different from that in the Union Jack.

The Scottish Parliament voted to change it in 2003, from Pantone 280 to the marginally lighter Pantone 300.

Talking to a friend about her family's trip on Eurostar, before which they stayed overnight in a hotel, I learn that:

ME (Rochester[4]): There is a village in Kent called Dunkirk.

This follows a few moments' confusion as Catherine tries to explain which side of the Channel they were on which night. But no, it turns out that as well as the famous Dunkirk there's also one over here. The name arose because in centuries past a Flemish person from the Continental Dunkirk came and settled there. The most delicious accidental discovery, though, comes as I'm waiting to get my hair cut. The place I use is in London (in the postcode Evelyn Waugh's friend had such problems with), and prides itself on giving the clientele something better than old copies of *Hello!* to peruse. The reading matter, often of an alternative bent, is changed frequently. Today it includes *The Complete Guide to Ferrets*, a book whose size and attention to detail leaves not the slightest doubt as to its title's accuracy. I'm flicking through it, thinking that yes, the book's presence is a nicely post-modern joke but there really isn't anything of interest to be found, when wham, along comes what has to be my first London fact:

SW (London South West): Some of the TV cables at Buckingham Palace for the 1981 wedding of Prince Charles and Lady Diana Spencer were installed by a ferret.

[4] The initials originally came from 'Medway towns'.

The cables had to be fed through a narrow underground duct. Conventional methods had failed, so the trusty ferret was fitted with a harness to which a very light but very strong line was attached. Then, lured by a piece of bacon, it scuttled through the duct. When it emerged at the other end engineers were able to attach the TV cables to the line and pull them through. These furry heroics push aside a long list of SW trivia, some of it from the same royal residence, such as the Queen's trick for preventing her dresses blowing up in strong winds à la Marilyn Monroe: she has lead curtain weights sewn into the hems. Down the road at Parliament was the ancient law (it survived until 2013) which forbade 'being an incorrigible rogue'. Further afield in SW – the only London postcode, incidentally, to straddle the Thames – there is the Balham pub where a man called John Sullivan once witnessed a guy stand up from his leaning position against the bar to get a light, then lean back without realising that in the interim the bar flap had been raised. He fell clean through the gap, and decades later when Sullivan became the writer of *Only Fools and Horses* the memory provided him with his most famous scene. Then there was the 1992 Men's Singles final at Wimbledon, during which Goran Ivanišević was warned for swearing, a warning that must really have irked him because he was doing it in Croatian – the umpire only realised because TV viewers had rung in to complain.

The project, I realise after a few weeks, has energised me, made me less inclined to put things off. For instance, I live about an hour from Cambridge, visit the city quite regularly and often end up walking past the Eagle. This is the pub into which DNA pioneers James Watson and Francis Crick ran to announce to some 1953 lunchtime drinkers that they had 'discovered the secret of life'. A plaque outside reminds you of the fact. 'Must go in one day,' I tell myself every time.

And have I ever got round to it? Of course I haven't. Visiting Cambridge the next time, though, I go in for a pint. It's one of those sprawling seventeenth-century buildings with different rooms opening off each other, including one at the back known as the RAF bar because its ceiling bears graffiti from Second World War pilots. The drinkers this midweek afternoon include tourists, students and a meejah academic I recognise from the telly. Turns out his bow tie isn't an onscreen affectation after all. I don't learn anything new, nothing I can put down as my CB fact, but it's genuinely moving to sit here, reflecting on what happened that day. It seems so recent, so immediate (you say that sort of thing about a gap of 60 years when you've reached 42). Momentous, too. There is a long and ignoble tradition of people in pubs suddenly claiming to have uncovered a fundamental truth of human existence, but for once these guys were telling the truth. Actually I *do* learn something new: it was Crick rather than Watson who made the announcement. There's a quote from the latter (who was American) painted on the wall. The 'secret of life' boast, he says, 'struck me as somewhat immodest, especially in England, where understatement is a way of life'.

The spirit of adventure continues on a trip to see my parents in the Midlands. In the same way I've always meant to pop into the Eagle, my partner Jo and I have always meant to visit Stratford-upon-Avon. It's just far enough from my parents' house to require a special effort. Inspired by the project, I insist that today will be the day we make that effort. My mother, God bless her, volunteers to look after our son Barney, and an hour later we're there. Stratford certainly trades on its most famous resident: there are restaurants or cafés called the Encore, Act V, Hathaway's, and even a curry house called Thespians. Jo and I can't recall if Shakespeare is actually buried here. In these days of smartphones doubt never lingers for long, so having established that yes, the authorial bones really do reside in Stratford, we walk along the river to the Holy Trinity Church and take a peek. William, Anne and their daughter Susanna are here, the playwright's stone helpfully marked out by a tasteful piece of blue cord draped round its edges. There are information boards telling you about his life. Anne, it seems, was pregnant when they got married.

Back outside we pass a young girl who has noticed a date on a gravestone. 'Eighteen sixty-two!' she says to her father. 'That's two thousand years ago!' Further along the river is the RSC itself, where the war on procrastination continues. There's a sign announcing guided tours of the theatre.

'We should do that one day,' says Jo.

'Piffle,' I respond, in a vague attempt at Shakespearian badinage. 'We shall do it now.'

There are ten of us on the tour. Our guide, a tall, wiry man in his sixties, exhibits just the right mix of knowledge, enthusiasm and interestingly shaped ears. By the end of the hour-long tour he will even have rescued the two pre-teen sisters from early resentment at their parents' choice of Sunday lunchtime activity. We're shown all over the building, seeing how a hundred million pounds was spent a few years ago in updating the 1930s structure. Our guide pulls back some black curtains in the passageway outside the auditorium to reveal cubicles containing mirrors and tables. 'Sometimes when actors need a quick change,' he says, 'there isn't time for them to get back to the dressing rooms upstairs, so they use side exits from the stage and meet their dresser here.' To speed things up costumes are often held together with magnets instead of zips. On one occasion a wire coat-hanger accidentally got magnetised, and an actor had to perform a whole scene with it stuck behind his head.

It's hard not to suspect, as Guide leads us enthusiastically around, that he wanted to tread the boards himself. He certainly knows the plays well enough, often including quotes from them in answers to our questions. And he's an engaging performer: his Laurence Olivier impression is highly entertaining, no less so for sounding nothing at all like Laurence Olivier. But the real reason I love him is that he continually peppers the tour with Shakespearian trivia. This, it dawns on me, is the solution to a problem: my CV research hasn't been going very well. Coventry, you see (and I'm allowed to say this, having gone to school there), is a fairly uninspiring place. Even 'Ghost Town' by local band the Specials, supposedly about their home city, was actually written in reference to the 1981 riots in Bristol and London. There's 'sent to Coventry', of course, but no one seems to know where that comes from.[5] In desperation I even Googled the words on a manhole cover in my local Suffolk town: 'Savage Nuneaton'. Peter Savage Limited, I learn from their website, 'has the UK's largest range of manhole covers, access covers and gully gratings'. Oh well. The words remain in my imagination as how Noël Coward would have met an enquiry about the town. 'Nuneaton? Very savage, Nuneaton.'

Today, though, solutions to the CV problem are flung at me like so many arrows of outrageous (good) fortune. Not every one is particular to this postcode: all theatres in Shakespeare's time, for instance, used sheep's blood for their fight scenes.[6] There's only one Shakespeare play whose title contains the name of a country: *Hamlet, Prince of Denmark*. Nowhere in the original

---

[5] Possibly the Civil War, when captured Royalist troops were imprisoned there.
[6] Alfred Hitchcock used chocolate syrup for *Psycho*: because the film was in black and white he was more bothered with consistency than colour.

stage directions for the balcony scene in *Romeo and Juliet* will you find any mention of a balcony. (This could have saved one actress a lot of trouble in a 2003 production in Malvern: she fell off it.) But as we stand in the glass-panelled room overlooking the stage from which sound and lighting is controlled, Guide finally does us proud with a venue-centric fact:

CV (Coventry): The sound effect of cannons for a 1963 performance at the Royal Shakespeare Theatre in Stratford was a recording of cast members exploding inflated crisp packets.

Heading back home, I realise that it's time to plan my first proper research trip. Somewhere not too far away – let's leave the lengthy Celtic jaunts as a treat for later. A pair of compasses are applied to the map, and the perfect candidate soon presents itself. It's somewhere I've always wanted to go, on account of it being a legendary British institution, an icon that in its relatively short lifespan (it wasn't even built when Watson and Crick discovered DNA) has entered the nation's very consciousness. Indeed it has come to *define* the nation, or at least a particular divide within it. It has even – the ultimate compliment in modern Britain – become rhyming slang, though for something it probably doesn't like being rhyming slang for. It lies in the NN postcode: the land of Victorian cop car chases beckons.

The trip is arranged for a fortnight hence. Before that, however, I have an appointment in London.

If you head north from Farringdon Tube station along Farringdon Road, you soon become aware that the ground is sloping noticeably uphill. This is only to be expected, as you are heading away from the Thames. Indeed underneath you is the now buried Fleet, one of London's subterranean rivers that feed their more famous cousin. The climb gets particularly steep as you head past the *Guardian*'s old offices, but levels out as you reach the busy junction with Rosebery Avenue. And there, on the far side of that junction, is an enormous building whose name reminds you, should your legs not be doing the job already, that you've reached the top of a hill. You are now looking at Mount Pleasant.

'The Mount', as it's known to its thousands of employees, is London's main postal sorting office. The picturesque name was chosen in 1879 when the Post Office took over the site that had previously housed Coldbath Fields Prison, renowned for a grim regime which forbade inmates from speaking and made them spend hours on the treadmill. As I approach on a chilly but bright December morning the sorting office looks massive, all the more so because of its elevated position. Turning left, I walk along the frontage facing on to Mount Pleasant itself, a small side street sloping down from the summit at the main crossroads. A group of sorting staff stand outside the main entrance, smoking and comparing National Lottery tactics. Further down the hill a huge basement area becomes visible, and I stop to peer through the windows at row after row of neatly parked six-foot-tall wire cages. Some are empty, some contain large plastic mailbags, themselves empty. There is no one to be seen. Clearly this area operates during the early morning, and today's work is already over. Oh – not quite: as I watch a woman appears, wearily dragging two full sacks from one side of the space to the other. It takes her the best part of a minute, a living portrait entitled 'Last Job of the Day'.

The street slopes down still further, away from the traffic rumbling past on Rosebery Avenue up above, until you reach the end of the building. Past that is a large patch of waste ground, some of it used as a car park, but with nothing to block your view all the way to the Channel 4 News building and its neighbours on Gray's Inn Road. This is on the same level as Rosebery Avenue, so that standing here you're in a dip. I love it when a great city does this, presents you with a quiet corner, a secret space hidden away from the bustle and noise. It makes anything you find there all the more special. And so it is today. Because turning right into Phoenix Place, I discover, halfway along the back of the Royal Mail building, the BPMA – the British Postal Museum and Archive.

This collection is housed in a large, modern room, and consists mostly of books. It also has some Perspex cabinets containing temporary exhibits. One of the current displays relates to postal security. There's a rather fetching tweed hat which, the label explains, disguises a hard inner casing – the garment was worn by members of the Post Office Investigation Department. Next to it lies one of their logbooks from 1965, recording various dastardly deeds. One offence crops up more than any other: 'letters of an obscene character'. What counted as obscene then? The Sixties were halfway gone – surely even the Post Office had started to swing by then? As I'm pondering the question some footsteps gently disturb the hush of the room (there's only one person working here today, an elderly chap seated at the table in the middle of the room studying old leather-bound business directories). Turning round, I'm confronted by the man I've come to meet: the BPMA's communications manager, Harry Huskisson.

In his mid-twenties, with a trim, dark beard and fashionably unkempt hair, Harry is proof made flesh of something that the project's early research has already hinted at: everyone loves the post. It's not a dusty old segment of social history, it's a vibrant part of our country and its tale. We all thrill to the thud on the doormat, love stories about what thudded on to other people's doormats in centuries gone by. Even now that email has taken over, Postie still has a role to play. Talking about my university days to someone who was born after those days had ended, I described the joy of peering into your padlocked pigeonhole and finding a letter or postcard from back home. 'Of course you never got that,' I said. 'No, I did,' came her reply. 'In my case it was the latest DVD from LoveFilm, but still, it's important. If all your communication was electronic, how sad would that be?'

Harry hasn't been in his job for long, having moved from communications work in the City. 'This is so much more fun,' he says. 'After trying to make a bank's quarterly results sound interesting, the stuff I've got to work with here is a dream.'

As instant evidence, we start by talking dirty. I ask Harry what counted as obscene in 1965.

He peers at the logbook. 'I'll have to look into that. Of course it changes in different eras. You know when *Ulysses* was first published we used to intercept copies sent by post? There was a special rate for sending books, but you had to leave the title showing. *Ulysses* was classed as obscene.'[7]

To avoid disturbing the chap at work, Harry and I retire for our discussion to a coffee bar round the corner in Exmouth Market. Within minutes it's clear that this aspect of the project will take more than a single visit to the archives: before the barista has even applied the cocoa to my cappuccino Harry has mentioned the M in RMS *Titanic* (even though she was primarily for passengers, the liner's letter and parcel work made her a Royal Mail Ship), the old rule that you could post a dead animal unwrapped 'as long as it didn't leak', and

---

[7] Many would argue it should have been classed as unreadable. James Joyce used 29,899 different words in it. The entire works of Shakespeare only contain 29,066.

Tony Benn's efforts to take the Queen's head off our stamps.[8] So Harry and I decide that, to introduce some discipline over the caffeine, we'll start with the stuff relating to the project's very raison d'être: postcodes themselves.

'They were needed,' he explains, 'because London was growing so massively during the nineteenth century. The huge increase in population meant a huge increase in the number of letters. And people weren't very good at addressing them properly. Though even if they had been, you still had the problem that lots of streets in London had the same names. A committee was set up in the 1850s to look at renaming them, but that idea got vetoed by wealthy families – lots of them lived on streets named after their ancestors.'

So instead Sir Rowland Hill formed his ten districts, oc-cupying a circle with a radius of 12 miles centred on the main post office near St Paul's Cathedral. (The building is still the world headquarters of the GPO's successor British Telecom – a statue of Sir Rowland stands outside it.) Then, as we've seen, in 1866 Anthony Trollope merged NE with E. Decades later the two letters would reappear, blinking in the light after tunnelling their way to Newcastle, though there was just time in their brief London existence for them to feature on road signs in Hackney (you can still see one on Victoria Park Road). In 1868 Trollope repeated his abolition trick, splitting the 'S' territory between SW and SE. This victim would also head north, eventually finding a home in Sheffield. Only four other non-London areas can boast a single-letter code: Birmingham, Glasgow, Liverpool and Manchester.

---

[8] You'll have noticed that he failed. What you might not have noticed is that the Queen is wearing a robe. This was added at her own request, as although she liked every other aspect of the design she felt her bare shoulders should be covered up for decency's sake.

'We have to point out that Trollope didn't just get rid of things,' says Harry. 'It's because of him that Britain has post-boxes. He saw them on his travels in France and Belgium, and decided to bring the idea back here.' They were around even before postcodes, the first three cast-iron ones trialled on Jersey in 1852. 'Obviously the idea was a success, and they were installed all round the country. At first they were coloured green to fit in with the countryside. The trouble was they fitted in *too* well – people couldn't find them. So the Post Office painted them all red.' The colour question leads us to telephone boxes, also the responsibility of the GPO. Harry and I trade facts. Mine is that early phone boxes were made tall enough for a man wearing a top hat to use them, Harry's is that after a while they all had to be made with sloping floors because people were using them as urinals.

Basic postcode systems gradually spread to other cities, but it was another century before things really got going. Technology was the driving force: machines were coming into existence which could automatically sort huge numbers of letters. (At first this was achieved by the machine 'reading' blue phosphor dots printed on to the envelope. These days it's done by bar-code.) But the machines required codes more sophisticated than just points of the compass and the odd number. A 1959 experiment with six-digit codes in Norwich failed because not enough people used them. In 1966, however, the Post Office got it right. Starting in Croydon, they introduced the system that survives, with a few modifications, to this day.

'A nice little quirk,' adds Harry, 'is that within a postcode area the districts work alphabetically, not geographically. The number "1" is always the main sorting office, but after that it goes by letter. So in East London, for instance, you'd think E2 would be next to E3, then E4 and so on. Well, as it happens E2 is Bethnal Green and E3 is Bow, but that's only because the alphabet goes like that. For E4 you jump way out to Chingford in Essex. Walthamstow is E17 because it's near the end of the alphabet.' So the band named after their home turf may have come from the big bad city, but numerically they ranked well down the list. Sorry lads.

As so often, something invented so mankind could master a situation has ended up becoming mankind's master. Some postcodes, for instance, cross national boundaries, which has led to people in Wales and Scotland getting the wrong channels when they sign up with Sky. Many drivers are now incapable of finding a destination unless they have that all-important postcode typed into their satnav. So commonplace is the habit that devious marketing types at a North London shopping centre ask visitors to the Christmas grotto for their postcode on the pretext that Santa has a satnav (lots of junk mail coming their way in January).[9] But the worst type of postcode-enslavement occurs in insurance. Many people have been unable to obtain house cover because, as far as the insurance company is concerned, their newly built house doesn't exist. That is, it doesn't yet have a postcode. And these days, if you're a house and your name's not on the list of postcodes, you're not coming in. The list stands at 1.7 million and counting, with 2,750 new codes added every month. (Around 2,500 are, to use the Royal Mail's rather dramatic term, 'terminated' each month.) But it's not enough for the Royal Mail simply to assign a new property its postcode – the insurance companies' computers have to take that information on board. Computers being what they are, these can be two very different things.

---

[9] The Sandringham estate's website claims that its Visitor Centre has no postcode. Drivers are advised to use that of the hotel over the road. Hopefully the nation has just enough navigational skill left to do the rest of the journey unaided.

There are other more entertaining ways in which postcodes worm their way into our daily lives. Perhaps it's because I work with words for a living, and perhaps it's also because I'm one of those people who like categorising and classifying (I believe the technical term is a 'man'), but my postcodes have always acted as minor playthings. The first one I had on moving to London ended '0BE'. The zero, of course, looked like an 'O', so it seemed a very grand address. Later, when I lived in Marylebone, my postcode began 'W1N'. The number-for-letter swap happened again, and even if nothing else was going right my post would guarantee a 'winning' start to the day. Then the Royal Mail changed all the codes in the area. 'W1N' was replaced by 'W1G'. It seemed a very cruel joke.

It was while living in that flat that I wrote my first novel. Showing an early aptitude for the principle that the last thing you want to do when you're writing a book is write a book, I decided that working at home wasn't on: I needed an 'office' to give the enterprise an air of discipline. Walking there would also get the endorphins, and so the inspiration, flowing. The chosen venue was the café in the Piccadilly branch of Waterstone's. As my flat was only a few yards south of the Marylebone Road, which is the boundary between W1 and NW1, and Piccadilly is the start of SW1, my walk comprised the entire length (or rather height) of a postcode. These days, out in Suffolk, my code ends 'NZ', and whenever giving my address to people over the phone I finish with '...for New Zealand'. As witness for the 'It's Not Just Me' defence, my friend Andrew also toys with his postcodes. His current one ends '5EA', which always makes him think of the sea, while as a child his last three characters were '2RT'. 'That's the thing about you,' someone once told him, 'you're too arty.'

But Harry's field of responsibility stretches much further back than the century and a half since postcodes first reared their heads. You could say it goes all the way back to 27 BC, when the Emperor Augustus Caesar first set up a postal system to get messages across the Roman Empire.

'They used messengers on horseback,' explains Harry. 'Of course the messengers needed to rest once in a while, and outside the resting places there were posts for them to tie their horses to. That's where we get the word "post".'

I'm beginning to like Harry. He's the sort of person who provides the best sort of answers: the ones that make you wonder why you never stopped to ask the question in the first place. We get on to the Post Office's strange rules. 'There used to be all sorts of them,' he says. 'Like the one giving you a reduced rate if you posted an envelope unsealed. That was because of the Printed Paper Rate, introduced in 1892 to allow newspapers, pamphlets and circulars to be posted for only half a penny. But you had to leave the envelope open so checkers could make sure you weren't sending anything else.' Although this rate was abolished in 1969, some people still send their envelopes unsealed. 'We wish they wouldn't – they can mess up the sorting machines. I have heard of people leaving the envelope open so postal workers can see there's nothing worth stealing in there. A bit like leaving your glove box open so car thieves can see it's empty.'[10]

Another quaint tradition was the human letter: you could pay the Post Office to post *you* to an address. On 23 February 1909 two suffragettes used this service to gain attention for their cause. Presenting themselves at the East Strand post office, they paid the requisite 3d and asked that their telegraph messenger boy, one A. S. Palmer, deliver them to 10 Downing Street, where they wished to speak with Mr Asquith, the Prime

---

[10] In Poland it's seen as bad luck to seal the envelope of a birthday card – it means the recipient won't live to open it.

Minister. Palmer duly did as ordered. There's a photograph in the archive of him standing outside the famous front door, presenting some sort of form to Asquith's butler. The two suffragettes, Miss Solomon and Miss McLellan, are facing away from the camera, so I can't vouch for how they looked, but if the bonnets are anything to go by I certainly wouldn't have argued with them. The butler was having none of it, though. As Palmer reported to his bosses: 'I took the Ladies to Mr Asquith's house but the police would not let them go in. I went in but the butler would not sign the form because he did not have the letters to sign for, because the ladies themselves said they were the letters. And Mr Asquith refused to see them.' I like this. Other countries have revolutions. We have the Prime Minister's butler debating whether a woman is or is not a letter.

Our coffee cups long since drained, Harry and I agree that unless we're going to spend the whole of Christmas and New Year in this café we should probably leave any further discussions for another day. He has, anyway, further research to do on topics we've touched on. For example, he's going to get me a look at a particular postage stamp from the 1970s, unissued because the event for which it was designed never came to pass. (It's incredible that anyone ever thought it might – this is why I'm so keen to see the stamp.) For now we go our separate ways, Harry to his office, me to the archive room. Here, within minutes, I'm lost in books like *The Humour of the Post Office* by Albert Montefiore Hyamson (1909) and *The Royal Mail, Its Curiosities and Romance* (J. W. Hyde, 3rd edition, 1889). They're absolute gems. I learn about the tradition of 'puzzle addresses', deliberately cryptic ones designed to test the ingenuity of the Post Office. Instead of just throwing the envelopes away, or returning them with an instruction for the sender to get a life, the Post Office rose to the challenge, establishing a staff of experts whose job it was to solve the puzzles. One envelope had, where the name of the town should go, a drawing of a swan followed by the letter 'C' (Swansea). Another was addressed simply '25th March, Clifton' – it was successfully delivered to Lady Day of Clifton. Meanwhile the experts worked out that 'that beautiful city, which charms even eyes familiar with the masterpieces of Bramante and Palladio, and which the genius of Anstey and Smollett, of Frances Burney and of Jane Austen, has made classic ground' was Bath. One envelope was addressed: 'To the gentleman who looked at a house near Cleobury Mortimer a little time ago, Bilston, Staffordshire.' It got there. Other wags wrote their letters in tiny handwriting on the back of a stamp and mailed it. Here the Post Office's patience did snap: they introduced a minimum as well as a maximum size for a letter.

The Post Office also did us the favour of keeping a file of letters sent to Father Christmas. One read:

Dear Santa,

When I said my prayers last night, I told God to tell you to bring me a hobby-horse. I don't want a hobby-horse, really. A honestly live horse is what I want. Mamma told me not to ask for him, because I would probably make you mad, so you wouldn't give me anything at all, and if I got him I wouldn't have any place to keep him. A man I know will keep him, he says, if you get him for me. I thought you would like to know. Please don't be mad.

Affectionately,
John

PS – a Shetland would be enough
PS – I'd rather have a hobby-horse than nothing at all

The book that most touches my heart, though, is *Thoughts of a Postman* by the unlikely sounding Manly Ritch. A collection of poems, it was published in 1923 by (and here's our first clue to the poems' quality) Manly Ritch. He trod the rounds in Greenwich, Connecticut (the BPMA don't limit themselves to British postal history). There's no record of how many publishers turned him down, but eventually Rich presented himself at the Ferris Printing Company in New York City and paid to have the job done himself. A picture of the author precedes the title page, his grey single-breasted uniform neatly buttoned, his peaked cap perfectly centred, his tidy moustache allowed to reach the ends of his top lip but not a millimetre further. I'd guess that at this point he was in his late forties, maybe early fifties. The air of duty emanating from the photo is matched in the single stanza underneath, which ends 'so unless health should fail, I'll deliver the mail, Till "the Grim Reaper" calls'.

Hands up: I start reading the poems because they're terrible. So terrible they're brilliant. The first one, 'Prelude', includes the lines:

Now I don't call my book 'Poems' –
I wouldn't be so vain –
If it's poetry you'll know it;
If not it will remain
The thoughts of a rhyming postman
Who works hard ev'ry day.

'The Call of the Farm' is, in its entirety: 'O, I want to go back/ Up a little old track/To a farmhouse I know of in Maine/Tis not much to see/But it means Home to me/And I long to be back there again.' Surely here we've discovered America's answer to William Topaz McGonagall?[11] Manly treats us to his thoughts on the plan to introduce Daylight Saving Time: 'Now don't you think we should agree/And stand by the majority?/ This thing will not be settled until it's settled right./If you're a law-abidin' man/You'll scrap the "daylight savin'" plan...' The titles alone give a clue to his mindset: 'Incapacitated'... 'Hope for the Best But Prepare for the Worst'... 'The Bible – Have You Seen It Lately?'... 'The Postman's Trusty Ford'...

But then you notice the poem called 'To My Wife'. It ends: 'And she is just as much my wife today/As e'er before. Why, "she is just away!"/I feel that she has gone to my new home/ To have things ready for me when I come.' Your hunch is confirmed when you find the poem 'In Memoriam: Mary Moody Ritch'. It relates the history of the couple's relationship, from their first meetings onwards: 'Until you spoke those precious words/That night I bent above you/Twas like the singing of the birds/I heard you say "I love you".'

'OK', you're saying, 'we feel sorry for the guy in his bereavement – but that doesn't mean his poems aren't terrible.' Maybe not. But it isn't just sympathy that's changing my mind about Manly. It's his poem 'My Work'. Not only does he set himself the extra challenge of making the first letters of each line spell out 'MANLY RITCH POET', he also finishes with:

Putting aside all thoughts of pleasure or
Of rest, I'll work away until I'm dead;
Each little rhyme of mine may then be read;
That is my hope. Is it worth striving for?

[11] The Scot's poem about the 1879 Tay Bridge disaster is legendarily bad. '[Y]our central girders would not have given way/At least many sensible men do say/Had they been supported on each side with buttresses/At least many sensible men confesses.'

Well, Manly, the answer seems to be yes. I'm sitting here 90 years later, doing exactly that. And OK, perhaps I'm enjoying your poems for reasons you wouldn't be entirely chuffed about. The only reason I found them at all is that you were a postman and this is a postal archive. But that's not the point. Poems, like letters, are more than mere words on paper: they're two humans connecting. You've connected with me, someone who was born (surely?) after you died, thousands of miles away on a different continent. It's the power the written word has to touch someone a long way away. And that's what not just your poetry but your job was all about.

It comes to pass, then, that the first proper field trip takes place a couple of weeks before Christmas. Packing an overnight bag, I set off for a British institution, a place that – in one sense, though not the geographical one – lies at the nation's very centre.

From my Suffolk village I drive north towards Bury St Edmunds, where I join the A14 and head west. Passing Newmarket I remember the other night in the pub, when my friend Martin, who like me occasionally sets the questions for the weekly quiz, reported a great piece of trivia: Newmarket is the only racecourse in Britain to span two counties. Bingo, I thought – that's CB (Cambridge) sorted. Cruel disappointment, however, lay in store. It turns out there are two separate courses at Newmarket, one in Suffolk, the other in Cambridgeshire. Neither spans the boundary. Not good enough: CB remains a vacancy. Further down the A14 is the signpost for the village which has surely the most English place name there could possibly be: Titchmarsh.

By now we're in the destination county (Northamptonshire), and also the destination postcode: NN. Turning on to the A43 I head towards the county town itself, but resist the delights of

Northampton and skirt its ring road to find the thundering, roaring beast that is the M1. Within moments my northward momentum has taken me past junction 16. Shortly thereafter, and just before I would have reached junction 17, I see, through the misty, almost drizzly greyness of this Wednesday afternoon, the sign that I've been waiting for. Most people see this place as a break in their journey. For me, today, it is journey's end. This is Watford Gap service station.

Motorway services have always fascinated me. It's the 'cocoon' element that makes them so compelling, the fact you're trapped there, suspended in an artificial bubble for as long as you pause your journey. A service station is a cross between a desert island and the *Big Brother* house, though thankfully filled with ordinary people rather than transsexuals yearning to be pop stars. All these people spend a short time together, normal individuals in an extraordinary environment, a bit like Tom Hanks stuck in an airport in *The Terminal*. A service station, in other words, is that most exciting of things: a human zoo.

Watford Gap isn't just any service station – it's the *original* service station, the first one on Britain's first motorway.[12] Watford Gap opened on the same day as the M1 itself, 2 November 1959. For two thousand years people have been coming this way, the word 'Gap' referring to the natural break in the line of hills here that provides an easy routing option for all kinds of transport. The Romans put Watling Street through it (these days it's called the A5), while the Grand Union Canal and the West Coast Mainline railway both snake nearby as well, all of them lying like cables tied together at a rock concert.

---

[12] Let's not get involved in any 'Preston by-pass' pedantry – yes, the two-lane stretch opened in 1958 and has since become part of the M6, but it was only eight miles long. The M1 was the first proper, full-length motorway.

The Watford in question is a tiny village a few hundred yards away, rather than the town in Hertfordshire.

The services may have opened on 2 November, but the buildings housing the restaurants weren't quite ready (welcome to Britain, folks). So for the first few weeks food was sold from disused sheds left over from the site's previous incarnation as a farm. When the proper facilities did open they boasted hostesses to welcome you and waitresses to serve you at your table. Motorists, however, proved reluctant to stump up the associated prices, so out went the staff and in came the self-service trays. Nevertheless, just as the M1 revolutionised travel, Watford Gap revolutionised the breaks you took from that travel. When the Sixties kicked in, its stars dropped in. The Beatles, the Stones, Cliff Richard, the Hollies, Dusty Springfield, Gerry and the Pacemakers and a host of others rested up at the service station between gigs. Eric Clapton remembers his band the Yardbirds being a bunch of lads who wanted nothing more than to 'get in a van and go up the M1'.

But the glamour eventually faded. By 1977 Roy Harper was writing a song called 'Watford Gap', including the line 'Watford Gap, Watford Gap, grease on the plates, it's a load of crap'.[13] These days service stations are seen as necessary evils at best, naff and depressing at worst. When the media run stories on the M6's Tebay Services becoming a holiday destination in their own right, they do so in mocking tones. Tebay has a caravan park, a duck pond, a butcher and easy walking access to the Lake District. Interviewed by the *Daily Mail*, 73-year-old Doris Short commented that she sometimes walks

---

[13] He not very cleverly tried to release it on EMI, one of whose directors was also on the board of the company that ran the service station. The song was dropped from the album. But modern rhyming slang continued to make Harper's point for him.

to the southbound side for a coffee: 'That's a nice outing.' The fictional character who spent an entire series living in a service station hotel could only have been Alan Partridge. As part of the research Steve Coogan, his producer Armando Iannucci and writer Patrick Marber went to stay in just such a hotel for 24 hours. They found themselves unable to last the distance. 'It was coming up to Valentine's Day,' recalled Iannucci, 'and they had a poster up extolling their "romantic package" that said something like "£50 gets you a candlelit dinner for two, with complimentary half-bottle of champagne – *not to be taken into the main bar area*".' Although this broke their resolve, the experience did make them realise 'there was some depth to this situation – a kind of social X-ray of male middle-aged Middle England – that we could explore'.

That's exactly why I'm here. I've chosen Watford Gap as my service station not merely because it's the most famous one, nor because (inexplicably) I've never been here before, but because it's the very middle of Middle England, the point accepted as Checkpoint Charlie for the North/South divide. Indeed one of the first things I see is a spoof sign the authorities have recently erected, its arrows pointing in opposite directions to 'The North' and 'The South'. The second thing I see is the Days Inn hotel, a modest two-storey building that tonight I call home. I only see it, though, by peering across six lanes of traffic and a central reservation: it's on the southbound side of the services. There's always one thing you forget to check, isn't there?

No real bother – a slip road and a B-road deliver me to the other side in seconds. Soon I'm checking into the hotel, whose reception hatch is staffed by a friendly local girl, her accent pleasingly similar to the East Midlands one that elongates 'o' sounds so beautifully. She asks if I'd like to buy a voucher that gives £10 worth of food at the restaurant next door for £7.50.

Seeing as for the next few hours I'm something of a captive audience foodwise, it seems silly not to. In fact I buy two, one for dinner, one for breakfast. She fills out the vouchers by hand and hands them over with my key. The ground-floor room is large and basic, with a sign in the bathroom warning guests that 'the towel rail will become hot when switched on', which is reassuring. The room's on the side of the building facing away from the motorway. From in here the traffic sounds like an ocean wave that never quite breaks against the shore.

Back outside for my first proper recce. Watford Gap is not a large service station. Each side has one main building and a BP Connect petrol station (plus, on this side, the hotel). Joining the sides is a footbridge, which unlike at more modern services is open to the elements rather than enclosed. You approach it at either end via one of those long sloping ramps that makes you turn back on yourself halfway up. Always frustrating but, given the number of times I'll be crossing it, probably the kinder option for my knee joints. Entering the main building I give a wide berth to the sales team holding cardboard bags full of make-up, and take my retail bearings. Straight ahead is Costa, to the right is WHSmith, to the left a restaurant called Restbite. Getting a tea from the first of these, I sit down. The small man at the next table is on his mobile phone. He has cropped hair and an Ulster accent. 'Right... Yeah... yeah... right... OK, thanks.' He ends the call, then immediately makes another. 'Chris? That shop closes at four thirty, right? Not four twenty-five... I *know* you're out of that shop... Four thirty, right?... I don't care. Put your watch back five minutes. That way you'll get it right. Right?' He hangs up without a goodbye. Chris, you sense, has got the message. I know I would have done.

Piled outside WHSmith is a large stack of next year's diaries, on offer at £1.99. Elsewhere in the building, I find, are Fone

Bitz (accessories of all kinds), vending machines offering cheap plastic toys, a row of coin-operated massage chairs and the Jackpot 500 room full of fruit machines. The last one reminds me of Jack Dee's comment on seeing a driving game at a service station ('Why not just carry on driving and throw 50p out of the window every minute?'), while the experience as a whole affirms the creed that seizes anyone entering a motorway service area: 'I spend, therefore I am.'[14]

I cross the bridge to the northbound side. The darkness is almost total now, and as the cars howl past below their head-lights pick out a drizzle so light I hadn't felt it. The entrance is guarded by another make-up team. After deploying more eye-avoidance skills, I loiter nearby and observe them at work. They're more skilful than their colleagues over the road, and a couple of them, a man and woman in their late twenties, are a decade older than the rest. Clearly in charge, they might also, judging by the body language, be an item-in-the-making. The team's real stroke of genius is their opening line. Not 'excuse me, would you be interested...' or 'could you spare a moment...', but: 'Did you get one?' The implication is that somehow there's been an error, that you've missed out on something. People are arrested by the sentence, stand there in confusion for a second or two, and this gives the seller their 'in'.

There's clearly been a party in McDonald's recently: five brightly coloured helium balloons are trapped in the roof girders, their ribbons wafting helplessly. Nearby is this side's Christmas tree, taller at ten feet than the southbound's, though both are artificial. Outside it's getting foggier, which adds to the 'trapped in a cocoon' feeling. This in turn heightens the

[14] I buy a new road atlas in Smiths. 'Would you like a chocolate bar with that?' asks the woman on the till.

surreal nature of everything. The nagging little imperfections you get throughout modern British life become, in this setting, positively sinister. Outside WHSmith is a display of cheap slippers in the shape of pandas, frogs, rabbits and the like – it's labelled 'AMINAL FOOTWARMERS'. The sign isn't a hastily scribbled one, either: it's printed and laminated, meaning none of the people involved in its production noticed the mistake. (Just as no one responsible for the wall-mounted Perspex sign in my hotel noticed the line: 'No not re-entre the building'.) Outside the female toilets a notice proclaims: 'Male cleaner on duty – thanks'. What's he thanking them for? You dread to think. Meanwhile the condom machine in the gents sells something called 'Sexual Performance Supplements'. They're available in 500mg capsules and contain, the machine boasts, 'herbal extracts, amino acids and caffeine which may improve your sexual performance'. I like the 'may': you can always spot a lawyer's touch. One brand is called 'Male Angel'. Another is 'Menhancer'.

The surreality continues back outside. A flash high-performance sports car bears the private registration plate 'THE 515'. I hang around waiting for a gown-clad Oxford don to return but no one appears.[15] A lorry filling up with fuel bears the legend: 'PANIC – The Complete Transport System'. All in all Watford Gap feels like a place where nothing is quite right. A cheap-suited businessman sports a midlife-crisis ponytail. You see plenty of those, but tonight I find myself wondering if he's a spy in disguise, the ponytail hiding the

---

[15] Come to think of it, car registrations rival postcodes in their scope for wordplay. One I often saw in Marylebone bore the plate '1 ANU'. It must have been a diplomatic car, maybe for Antigua: the letters are the code for the island's airport. One day someone is bound to make the obvious addition with a marker pen.

wires from his recording equipment. Clearly it's time to settle my nerves with some food, so I return to the southbound side and enter Restbite. The dinner options all look appetising enough. I plump for the chicken tikka curry with rice. It has to be an apple juice to wash it down, as nowhere in the services can you buy alcohol of any kind. (Shortly after my trip England will get its first motorway pub, the Hope and Champion at Beaconsfield services on the M40.) All together this comes to £9.89. I proffer the £10 voucher. The woman on the till files it in the compartment next to the fivers, then pushes the drawer shut. It gives the usual 'ping', while she utters a 'thank you' and turns to go.

'Er... excuse me.'

She turns back. 'Yes?'

'My change?'

She looks puzzled.

'It came to £9.89. That was a £10 voucher.'

'You don't get change from vouchers.'

'Sorry?'

'You don't get change from vouchers.'

Again, this sort of petty retail vindictiveness happens all the time these days, but here, tonight, the illogicality feels threatening.

'So if I'd paid with a tenner, I'd have got the 11p back?'

'Yeah.'

'But because I paid with a voucher that was *worth* a tenner, I don't?'

'That's right.'

She's visibly uncomfortable now. And while I hate the argument that says 'You shouldn't take it out on the staff, they're only doing their job' (who else can you address your complaint to?), equally I don't want to be the sort of person who lets himself get this bothered by 11 pence. 'That doesn't seem very sensible, does it?' I say.

She shakes her head. 'No, it doesn't.'

And leaving it at that I turn to get my cutlery. The chicken tikka is good, though there's not very much of it. Can't help thinking of Alan Partridge smuggling a larger-than-regulation-sized plate into the service station buffet. The restaurant is quiet this evening – only a couple of the other tables are occupied, one by a woman in a coat made, apparently, from an entire duvet. My reading matter comprises some research notes on motorways. The M2, it transpires, is the only British motorway that connects with none of the others. The M6 is the longest, stretching 232 miles from the Catthorpe interchange in Leicestershire to just short of the border with Scotland, where it produces its passport, becomes the A74(M) and proceeds to Glasgow. The widest bit of motorway is the M25 near Heathrow, offering no fewer than six lanes in each direction. If you want to reach for the skies, meanwhile, head for the M62 in the Pennines – the section near junction 22 is, at 1,221 feet, the highest motorway in the UK. It's located, appropriately enough, at Windy Hill.

The two hours' free parking you get at service stations, I learn, are a legal requirement. Go a second over, mind you, and you'll be snapped by enforcement cameras. They automatically read the number plates of every vehicle entering and exiting the service areas, so the computer knows exactly how long you've been there. There are also cameras monitoring the gates leading directly into service areas from minor roads. Breakdown trucks are allowed to use these, something Jo and I discovered when we were rescued by one. Being driven through the gate felt like taking part in a presidential motorcade. One of the earliest service stations (1965) was Forton on the M6 in Lancashire, designed by the architect Sir

Thomas Penberthy Bennett. As if his name wasn't splendid enough in itself, at the Ministry of Works during the Second World War he rejoiced in the title 'Director of Bricks'.

But it's the M1 itself that provides the most interesting reading. Britain took time getting used to its first motorway. Early drivers stopped in the left-hand lane to have their picture taken on the exciting new road. Some pulled over on to the hard shoulder and had a picnic, while one family even did so on the central reservation. A couple reported that their car had been stolen from Leicester services. The policeman asked them where they were headed, and when they told him he politely suggested they might like to go and look in the northbound car park: this was the southbound one. That said, the drivers weren't totally to blame. The road itself had to take some of the responsibility. The hard shoulders, for instance, had been built just eight feet wide, meaning cars entering them at any speed frequently rolled off the other side into a ditch. And long stretches of the M1 were perfectly straight, which didn't aid concentration. Later motorways had curves included even where they weren't necessary, simply to keep drivers alert, as well as to keep their speed down. On the day Transport Minister Ernest Marples opened the M1, he proudly announced to the gathered dignitaries that it 'heralded a new age of road travel in the scientific age'. Then he watched as the first public users put their pedals to the metal and floored it into the distance. Turning to a colleague, Marples whispered: 'My God, what have I done?' Things weren't helped by the complete absence of a speed limit. Thrusting young motorcyclists earned themselves the nickname 'Ton-Up Boys'. Even they were left standing, however, by Jack Sears and Peter Bolton, two competitors in the 1964 Le Mans 24-hour race who used the M1 as a practice track. The chaps got their AC Cobra Coupé up to a breezy 185 mph.

Dinner over, I spend the rest of the evening monitoring events on both sides of the services. Watford Gap, it's becoming clear, hasn't really made it into the twenty-first century, not in spirit. Everything's been modernised but it still feels dated, the date in question being the drab Seventies, with elements of the corny Eighties. The smallness doesn't help – compared to some of the M25's mega-services this seems like a collection of huts, and not a very big collection at that. But working Britain still stops off, the men (it is almost all men) in their yellow hi-vizzes and their steel toe-caps. An Asian guy with a greying goatee, wearing a bobble hat and a red Ferrari fleece, blows on his tea to cool it down. The AA rescue a broken-down motorist. Several drivers shun the facilities completely, staying in their cars to talk on their mobile phones. Then the lorries begin to park up for the night. They've come from Hatfield and from Spain, they bear the logos of FedEx, Laura Ashley and – of course – Eddie Stobart. There's also a Hovis lorry, which reminds me of another fact:

SP (Salisbury): The famous 1973 'schoolboy pushing his bike up a steep Northern hill' Hovis advert was actually filmed in Shaftesbury in Dorset. It was directed by Ridley Scott.

I like the thought that the advert was the work of the same man who before the decade was out would be making an alien appear from John Hurt's chest. It also left us in the position where a cultured person is defined as someone who can hear Dvorak's New World Symphony without thinking of bread.[16]

---

[16] The bread's name is shortened from '*hominis vis*', Latin for 'the strength of man'.

At just gone nine a jabbering squadron of schoolchildren explode into the northbound building, a couple of dozen early teenagers still at that stage where they stick to their own genders, though amidst the shrieks and laughs there are several glances. Clearly there's been a full-on Big Day Out to London, and this is the rest on the way home. Bladders are emptied, fast food and fizzy drinks purchased, then it's back out to the coach. After this brief injection of life-affirming energy, the services revert to their monastic dullness. The only sound is the constant beeping from the McDonald's ovens, alerting staff that various items are ready.

At eleven o'clock, after crossing the bridge several more times, I decide to call it a night. Venturing out of the north-bound building for the final time, I'm confronted by a steam train. A proper, genuine, wheels-taller-than-I-am steam train. Has it hopped a couple of hundred yards west from the main-line? No, it's on a lorry, a specialist transporter whose cab bears the legend 'Off the rails!' Bits of the lorry's chassis are so high that the driver can stand underneath it for a pee, thereby saving himself the walk into the services (I know this because he does so as I pass). Even I, who know nothing about trains, can see that this is not just a thing of beauty but a miracle of engineering. Having positioned myself so the driver is out of view, I stand to admire the dark green train, trying to work out which of the highly polished pieces of brass and steel down the side are connected to which other pieces, and how the whole thing works. Failing, I content myself with savouring the general effect, and reflecting how sad the train looks, dependent for its movement on a big, bland lorry, albeit one that's been individually designed to provide it with maximum comfort. Road's victory over rail in a single image.

Up on the bridge I stop for one last look at the traffic below. Motorways at night are always reassuring: no matter what the hour, no matter how silent and becalmed and gone-to-bed the rest of the landscape is, these carriageways always have at least a few cars on them, evidence that the country is still ticking over. They're Britain's vital signs. This *particular* motorway at night, moreover, always reminds me (appropriately enough, given the vehicle in the southbound car park) of the Great Train Robbery. The M1 was four years old when Bruce and the boys liberated the cash from the Royal Mail's overnight Glasgow to London service. The point they chose, Bridego Bridge, lies a few miles west of the motorway. It's now pretty well accepted that if the gang had driven back to London straightaway, instead of hiding out at a local farm, they'd never have been caught. Instead of providing the police with a house full of fingerprints (including the Monopoly board on which they'd played with the stolen banknotes), they'd have been tucked up in bed at home before breakfast time. Even without clocking up the ton-plus speeds that would then still have been legal.

As the car lights pierce the now-thinning fog (red ones to my left, white ones to my right), I think of how different that story would have been. There'd have been no Ronnie going over the wall, no Buster on the beach at Acapulco. Instead the Great Train Robbery would have been Britain's most famous ever unsolved crime. It's the evening's final blob of strangeness, its last view of a world where things just aren't quite right.

The next morning finds Watford Gap services and the fields surrounding them awash in bright winter sunshine. Stepping out from the Days Inn I actually have to shield my eyes from the glare of nearby windscreens. Restbite provide a Traditional Breakfast for £6.59, some Extra Toast for £1 and a Coffee for £2.35, making £9.94 in total, so this time I only miss out on six pence worth of change. The staff clearing away trays chat to each other in Polish. A man at the next table boasts to a colleague about his frequent business trips to America. Every sentence is peppered with the word 'bucks'.

It's time to take my leave of Britain's first motorway service station. In tribute to all the lorry drivers I buy a Yorkie bar for the drive home, then head for the exit. Passing the make-up team I realise that one of the women's faces looks familiar.

'Excuse me...'

She turns, an eager smile betraying astonishment that someone has approached her for once, rather than the other way round. 'Yes?'

'Weren't you staying at the Days Inn last night?'

She nods. 'Oh yeah – you were there as well, weren't you?' Her accent is broad Yorkshire. Only now do I see that underneath the copious foundation, mascara and lipstick is a girl barely older than the ones who invaded the northbound side last night.

'So you work two days in a row? They put you up, I mean?'

'Yeah, we get a couple of rooms.'

The maths confuse me. She can't mean two rooms each – why would the firm do that? 'But there are loads of you, aren't there?'

'Just the six. We share three to a room. It's a good laff.'

Assuming their rooms are the same as mine, that's two in the bed and one on the extra-long sofa. I remember the body language of the two older ones from the northbound team. Best not pursue this line of thought any further. 'Must be a bit strange, working here then not going home?'

'Nah, it's good fun.' She's obviously completely sincere. 'We call it a "road trip".'

Not quite what Jack Kerouac had in mind, but still. It turns out the team are from Leeds. We chat for a few moments longer, but something isn't right in the way she talks about their stay.

'Er – it is just the two days you're doing, isn't it?' I ask.

'Nah. Six.'

'You're here for *six* days?'

Again the smile, again the cheeriness. 'Yeah.'

'You're living at Watford Gap service station for six days?'

'Yeah. It's good fun.' Her surprise at my surprise is its own comment on youthful optimism. As with the schoolkids last night, the display of sheer vitality you possess simply by virtue of not yet being twenty proves infectious. Just to know that this girl exists, that she's excited by the prospect of spending nearly a whole week in a motorway service station, and a not very well-appointed one at that, inspires me. There will be a spring in my step for the rest of the day because of this girl.

The quickest way home would, of course, begin with the M1 itself. But before engaging in multi-lane travel, I instead take the slip road, the one leading to the village of Watford. There, turning left at the fourteenth-century church of St Peter and St Paul, I park up in a lane and consult an Ordnance Survey map. The footpath I need stretches away from the village across the rich green Northamptonshire landscape. Heading for the gap between two of the many groups of trees, I'm preceded by both my lengthy shadow (the sun's low in the sky at this time of year) and my breath condensing against the cold air. Once you're through the gap the ground dips towards a hollow. Crossing the footpath up ahead is a train line, not the West Coast Mainline but a smaller one running east to west. It was built by the London and North Western Railway in 1877. Lord Henley, who owned the land, agreed to the tracks crossing his turf only on condition that the bridge over the hollow was of a particular design. It's this bridge I've come to see. It is known as Pulpit Bridge.

Lord Henley, as well as being the landowner, was a lay rector. The bridge, which is only fifteen feet or so high, was built so that each of the four corners up at track level resembles a church pulpit. They, like the arches running between the supporting stone columns, are made of intricately fashioned iron, painted a lovely dark green to fit in with the countryside. (As is the London Midland train that pootles past on its way to Long Buckby.) Also on the arches, immediately below track level, are four copies of the Henley coat of arms, an ornate blue 'H' with a red crown over it. The whole thing is in fantastic nick, and were Lord Henley around today he'd be justifiably proud. He might also, however, try to stop the train: he was allowed to do that in his day. Being the MP for Northampton he was up and down to London a lot, and had the right (like lots of local bigwigs back then) to use the bridge as a private railway station, rather like a modern 'request' bus stop. Imagine their faces if they returned today and encountered the *Daily Telegraph*'s parliamentary expenses team.

After passing under the bridge to admire it from both sides, I start back towards the village. This field used to be the 'North Ride' across Watford Park, and as the landscape is unchanged since Lord Henley's time (not a modern building to be seen) it's easy to imagine him and his chums galloping their horses here. Or it would be, but for one thing. The landscape isn't *quite* unchanged. There are no modern buildings to be seen, but there is a modern structure. Less than a mile away to the right, peeping at several points through gaps in the trees, is the M1. Its constant rush seems louder here than it did in the service station, where your brain obviously filters out the noise. I've been wondering whether Pulpit Bridge might pip Watford Gap to the title of NN fact, but charming and quirky as it is, I know, standing here now, that one particular fact about the services has to be the winner. Because it's a fact that takes you back in time.

Travel, at its best, moves you not only from A to B but through the fourth dimension as well. You see things as they are, compare them to how they were, and really feel that you've learned something about your country. Coming here to sample Watford Gap, get a feel for the service station in its middle age, the thing my mind keeps returning to is a picture of Keith Richards there in the 1960s. It's early enough in the Stones' career for him to be wearing a collar and tie, though the defiant expression is already in place as he stares into the camera lens, ignoring the man trying to engage him. Behind Keef is a glass cabinet containing trays of sausage rolls, cling-filmed sandwiches, individual jam tarts. The woman behind the counter wears one of those white paper hats that used to perch miraculously on the back of the head without falling off. Tea is sixpence.

Fast-forward to a story I heard recently about Mick Jagger. At a lunch in Oxford he fell to talking with another guest, and got progressively more and more fascinated with the subject under discussion. As the afternoon wore on Jagger realised he was getting close to the point where he would have to leave: he was being driven back to London for an evening engagement, one that it was impossible to get out of. So, excusing himself from the conversation for a moment, he called his office. They were instructed to cancel the car, and order instead, for the last possible moment, a helicopter.

Now that rock stars can live like this they don't stop off at Watford Gap services any more. Yet in the 1960s, as we saw earlier, you couldn't order your egg on toast there without falling over one. When it wasn't a Stone it was a Beatle, all referring to the services by their then name of the Blue Boar (the company which ran them). The idea that this was how legends travelled seems incredible now, and makes you realise just how much Britain has changed. And so the fact for this postcode has to be one that commemorates this long-departed era, and puts down a marker for a country that was radically and beautifully different:

NN (Northampton): When Jimi Hendrix first arrived in Britain, he heard so many fellow musicians referring to the Blue Boar that he assumed it was a trendy London club.

2

A TRIP TO PLUTO

The New Year dawns in a blaze of planning, and indeed a blaze of facts. The sense of anticipation you get at the beginning of every January – wondering what the next twelve months will bring, where they'll take you – is heightened this time round by that map on the wall. At many points during the final tinsel-strewn days of the old year I'm to be found gazing at it, dreaming of adventures in store. And, as ever, marvelling at Britain's place names. Who would have guessed that, lying a few miles apart from each other in SY (Shrewsbury) territory, are a Cockshutt and a Clive?

The venue for the next field trip presents itself fairly easily, on account of the fact that it is (a) a much-talked-about, much-written-about part of the country I've never really explored and (b) somewhere that will bag me not one but four, count them *four*, postcodes in one go. In the meantime home-based research continues apace, both actively and passively (in other words when I'm looking for facts and when I'm not). An article on the day-to-day running of Parliament reveals that:

MK (Milton Keynes): Acts of Parliament are still written on genuine vellum, the authorities spending £130,000 per year on the stuff.

The firm which supplies it is based in Newport Pagnell. The pieces of vellum,[1] once they've had our representatives' words of wisdom added to them, are rolled up and stored in a room at the Palace of Westminster which is maintained at a steady 16.5 degrees centigrade. There was a move in 1999 to end the centuries-old tradition, but MPs voted it down. And so modern legislation continues to pile up in skinny form, joining such legends as the 1782 Land Tax Act, the longest act ever at a quarter of a mile. If you were to unroll that outside Parliament it would be longer than Parliament.

While we're in a political vein, let's head to Bewdley, whose MP for nearly 30 years was Stanley Baldwin:

DY (Dudley): Stanley Baldwin is the only British Prime Minister ever to serve under three different monarchs.

His second spell in the post (1935–7) covered George V, Edward VIII and George VI.

Heading north, we pass through...

DE (Derby): A Frenchman, observing a nineteenth-century football match involving hundreds of players in Derbyshire, remarked: 'If the English-men call this playing, it would be impossible to say what they call fighting.'

---

[1] The word comes from the Old French '*velin*', meaning calf skin, though any animal can be used – modern vellum is made from calf, goat or sheep. Parchment is pretty much the same stuff, just with an extra layer of fat trimmed away.

... and arrive at Stoke-on-Trent. It's supremely tempting to award this area to Lee Streeter of Stafford, for the 2012 incident in which he texted everybody in his address book offering cannabis for sale: two of the numbers, he realised too late, belonged to police officers who had helped him after a car accident.[2] But ST, I decide in the end, can only belong to JCB:

ST (Stoke-on-Trent): The perfectionist Joseph Charles Bamford, founder of the digger company that bears his initials, was so happy when an exasperated French businessman said the initials stood for 'Jamais Content' that he had the words displayed over the entrance to his factory.

Don't worry, though: all you 'dumb criminals' fans can get your fix further north, just over the border into Scotland. It is only 'just', mind you: the DG area, standing for 'Dumfries and Galloway', also includes a few English addresses in Cumbria. Not for nothing did this region come to be known as the 'Debatable Lands', disputed for centuries between the two countries. The general atmosphere of lawlessness made it fertile hunting ground for the Border Reivers, criminals who raided the territory and stole from it.[3] Enemies called them 'devils', and one particularly deep and well-hidden valley which they used for storing half-inched cattle became known as the Devil's Beef Tub. However, our story concerns a more modern criminal: Buck Ruxton, the Lancaster doctor who in 1935 strangled his habitually unfaithful wife. He also had to strangle their housemaid to prevent her revealing the crime. Ruxton

---

[2] In case you're wondering: 18 months.

[3] 'Reive' meant 'to rob' – it gave us the modern word 'ruffian'.

then dismembered the two bodies in his bathroom to disguise their identities, wrapped the various parts in newspaper and drove up to Scotland to dispose of them. Coincidentally the stream he chose, north of the town of Moffat, was only a couple of miles from the Devil's Beef Tub. It was to become known locally as 'Ruxton's Dump'.

The case was one of the first in which forensic evidence played an important role: scientists superimposed a photograph over the X-ray of a skull, while entomologists were able to estimate the date of death from (brace yourself) the age of maggots found in the bodies. But even without the *CSI* brigade, Ruxton hadn't exactly helped his own cause. The newspaper in which he wrapped the body parts was a special edition of the *Sunday Graphic* sold only in Lancaster and Morecambe. Fair enough, you might say, easy mistake to make. What wasn't so clever was knocking over a cyclist as he drove home. A police officer stopped his car and made a note of the registration number, crucial evidence later on when Ruxton denied ever having gone to Scotland. None of this, however, is the fact I'm going to select from the story. I'm plumping for one of its bizarre footnotes – which actually gets filed under a different postcode:

PR (Preston): The bath in which 1930s murderer Buck Ruxton dismembered his victims is now used at the stables of Lancashire Police's mounted division as the trough from which their horses drink.

Until not so long ago, a very helpful chap at the stables informs me, it was also used in the initiation ceremony for newly qualified officers: they were given a cold bath in it. Making this choice for the PR fact means I have to apologise to Napoleon III. Until now he was favourite for the nomination, or rather Lord Street in Southport was – this was where Napoleon lived in the 1840s before returning home to become French Emperor. The wide tree-lined street gave him the idea for the boulevards he introduced to Paris. Mind you, the choice also leaves the DG field open. The aforementioned Moffat stakes an early claim with its Star Hotel, which at only 20 feet used to sit in the *Guinness Book of Records* as the world's narrowest hotel. But it has since lost out to a five-footer in Spain (slacker), so instead we turn to another hotel, the Ellangowan in Creetown. It was here that Britt Ekland's famous naked dance in *The Wicker Man* was filmed. Except it wasn't *totally* the Swedish actress's dance:

DG (Dumfries and Galloway): Britt Ekland was furious at being replaced by a body double in *The Wicker Man*, as the replacement bottom was larger than hers.

In fact the movie as a whole was an unhappy experience for the second Mrs Peter Sellers. Scotland in October isn't the balmiest of places, but as the film was set in summer the cast weren't allowed to wear overcoats. Indoors, the legendary scene got her even angrier. 'For me,' she explains, 'anything below the waist is private.' So although she was prepared to show her breasts, her bottom was off-limits (surely the reverse of what you'd expect?). Even though Ekland claims her agent had made the situation 'very clear', it still came as a surprise to director Robin Hardy, who was forced to scrabble around for a stunt posterior. Eventually a stripper from Glasgow was brought in, though on a day Ekland was away from the set. The first she knew about it was when the film came out. 'Her bottom was much bigger than mine,' she complained. 'It was ridiculous.'

Back in England, meanwhile, it's time to dispatch a myth:

HX (Halifax): The Halifax Gibbet, a device for decapitating criminals, was in use in the Yorkshire town centuries before French revolutionaries 'invented' the guillotine.

This story is one huge example of the fun to be had from poking around in a tale you thought you knew. For a start, the man I'd always taken to be the inventor of the guillotine, French physician Joseph-Ignace Guillotin, was not only not the inventor, he didn't even support the death penalty. It was named after him because he proposed a device to cleanly and painlessly decapitate the condemned person, a move he hoped would be the first step towards the abolition of capital punishment.[4] But even Antoine Louis, the man credited with the instrument's design, wasn't the first to put his head to the problem of taking off other people's. In Halifax, the Gibbet had been in use for ages, certainly since the 1500s and possibly earlier. A replica stands in the town now, and if it's not a guillotine in everything but name then I'm a *pain au raisin*. Two parallel pieces of wood, 15 feet tall, supporting a 4-foot 6-inch block containing a 7-pound axe blade. The blade was secured by a rope, which was in turn held in place by a pin. When the pin was removed, the blade descended. Executions were communal events back then – every person in the crowd would take hold of the rope, or at least (in the words of a 1586 witness) 'putteth forth his arm so near to the same as he can get, in token that he is willing to see true justice executed'. Then they pulled together to remove the pin. Unless, that is, the offender had been convicted of stealing an animal. In that case the stolen animal (or one from the same species) had the rope tied to it and was then driven away.

[4] Bad luck, Joseph – France carried on using the guillotine until 1977.

Down in Gloucestershire there's yet more inventiveness. Thankfully it's of a less gruesome nature, though does still involve sharp blades. In 1830, Edwin Beard Budding of Stroud, after visiting a local mill and seeing the machine used to trim nap from woollen cloth, went away and came up with the lawnmower. Two of his early models were sold to London Zoo and Oxford University.[5] Gloucester itself, via the composer John Stafford Smith, gave America the tune for 'The Star-Spangled Banner', but it's out to the badlands of GL9 that we journey for our fact. Here is to be found the village of Badminton, and in particular Badminton House, the home these past few centuries of the Dukes of Beaufort. Not only does it host the famous horse trials every year, it also gave its name to a sport which the army brought back to Blighty from India in 1873. First played at a party given by the Duke, badminton soon became all the rage. It isn't the fact that today's top players can propel the shuttlecock at 200 mph that amazes me – it's what that shuttlecock is made from:

GL (Gloucester): The shuttlecocks used in professional badminton are made with real goose feathers, which are always taken from the bird's left wing.

These, apparently, ensure a better flight, though no one seems to know why. They are plucked while the goose is still alive, causing it incredible pain. I'd never realised that

[5] Just to prove what we've been saying about nineteenth-century inventors, Budding is also one of the men credited with the adjustable spanner. As the other contender, Richard Clyburn, was also from these shores the tool is known in France, Germany, Spain, Italy and several other countries as the 'English key'.

badminton might be on the hit list of the League Against Cruel Sports.

There's one other bit of 'on the ground' research before the field trip proper, and it concerns a geographical curiosity. It's the subject of some dispute, though this doesn't bother me, as either way round it's going to provide a fact for the PE (Peterborough) postcode. Enquiries lead eventually to a very helpful gentleman at Lincolnshire County Council, who is happy to email me an ultra-large-scale map of the area in question. Having printed it out, and made time on the way back from a trip somewhere else, I find myself on a bright January day parking up in the Rutland village of Tinwell.

One of the winding lanes that led here (I'm now a stranger to fourth gear) contained a 'Welcome to Rutland' sign which was crying out for the slogan 'England's smallest county' to be added underneath. Just as well no one has, as that title doesn't actually belong to Rutland, or at least not all the time: it drops to second smallest whenever the tide comes in on the Isle of Wight. It is true, however, that Rutland is the only county in England without a McDonald's. And it's undeniably beautiful. Many of the cottages here are built from a local light-coloured sandstone that in today's sunshine prompts pleasant memories of crème brûlée. Opposite the church in Tinwell is a building made of the same stuff, with a ten-foot arch over one doorway in the shape of a horseshoe. Closer inspection reveals that it is indeed Tinwell Forge, still operating as a blacksmith's business to this day. *My* business, however, lies in the opposite direction, down a footpath leading through the churchyard and out into open country.

Within fifteen minutes I'm following a stream that meanders south-eastwards towards the A1. This is reminiscent of looking at the road's bigger sibling the M1 from that field in North-amptonshire, but this time I'm going to get a lot closer to the traffic: directly underneath it, in fact, as the path and indeed the stream pass below an elevated section of the road. Once I'm through into the field on the other side I turn immediately to the right, and hug the bottom of the 30-foot bank that slopes up towards the road. So you can get your bearings for the next couple of paragraphs, the A1 is at this point running pretty well north–south, while the footpath that took me underneath it ran east–west.

As I walk along I see that the bank is peppered with bits of litter that have either dropped or been thrown from the road above. There's a huge plasma TV screen which has literally fallen off the back of a lorry (unsurprisingly it's smashed beyond use), while a label fluttering from a tree branch reveals that there's a variety of potato called Piccolo Star, and a field in my home county of Suffolk known as Crotch Top. After a couple of minutes I reach another stream, also running east–west underneath the road. The litter alongside it includes empty cans of spray paint, and the huge concrete wall supporting the carriageway bears several graffiti tags, as well as, in foot-high letters, a crucifix and the phrase 'Forgive my sins, Father'.

Time to consult the map. I walk east along the stream for a few metres, then stop, choose a point where the stones lining its banks have fallen into the water, and clamber across them to the other side (the stream is *slightly* too wide to confidently make it in a single jump). Then I walk along the southern bank for 25 paces, which happens to bring me up against a tree that has semi-collapsed, various of its branches and sub-trunks dangling in the water. They are at the same time an obstacle and the means of getting across that obstacle, so soon I've managed to recross the stream and am once again standing on the north bank.

Why this curious manoeuvre? Well, by completing it I have stood in four English counties within a couple of minutes. They were, in order: Rutland, Northamptonshire, Cambridgeshire and Lincolnshire. This was the geographical curiosity in question: some people try to tell you that the counties meet at a single point, the only point in England where four counties do so.[6] But it's not quite true. It's very *nearly* a quadpoint (as mapheads label such places), with the counties as listed just then being to the north-west, the south-west, the south-east and the north-east. But actually Rutland has been 'pulled' slightly to the left and Cambridgeshire slightly to the right, meaning that there are in fact two tripoints a few yards apart. Between those two points the stream forms a county boundary, Lincolnshire to its north, Northamptonshire to its south. And so:

PE (Peterborough): The boundary between Lincolnshire and Northamptonshire is, at 19 metres, the shortest county boundary in England.

And I have walked the lot of it.

'Try tapping.'

'What, here?'

'Anywhere.'

I rap my knuckles against the wall. They produce a totally dead sound. Not even a hint of an echo.

'Every time you hang a picture here,' says Hugh, 'you wear out a drill bit.'

'From one single hole?'

He nods. 'It's 1943 concrete. It's not getting any softer. In fact it carries on getting harder.'

Late January now, and I'm standing in the living room of Hugh Sheer's bungalow in Greatstone. It's the first stop on

---

[6] There are several dozen points where three counties meet.

my field trip to Kent, famous as the 'garden of England' but somewhere I've not really visited that much, certainly not enough to form a proper impression. The phrase always puts you in mind of lush, fertile countryside, fields and meadows and pastures bursting with greenery, a landscape rich in both senses of the word. One of my previous Kent outings was to Chartwell, the country residence of Winston Churchill (now owned by the National Trust), where the surrounding area certainly did fit the image. As did the Lamberhurst home of another Tory PM, Margaret Thatcher. Admittedly I've only seen it in documentaries, and the footage only shows the garden rather than the country beyond it, but everything about it says 'well-heeled'. Maggie prunes the roses as Denis stripes the lawn, using a mower the size of a Ford Cortina. His impressively strong spin at the end of one length reveals a capacity for U-turns his wife never shared.

Another memory of Kent, though, is a Bank Holiday Monday afternoon in Rochester. Jo and I, then still living in London, had gone for a nice day out. Fools. The town's inhabitants showed us, with quite shocking candour, that Kent can mean lager as well as sherry, tattoos as well as twinsets, full-on fist fights in the street as well as bridge evenings. And just as the people can differ, so can the geography. Much of Kent is coastal and bleak. Looking out of Hugh's window, I know that if it weren't for the houses opposite, and the houses on the seafront road a few yards beyond that, I'd be looking at a shingle beach, a grey and blustery English Channel, a distinct lack of anything worthy of the name 'garden'. A couple of minutes' drive down the coast is Dungeness, the promontory so dry and inhospitable to vegetation that it's classed by the Met Office as Britain's only desert. If Kent really is the garden of England, this is the rockery.

So what has brought me here, to the very extreme of TN (Tonbridge)[7] territory? Operation Pluto, that's what, a chapter of the Second World War story which depended, in part, on the house I'm standing in now. Appropriately enough for the project, I had to make my first contact with Hugh by letter: I knew about the property's role in Operation Pluto from the literature on the subject, but not who lived there. So an envelope addressed simply to 'The Occupier' was posted. The next day an email appeared in my inbox. Hugh had a wealth of material on his home's former existence, which he'd happily share over a cup of tea and a bacon roll at a time of my choosing. Now retired from a career as a telephone engineer and a policeman, Hugh's days are his own. Here we are then, him in his V-neck pullover inviting me to tap the wall, his wife Shelia supervising the delicious sizzling sounds emanating from the kitchen.

Pluto wasn't an initiative to raise the country's morale by playing Mickey Mouse films – the letters stand for 'PipeLines Under The Ocean'. As Hitler began to find himself on the back foot, and the Allies realised the time was coming for them to invade France, minds turned to the question of how to fuel all the vehicles that would be taking part in D-Day, before (with any luck) surging further across Europe. Sending boats laden with petrol across the Channel would have been asking for German bombers to do their worst. Instead the British

[7] No, the initials don't denote Tunbridge Wells, though confusingly TN1 – '1' normally belonging to the place that named the postcode area – *does* cover Tunbridge Wells. Tonbridge is TN9 to TN12. It's enough to make you Disgusted. The mythical creature first appeared in the *Tunbridge Wells Advertiser* when 1950s staff made him/her up to fill their empty letters column. Framed in Steve Coogan's downstairs loo is a letter to the BBC from someone in Tunbridge Wells, complaining – in all seriousness – about *On the Hour* sports reporter Alan Partridge being given his own Radio 4 series.

planned a scheme which, when I first read about it, and being a man whose engineering expertise begins and finishes at the simpler end of the Lego range, had me convinced that I'd misunderstood an entire paragraph. But no, that was exactly what the British did: they laid a pipeline along the seabed all the way from Kent to Boulogne. Not just one, either – 17 of the things. Plus a further four going from the Isle of Wight over to Cherbourg. The petrol was sent through those pipes, up to a million gallons of the stuff a day.

How do you get that much petrol flowing? You can't stand on the beach at Dungeness tipping it in from jerrycans. You need to pump it. Which is where Hugh's Art Deco bungalow came in. It had been built in 1936, one of five on this road, all in the same style, three on this side, two opposite.

'As you can see,' says Hugh, 'the whole area's been developed massively since those days. But back then these five dwellings were the only thing round here. As soon as the war started the area was cordoned off, including the beach. The residents had to have ID cards to get through. Then finally in 1943 the government said, "That's it, we're requisitioning the houses, off you go."' Even if German planes couldn't bomb pipelines under the Channel, they could certainly bomb the pumping stations sending petrol down those pipelines. The stations, therefore, had to be disguised to keep the whole set-up a secret. 'That's what the military wanted these houses for,' continues Hugh. 'You don't build a pumping station and write "Operation Pluto Pumping Station" on the roof. You use a house, keep it looking exactly *like* a house. And you do everything as quickly and unobtrusively as possible. They ripped a hole in that wall round the side there, got all the pumping equipment in, then resealed it straight away.' Later Hugh will show me the faint line on the external wall that is the only sign this ever happened.

While the deception kept the outside of the bungalow looking exactly the same, inside it was all change. 'The whole lot was ripped out. Every internal wall. Iron girders were put across the top, then on top of those they put eighteen-inch thick arches of reinforced concrete, straddling the girders. Every thirty inches you've got a girder. And as you can see . . .' Hugh indicates the front window, 'they made the external walls twenty-four inches thick.' Plenty of room for pictures on this windowsill. 'That's concrete as well, with metal grilles built into it. Plus up there, running over the window, is a railway sleeper. We know that because we had that bit replastered a few years ago, and the builder found it. To this day, you could strip every internal wall out of this place and it would stay standing. You can arrange the rooms however you want. How many houses can claim that?'

There are other benefits, too. Hugh and Sheila moved here in 1986. The following year Britain was hit by the hurricane which weatherman Michael Fish assured us wasn't coming. 'Most of the houses round here took a real hammering,' says Hugh. 'We were OK, though. The only thing we suffered was a slate blowing off a neighbour's roof and coming through our window.'

The three buildings on this side of the road were pumping stations, while the two opposite were used as staff quarters. Other buildings on this stretch of the coast joined the fray as pumping stations, too, including a tiny church down on Dungeness. Underground pipes ran the few yards down to the beach, where they were buried under the shingle before linking up with the underwater pipes completing the route to France. For the oil in question it was the final stretch of a journey all the way from America. Shipped across the Atlantic to Birkenhead, it was then distributed to airfields around Britain using an existing network of underground pipes.

Among Hugh's collection of documents is a map given to him by a local historian who researched Pluto. A normal Ordnance Survey map of the area, it is marked in pencil with the exact route of the pipe feeding down through Kent to Dungeness. 'He did it with the help of a local Scout group. Every cross you see – here, for instance ... here and here ... is where the pipe went under a road or a lane. Those points were marked with stiles, in case they needed to locate the pipe later on.'

'Stiles?'

'Normal stiles, the ones walkers use for climbing over hedges. Or not *quite* normal. They used a subtly different design, so that no one spying for the Germans would notice the difference. But anyone who needed to know could recognise the design, and work out that that's where the pipe was running.'

Although Pluto was an extension of the land-based network already in place, the task of making pipes capable of stretching thirty miles along the seabed was a massive technical challenge. But this was Britain during the Second World War: challenges were there to be met. First into the fray was Arthur Hartley, chief engineer of the Anglo-Iranian Oil Company. He had the brainwave of adapting telegraph cable technology, which had been carrying messages along the seabed for decades. Strip out the core of a cable like that, he said, and you might have something you could pump petrol through. Several firms set to work on it, including Siemens, Johnson and Phillips, Pirelli and (seemingly determined to be mentioned at every possible turn in this book) the Post Office, whose experience in laying telegraph cables was vital. If you want a flavour of the different elements of society involved, try these names for size: lead-burners included the brothers Frank, Albert and Ron Stone, while Shell's chief chemist was

John Augustus Oriel. He contributed crucial expertise despite the damaged eyesight he'd suffered as a result of being gassed during the First World War.

There were lots of false starts, with pipes twisting, kinking, bursting and God knows what else-ing, but eventually a design was arrived at. The metal pipe had an internal diameter of just three inches, protected by external layers of materials such as jute and bitumen-prepared cotton. The authorities set about making it in three-quarter of a mile lengths, which could then be joined together. 'They trialled them in the Clyde and off the coast of Devon,' says Hugh. 'They tested them up to a pressure of five thousand pounds per square inch, even though they were only going to need one thousand two hundred when it came to it.' The figures involved are mind-numbing. One pipe was 50 miles long and weighed 4,000 tons. When the pipes were coiled up ready to be transported they had to be filled with water – otherwise they'd have crushed themselves with their own weight.

'How do you go about getting something like that down on to the seabed?' I ask.

Hugh reaches into a folder, producing a picture of something that looks like an enormous cotton reel. 'The Conundrum,' he announces. 'So-called because it was a *drum* with *cone*-shaped ends.'

There's a speck of dirt on the picture. I'm about to wipe it off when I realise it isn't a speck of dirt at all – it's a person, or rather four people, standing next to the drum. 'Blimey,' I say. 'How big was this thing?'

Hugh smiles. 'If you're wrapping dozens of miles of cable round something, it needs to be big, doesn't it? They built a few Conundrums – some were forty feet in diameter, weighed several hundred tons. That was empty. Then you had the extra weight of the pipes wrapped round them.'

The plan was to float the drum in the sea between two tugs, which would then pull it across to France. As they went the pipe would unwind itself and sink to the bottom of the Channel. An early effort involved HMS *Buster*, one of the navy's most powerful tugs, but despite her plucky name the vessel couldn't get enough speed up. An approach had to be made to Sir Hastings Ismay, Churchill's Chief of Staff, because the list of the biggest tugs was kept by the Prime Minister himself in a locked drawer. Soon HMS *Marauder* was on her way. Even she had difficulties. But then someone had the brainwave of spacing the two tugs further apart so that their wake flowed past the Conundrum rather than into it. This had been slowing it down. Eventually it was drums ahoy, and the pipes were on their way to France...

...where the final problem awaited. Namely pulling the pipes ashore. The winches the engineers had been planning to use turned out not to be strong enough. Then a naval officer remembered his childhood, watching steam-powered ploughing engines at work on a farm. A quick phone call to the Ministry of Agriculture and Fisheries, and half a dozen engines were dispatched. After the success of the D-Day landings had established that war traffic was going to be very much a one-way affair from then on,[8] the pipe network was extended right across the Continent into Belgium, Luxembourg and even Germany itself. It was in use until well after Hitler had been defeated. Then, because there was such desperate need for raw materials (especially lead) in post-war Britain, almost all the pipes were recovered and brought back home. An extra bonus, in the midst of petrol rationing, was the discovery that they still contained 75,000 gallons of fuel.

---

[8] Churchill had to be ordered by King George VI to abandon his plan of personally accompanying the first troops over to Normandy.

By now Sheila has completed operations in the kitchen, and the three of us are enjoying our bacon rolls.

'It must be wonderful,' I say, 'knowing that your home played such a role in the war effort.'

Hugh's collection of Pluto documents is the only answer this question needs. Sheila, though, points out the practical difficulties involved. 'When we had our extension built at the back we couldn't get the gas supply down there,' she says. 'But that's OK – we've got a stove in there instead. And,' she points to the two-foot-thick wall, 'the house stays nice and warm in winter. You don't lose much heat through something like that.'

It's strange, sitting in a perfectly normal room, with its ornaments and dining table and pictures of Hugh and Sheila's daughter and grandson on the wall, to think that this is the exact spot from which millions of gallons of petrol were pumped 30 miles across the Channel in total secrecy. Strange but, once you've got your head round it, an instant ticket back to a time when Britain was a very different place. 'Even after the war,' says Sheila, 'things happened down here that you wouldn't believe today. Like they used to play cards in the pubs for plots of land. That's why you sometimes see an empty space in the middle of new houses that have been built – no one knows who owns it.'

'There was one builder,' adds Hugh, 'who found a plot, built himself a bungalow, and the day he finished a bloke came up to him and said, "Thanks very much for the new house." It had been his land all along. He showed the builder the paperwork, said, "My deeds, my land."'

Conversation continues, and at one point Hugh mentions something that I know instantly has to be my TN fact. I think about it later, as I'm standing on the beach, gazing down at the one remaining piece of Pluto pipe that has been exposed among the shingle. Only the inner metal core remains, rusting away to nothing – for most of the dozen or so feet that are visible only half the pipe's circumference has survived. If you didn't know what this was you'd assume it was an old drainpipe someone had dumped here. If you do know what it is you stand in awe.

The light's beginning to go now, the wind blowing even harder and colder. Soon I'll be in the famous Pilot Inn down the road, enjoying chicken-and-ham pie and a pint of bitter, watching the regulars at the bar as they josh and banter and sup. Seventy years ago, it'll hit me, these would have been exactly the sort of men charged with building the Pluto pipes, sailing the tugs across to France, fighting (the younger ones at least) in the tanks those pipes had fuelled. But for now, I'm standing on the desolate and deserted beach, a broken length of metal pipe at my feet, thinking about the man who features in my fact:

TN (Tonbridge): A German spy who landed on the beach near Dungeness during the Second World War gave himself away by walking into a pub at nine-thirty in the morning and asking for a pint of champagne cider.

I assumed on the way down here that my fact would concern Operation Pluto itself, some nugget of engineering genius concerning the pipes or the way the military got them on to the seabed. But amazing as all that has been, the story from Hugh which captured my imagination more than any other was the one about Carl Meier. He and his companion Jose Waldberg travelled in the opposite direction to the petrol, from France to England, at a time in the war (September 1940) when such traffic had been far more common than it was by 1944. After a farewell party with their handlers in Le Touquet, the two spies were brought across under cover of darkness by fishing boat. Seven miles off the coast of Dungeness a rowing boat was lowered into the sea, Waldberg and Meier climbed into it and rowed themselves the rest of the way, coming ashore somewhere near the bit of beach I'm standing on now. Gazing out at the far from unchoppy water, my stomach lurches. Forget doing it at night, forget doing it in the knowledge that there are people on the shore who don't want you to succeed, and that if they catch you you are dead (not a figure of speech) – simply rowing ashore from seven miles out is a mammoth feat in itself. When Waldberg and Meier[9] reached land they hid their belongings and food in a disused lifeboat, stashing their wireless set under an overturned advertising hoarding. Later, when dawn came up, they moved the wireless to a safer place in a tree not far from the seashore.

By now Waldberg had developed a bit of a thirst, and the two agreed that Meier should walk to the nearby town of Lydd to get them something to drink, as well as some cigarettes. The implication seems to be that the thirst was the result of a hangover from their farewell party the night before. If it was, then Meier completed the pair's 'don't mind a drink or two' image by entering the Rising Sun in Lydd, whose front door was open but which was not, at 9.30 a.m., serving. Of course any local would have known that, but to underline the fact that he wasn't from round these parts, Meier asked the landlady for a pint of champagne cider. Mabel Cole explained that she couldn't help him and he'd have to come back later, but that he'd be able to get the cigarettes he wanted at Tilbey's Stores over the road. Meier thanked her and turned to go, banging his head on the low ceiling and breaking a light. By the time he

[9] Technically Meier was Dutch – but he had been born in Germany, and was a member of a political group working for union with the Fatherland.

returned to the pub later, the authorities (alerted by Cole) had sent an RAF officer to wait for him. Not having the required residents' pass, Meier was arrested. Under questioning he accidentally said that 'we' arrived last night: soon Waldberg was picked up as well. Three months later, on 10 December, the pair were hanged at Pentonville Prison in London. Waldberg was 25, Meier a year younger.

Something lying in the shingle a few yards from the pipe catches my attention. It's a passport, or rather the cover and title page of one. (It's at moments like this I'm glad I write non-fiction – put that sort of thing in a novel and no one would believe you.) In the gloom I have to use the light from my phone to read it. A quick web search reveals nothing untoward about the 46-year-old British owner: clearly he has simply lost the passport. But the ID document makes the story of Meier and Waldberg seem all the more real, as though it could have happened yesterday. If I was in a different mood, thinking about all this indoors where I was dry and warm, their incompetence might seem funny, part of the raw material that decades later inspired *Dad's Army* and *'Allo 'Allo*. Now, though, standing here, looking at the short length of pipe at my feet, the tale of the spies and that of Operation Pluto merge together in my mind to reveal a time – one not so long ago at all – when this nondescript stretch of beach on the Kent coast was a very different place indeed.

It isn't every bed and breakfast that supplies you with an individually sourced poem alongside your muesli and toast. But Alison Noyes, proprietor of the Watch Tower B&B on Dungeness, was interested enough when I told her about the reason for my stay to look up and print out 'The Counties', Carol Ann Duffy's response to the Royal Mail's 2010 announcement that they were thinking of removing counties from the addresses in their database and relying solely on postcodes instead. Of course the whole point of a postcode is that you don't need the county, or indeed the city, town or village – simply the house number and street will do.[10] But needless to say the burghers of just about every county in the land protested. I can't exactly blame them – my status as a Suffolk resident of an Essex postcode always has me inserting the county before the code. Duffy voiced her objection more artistically:

> *But I want to post a rose to a Lancashire lass,*
> *red, I'll pick it,*
> *and I want to write to a Middlesex mate*
> *for tickets for cricket*

...and so on. It doesn't surprise me that Alison knew about the poem. The shelves in my room are full of poetry books and novels, remnants of the lifelong love of literature that the younger Alison indulged by teaching in her native London, before deciding she should get a proper job and train as a solicitor. The new career didn't last long, hence the move to Kent to run a B&B. The property's name honours the fact that it was constructed circa 1810 as a lookout against Napoleon, though it's been extended and modernised since then, and even the central section (the only remaining bit of the original building) isn't particularly tall (the word 'Tower' was added in the twentieth century). But still, when Alison asks how my researches went yesterday, and I tell her about Pluto and the spies, our conversation soon turns to how close this bit of England is to France.

'I like being this close to the Continent,' says Alison. 'On a clear night you can see the headlights of the cars over at Cap

---

[10] In many cases you could even get away without the street – the average postcode covers just 17 addresses.

Gris Nez, which is the closest bit of France to England –
twenty-one miles from Dover. I've always felt very European,
but living here has really underlined it.'

As the German politician Ludwig Erhard once put it, 'without Britain, Europe would remain only a torso'. If that makes
us the head, it hasn't only been a case of the eyes picking out
car headlights – the ears came into play, too, during the Battle
of the Somme, when you could hear the artillery guns from
Kent (in fact from Hampstead Heath, too). Even the more
antiquated cannons used at the Battle of Waterloo were heard
in Sussex.

Another factor in Alison's identity is that she's Jewish.[11] As
we examine the map of Kent that will guide me on today's
travels (sniggering when we notice the place names Donkey
Street, Wheelbarrow Town and Ripple), she points out that as
far as she knows there are only four shuls (synagogues) in the
whole of the county.

'You'd have thought there'd be more, wouldn't you?' I reply.
'For such a big county. And especially as it's the first bit of
England anyone fleeing Europe in the Thirties would have
reached.'

'Ah, but they all headed for London,' says Alison. 'Jews like
big cities. They feel safe there.'

Eventually it's time to saddle up and head northwards along
the coast. CT (Canterbury) territory is calling. Appropriate
that I should leave TN by road – it was here in 1914, on
dangerous bends near Ashford, that Britain's first ever white
lines were painted. Near Dymchurch there's a field of sheep
whose trough is a modern white plastic bath. One of them is

[11] Her surname means 'of Noah', though she points out that as it's comprised of the words 'no' and 'yes' you could also see it as the ultimate in
ambivalence.

taking a drink, possibly with a view to hopping in afterwards for a quick scrub down. Then, after the village, a Martello tower has been converted into a private house (tasteful shade of ochre, modern glass section added on top). These thick brick structures, a bit like windmills without the sails, were built along the coast of south-east England to guard against (that man again) Napoleon. The British attacked one in Corsica in 1794, and its design so impressed them that they copied it and named it after the tower's home. Though they did so with the usual English skill at European languages: the place was actually called Mortella. Hythe shows how the nature of drama has changed round here these past 70 years – near a café called the Spitfire is a local newspaper board announcing: 'Phones Dead for Two Weeks'.

Next it's Dover, announced first by the increasing number of lorries on the road, then, as you round a corner and start to descend, the sight of the famous white cliffs. 'No promontory town or haven of Christendom is so placed by nature and situation,' Walter Raleigh told Elizabeth I, 'both to gratify friends and annoy enemies as this your Majestie's Town of Dover.' When a triumphant Duke of Wellington returned here in 1814 (having ensured that the Martello towers were never called into action), he parked himself at the Ship Inn and ordered 'an unlimited supply of buttered toast'.[12] These days the cliffs erode by a centimetre a year. Don't bother looking for the famous bluebirds, either – the breed is American (as was the song's writer), and is never found in the UK. The nature of returning

[12] Wellington also puts himself in the CT running alongside Augustus Pugin, designer of the Palace of Westminster – they both died in the postcode on the same night (14 September 1852), rather like JFK, Aldous Huxley and C. S. Lewis all dying on the same day. Pugin was at his home in Ramsgate, Wellington a few miles down the coast at his castle in Walmer.

Brits has changed as well: a recent report found that an average of ten cars a day emerging from English Channel crossings were breaking down under the weight of duty-free booze.

After Dover the signs read 'Sandwich', the town whose fourth Earl, as well as being the reason Hawaii was originally known as the Sandwich Islands when Captain Cook discovered them in 1778, invented the famous snack. The first ever filling was salt beef. It's tempting almost beyond resistance to go looking for the signpost near here which points to the tiny village of Ham as well as the more famous town, so that it reads 'Ham Sandwich'. But duty, in the form of Broadstairs, calls. No, not because the town gave the world Ted Heath, the man who denied that he had greeted news of Margaret Thatcher's resignation with the words 'Rejoice! Rejoice!' ('I didn't say it twice, I said it three times'). Nor because some steps down to the beach near here are the ones which inspired John Buchan to write *The Thirty-Nine Steps*. No, I'm in Broadstairs because it was home to the man who invented the bank holiday.

High on a cliff, looking down on the town and the sea beyond it, is Kingsgate Castle. The king in question was Charles II (his ship landed on this bit of the coast in 1683 after being caught in a storm), though the castle didn't come along until the 1760s, when it was built by the Whig politician Henry Fox. After passing through the hands of subsequent owners (one of whom we'll return to shortly), the castle was altered and enlarged in the early twentieth century, before being split into the 30 or so private flats that stand here today.

Two tall wooden gates now shield the building from the road. I've just got out of my car to read the notice on one of them (it makes passing mention of the hero of our story), when the gates swing open and the caretaker, a cheery middle-aged guy who mistakenly assumes I've come to visit one of the residents, waves me in from the far end of the long drive.

It seems rude to shout, so I drive down to explain the mis-understanding. When he learns why I'm here he's more than happy to help. 'Park up there, mate,' he says, pointing to a spot next to his own van. He leads me through the main archway containing the residents' noticeboard, and across the central courtyard into a wing whose hall displays various important-looking portraits, as well as a picture of the original gate in the original castle. There's also a huge framed sheet bearing the signatures of 1930s and 1940s tenants, most of which confirm those tenants' poshness by being completely illegible.

'Nick Faldo used to live here, you know,' says Caretaker. We step outside again so he can point to a window in the higher of the two storeys. 'That was his flat. He liked living here because he used to play a lot of his golf at Sandwich.'

I look round at the dark stone. 'Quite forbidding, isn't it?'

'Flint,' replies Caretaker, sighing. 'Leaks like a sieve.'

Remembering that he has a book about the castle's history somewhere, he goes off to look for it, leaving me standing in the main courtyard. I consult my notes about the man who owned the castle in the nineteenth century. Rereading them under the flint's forbidding gaze makes an already strange story somehow even stranger. Sir John Lubbock was one of those men who, in return for having been born to a very rich father and not needing to work for a living, seemed to see it as their duty to behave in an eccentric and bizarre way so the rest of us could have something to laugh at. Lubbock Snr had made a packet in the City, using some of it to buy a 3,000-acre estate near Downe, the Kent village to which, in 1842 when Lubbock was seven, Charles Darwin moved. The young John eventually became Darwin's friend, sharing as he did the famous man's interest in nature.

Lubbock's research, however, was a little more unusual than the famous naturalist's. His black terrier puppy Van, he became convinced, was intelligent enough to read. So he placed a strip of cardboard inscribed with the word 'Food' over the animal's empty bowl. To get fed, Van had to bring the strip to his master. I know what you're thinking: this doesn't in itself mean that the dog could read. True. But then Lubbock did away with the bowl, placing the 'Food' card in a line with nine others marked with different words. Van picked it out every time. He also learned to read the words 'Water', 'Bone' and 'Tea'.[13] Later the system was extended so that to request a walk Van simply had to bring Lubbock a card saying 'Out'. Sir John knew that this behaviour was exceptional: his wife's pet collie could never read a word.

Dogs, however, were far from Sir John's only interest. Bees excited him beyond belief, so much so that he kept a hive in his sitting room in order to observe their behaviour. To prevent them escaping into other rooms he constructed a tunnel leading from the hive's entrance to an open window. Also resident in the sitting room were Lubbock's ants. They lived in a glass box, spotted with dabs of paint so their master could tell them apart. He also named them, showing them off to visitors including William Gladstone, Randolph Churchill (father of Winston) and the Archbishop of Canterbury. In one experiment Sir John got the ants drunk using tiny drops of alcohol. The sober ones, he noted, would carry their pissed friends home.

Lubbock was keen that his children should inherit his love of nature.[14] The ideal starter pet, he reasoned, was the ferret,

[13] The dog, clearly tired out by all the reading, had developed a taste for lukewarm, milky tea.

[14] He himself was one of nine siblings. Three of his brothers played first-class cricket for Kent. Two of those three also played for Old Etonians in the 1875 FA Cup Final. Of course they did.

so he bought a pair from a London street vendor. On the train back to Kent, however, the ferrets gnawed through their sack under his seat and began terrorising the other passengers. Sir John gathered them up and locked them in his briefcase. Problem solved, though he did discover later that they'd eaten his parliamentary papers. He was MP for Maidstone, you see. (You could behave like this back then and still get elected. Happy days.) Lubbock's briefcase was once stolen, though the thief soon got rid of it when he discovered the contents. No, not ferrets. Bees.

Sir John, it's already clear, was someone prepared to stand out from the crowd, depart from the conventional wisdom. So when he proposed, within a year of being elected to Parliament, that workers should be given more holidays, he was ready to counter Benjamin Disraeli's objections that employers would lose money. He persuaded his own party, the Liberals, that the measure deserved support, and as they were in power at the time the Bank Holidays Act 1871 found its way on to the statute books. It gave everyone the day off on Easter Monday, Whit Monday, the first Monday in August and Boxing Day (Good Friday and Christmas Day were traditional breaks anyway, so didn't need to be included).[15] Needless to say, this proved rather popular. Some people called the bank holidays 'St Lubbock's Days', while one newspaper proposed the erection of a solid silver statue of a monkey (in tribute to Sir John's support for evolutionary theory).

All of which is thoroughly splendid, and an excuse to this day for excessive drinking and long queues in Homebase. But it doesn't answer the question many people asked Sir John at the time, and few of us stop to ask ourselves now: why are they

[15] This was for England, Wales and Ireland – Scotland got New Year's Day, Good Friday, the first Mondays in May and August and Christmas Day.

known as 'bank' holidays? Simple, said Lubbock, providing the answer that now becomes my 19th fact:

> **CT (Canterbury): The bank holiday got its name because employers would have ignored a vague title like 'general' or 'national' holiday – only by forcing the banks to close could you ensure that no business was possible at all.**

Down in the town itself, the good people of Broadstairs are going about their lunch hour. Prezzo is quiet, the Star of the Sea chippy is warming up, while the Royal Albion Hotel bears a plaque boasting that Charles Dickens wrote part of *Nicholas Nickleby* here. (The novelist lived in a different part of Kent, where he successfully campaigned for a postbox to be located right outside his house, thereby saving himself a walk to one further away.) Passing the florist whose community noticeboard advertises 'Pilates with Celia', I call in to the Cancer Research charity shop. To the accompaniment of Perry Como's 'Magic Moments', the two women behind the till chat about their dogs.

'Mine,' says the one with the strong Welsh accent, 'spends ages scrunching up the blanket in his bed. Goes round and round, he does, getting it *just* the way he wants it. It's only after he's done that he'll settle down.'

'Mmm,' replies her colleague. 'Mine used to make love to his.'

At a café round the corner, I make up for not seeing the 'Ham Sandwich' sign this morning by ordering one. A fifty-something couple sit at the next table, seemingly as British and middle class as it is possible to be. He peruses the menu: 'What's flapjack?' How can you have reached this age in this country wearing that much M&S and not know what flapjack is? His wife's response is unarguable: 'It's all oats and stuff.'

The road soon calls again. It leads through Margate, the town offering the Funshine amusement arcade and seagulls the size of baby llamas, but no Victorian pier. For a couple of decades after 1978 it offered only a derelict Victorian pier, a huge storm having all but destroyed the structure. Not long afterwards a demolition expert, Paul Burring, was brought in to finish the job. Unfortunately he reckoned without the engineering nous of Eugenius Birch, whose revolutionary piling technique in the 1850s had provided much more secure foundations than those enjoyed by previous wooden piers. Burring's first attempt at blowing up the remaining 34 metal legs was captured by TV cameras. He pressed the button. Water flew hundreds of feet in the air, but the legs stayed put. Burring tried again. He achieved nothing more than shooting a metal rivet through the window of the nearby Britannia pub, where it buried itself in the wall. At this point, according to a council official, Burring 'told us he could do it in one bang if we didn't mind bits of the pier all over Margate'. The council politely declined. Police insisted that any further attempts take place at high tide so that water could contain the debris. On one occasion high tide was at midnight: Burring woke up the whole of Margate, but again failed to shift the pier. Further efforts were hampered by the sea washing away charges, though one bang did cause the lifeboat house to list slightly. Only in 1998 was the pier finally vanquished.

Now I'm heading west, through Kent's northern extremities in the general direction of London. I pass through ME (Rochester) territory, joining the M2 motorway not far from Dunkirk, the village which provided the area's fact early on in the project, then it's briefly into the land of DA, whose main town concludes the old rhyme 'Sutton for mutton, Kirkby for beef, South Darne for gingerbread, Dartford for a thief'. The fact for this area is both surprising and disappointing, but I'm recording it as an acknowledgement that one's home country has faults as well as strengths. This doesn't stop you loving it – in fact no real love can be called complete unless it acknowledges imperfections. To understand why the fact has let me down so much, those of you who aren't familiar with the amplification arrangements of major rock bands must first take on board the meaning, to those of us who are, of the words 'Vox AC30'. When it comes to delivering the chunky power chords and soaring solos of the world's finest guitarists, this box of trickery is second only to the Marshall (the amp customised by Nigel Tufnel in such a way that any *Spinal Tap* fan in your life keeps making tiresome jokes about things going up to 11). It would take several pages to list the guitar heroes who have favoured the AC30 over the decades, but for now suffice it to say that watching Queen's legendary 1986 Wembley gig you'll see Brian May in front of a cliff face of the things. It was in Dartford that Tom Jennings founded the company which makes the amp. Even to see its name written down sends a pleasurable pulse through the eardrums. Imagine how far my crest fell, then, to learn why the legendary beast came into existence:

DA (Dartford): The Vox AC30 guitar amplifier was invented at the request of Hank Marvin, because the previous model (the AC15) was insufficiently loud to be heard over the screaming of early Cliff Richard fans.

I'm not going to comment on this. Recording the dark moments in your country's history is one thing, sitting around and moping about them is another.

Instead let us sail boldly on towards the final fact of our Kent crusade. It is to be found in the pleasingly named Petts Wood, deep in the heart of BR country, those being the letters denoting Bromley. As the word 'wood' implies, Kent has got all lush again by now, though seeing as we're into the sprawling monster known as 'Greater London' much of that lushness has been built on. Petts Wood survives, however, a few acres of greenery between Chislehurst and Orpington. The fact could have been that in 2009 the local branch of Woolworths was the last in the UK to close. Realising this, the manager bagged up the final handful of Pic'n'Mix and auctioned it on eBay, raising £14,500 for charity. But no, our destination is actually within the wood itself. Having parked on a nearby street I follow a footpath into the trees, which are so densely packed that within a matter of yards the sound of the traffic on the busy A-road has taken second place to birdsong. Which is fitting, because even though this is a late afternoon in winter, it makes it easy to imagine that I'm here on the early summer morning over a hundred years ago when a man called William Willett rode his horse through here. Just as I do today, he found himself all alone. 'What a pity,' he thought, 'all those people still in bed, missing out on this beautiful sunlight.' And this is how the idea came to him: British Summer Time.

It wouldn't sit very easily with Manly Ritch, one of whose poems, you'll remember, called for America's 'daylight savin' plan' to be abandoned, but Willett soon became a campaigner for clocks to be adjusted during summer so that more people could enjoy more light. His 1907 pamphlet 'The Waste of Daylight' proposed an advancement of the clocks by 20 minutes each Sunday in April, then a matching retreat during September. Sadly Willett died eight years later. Very bad (if you'll forgive me) timing, as the following year, on 17 May 1916, Parliament passed a simplified version of his plan, advancing the clocks by an hour on the following Sunday. The First World War had focused everyone's minds: any possible way of saving coal was attractive. (The Germans had already introduced a similar scheme.) After the war was over, the Summer Time Act 1925 made the measure permanent.

In a bizarre twist, William Willett's great-great-grandson is Chris Martin, the lead singer of Coldplay. This isn't, however, how their song 'Daylight' got its name, nor their song 'Clocks'. The Willett connection *is* the reason that a pub near here is called the Daylight Inn, but even this isn't my fact. No, for that I plough further into the wood, eventually coming to a small clearing. In its centre is a stone memorial, an oblong about eight feet tall, all four faces unsmoothed so it looks rather like a pre-historic grandfather clock. On one side, engraved in a beautifully simple font, is confirmation that this is a tribute to Willett, 'the untiring advocate of Summer Time', while on the other is a sundial. It's a vertical one, the figures engraved in the stone, the shadow (whenever there's any sun, which there certainly isn't now) cast by a triangular piece of metal sticking out at right angles.[16] Underneath the dial are the words 'HORAS NON NUMERO NISI AESTIVAS', meaning 'I will only tell the summer hours'. Yes, look more closely and you notice that the piece of metal, which should be centred so that at midday in GMT the sun produces a shadow on the 'XII', is actually positioned above the 'I'. In other words:

BR (Bromley): The sundial in Petts Wood, unlike almost every other sundial in the UK, is set not to Greenwich Mean Time but to British Summer Time.

[16] Hence 'sundial' being the answer to the old riddle 'Which timepiece has the fewest moving parts?' The timepiece with the most moving parts is the egg-timer.

FACTS ACROSS THE WATER

'We had a brilliant day. It was great. And you've got to expect a good punch-up at a wedding.'

As sentences in news stories go, this one certainly grabs your attention. The event in question took place in Bradford. The happy couple can't have expected their nuptials to produce the headline 'Wedding Brawl Started Over Pork Pie', but then, as the groom's reaction showed, he wasn't exactly bothered, either by the pork pie or the publicity. The item of food was used as a missile. The bride was, according to the shocked barman, 'devastated – her dress was ruined, she had a lovely big white gown and it had beer and WKD all over it'. Another woman had her ear and cheek bitten, and there were also contributions from a water pistol. It all makes for an amusing few column inches, though none of the details really merits the title 'fact'. Not that that matters, as the area is already sewn up, by a native of Cleckheaton:

BD (Bradford): Roger Hargreaves created the first *Mr Men* character when his six-year-old son asked him what a tickle looked like.

Nonetheless, the wedding story plants the idea that the news might be productive hunting ground. Sure enough, a few days later scientists make an announcement about something they've found on a beach:

NR (Norwich): The earliest human footprints outside of Africa, discovered near Happisburgh in Norfolk, date from over 800,000 years ago.

The prints – about 50 of them – were discovered several months previously, after rough seas had gradually uncovered a new layer of sediment beneath the sand. Twelve were complete enough to analyse, and two even showed details of the toes. The species involved, *Homo antecessor*, probably made its way to what is now Norfolk across a strip of land which still then connected the UK to the rest of the Europe. After studying 3D scans of the prints, archaeologists have concluded that they were left by a family group, possibly of five people, including an adult male who was 5 feet 9 inches tall. They were walking in a southerly direction, in other words upstream along mudflats in the estuary of an early River Thames (which then flowed into the sea further north than it does today). The experts think they were searching for seafood – lugworms, crabs, seaweed – and might have lived on an island in the estuary to protect themselves from predators, the steps having been left when they were walking from the island to the shore at low tide. In terms of taking me back into Britain's past (at least its human past), this is certainly the furthest the project will go. For ages I stare at the news story, examining the picture of one of the footprints. I was moved a couple of years ago when builders in the City of London unearthed a Roman dice, but this is even more affecting than that, showing the shape of one of my (to use the word in its broadest sense) ancestors. It's all the more poignant because the prints, after nearly a million years of commemorating those humans' existence, were washed away by the tide within two weeks of being uncovered.

Looking at the map to check on Happisburgh's location, my gaze falls downwards through East Anglia towards my own part of Suffolk, crossing two postcode areas as it goes. So I decide to tick those off the list now:

IP (Ipswich): The Nutshell in Bury St Edmunds is, at 15 feet by 7 feet, Britain's smallest pub.

Very nice it is too. I've had a drink in there, seated at the tiny table at one end of the bar. A couple of people sat in the windowsill at the other end, and there were three people standing. Hey presto, we'd filled it. Us and the black cat, that is – the dried corpse of one, uncovered during renovations. Builders used to brick up live cats behind chimneys, a move seen as good luck, for the property if not the cat. When it comes to my home patch of CO, I toy with the idea of linking it to NW. My local town of Sudbury has a plaque on a stone flower bed in the market square commemorating the square's appearance in *The Hundred and One Dalmatians*, the novel inspired when a friend of the author Dodie Smith commented that her own dogs of that breed 'would make a lovely fur coat'. In the book Pongo and the other dogs pause in the square during the search for their puppies, which have been stolen and brought to Suffolk. Passing the plaque one day I remember that their home was near Regent's Park, and that to hear the Twilight Barking telling them where the puppies are they stand at the top of Primrose Hill.

The 'linking up' idea is appealing, especially as it fits with the 'only by splitting a country up can you unify it' notion. But handing over two facts to the same novel seems excessive. And besides, CO contains another plaque that commemorates something rather more momentous:

CO (Colchester): After Captain Lawrence Oates died on Scott's ill-fated trip to the Antarctic, his mother polished his memorial plaque every week for the rest of her life.

And as she didn't die until 1937, that meant a quarter of a century. The day Oates said he was 'just going outside' was 17 March 1912 – his 32nd birthday. The following year his army colleagues unveiled a brass plaque in the church opposite his family home in the Essex village of Gestingthorpe, a couple of miles over the county border from Sudbury. Every week Caroline Oates polished the words '...when all were beset by hardship, he, being gravely injured, went out into the blizzard to die, in the hope that by so doing he might enable his comrades to reach safety'. What the plaque doesn't record is that as he left the tent Oates didn't even bother to put on his boots – he went to his death in his socks.

If CO and NW aren't to be linked by Dalmatians, however, they can be linked by walking. The type involved in Camden Town isn't quite as dangerous as that practised by Lawrence Oates – although it isn't far off:

NW (London North West): While demonstrating a new crossing aimed at reducing pedestrian road deaths, Transport Minister Leslie Hore-Belisha was nearly knocked down and killed by a speeding car.

It was only by 'standing stock still' that Belisha managed to steer clear of the sports car treating Camden High Street like a test track. Perhaps, went officialdom's thinking after this 1934 incident, some white lines painted on the road and a sign saying 'C' (for 'Crossing') weren't going to combat the road menace after all. (Deaths that year had totalled over 7,000, half of them pedestrians. The figure these days is about a third of that.) So metal studs were fitted on to roads to slow drivers down, and orange lights were fitted on to posts to draw attention to the crossings – the legendary 'Belisha beacons'. The politician's campaigning was opposed every potentially lethal step of the way by Conservative MP Colonel John Moore-Brabazon, who called the new legislation 'absolutely reactionary'. He conceded that fatality levels were high, but 'older members of the House will recollect the number of chickens we killed in the early days of motoring. We used to come back with the radiator stuffed with feathers. It was the same with dogs. Dogs get out of the way of motor cars nowadays and you never kill one. There is education even in the lower animals. These things will right themselves.' Moore-Brabazon's own number plate, FLY 1, revealed his true transport love: in 1910 he had become the first person in Britain to qualify as a pilot. The previous year, as a 'joke' aimed at proving that pigs could indeed fly, he'd put one in a waste-paper basket, tied it to his aeroplane's wing-strut and taken the unfortunate porker for a spin over Kent. Most authorities agree that this qualifies as the first ever live cargo flight.

Wanderlust has taken hold now, and I decide that the next trip needs to be further afield than the previous ones. Scanning the map for possible destinations, my eye is caught by somewhere in the UK's top left corner, so top left in fact that you have to say 'UK' rather than 'GB'. I've never visited Northern Ireland. That's it, then: plane tickets are booked, a hotel reservation is made. There's only one hotel it can be, the Belfast institution known to trivia fans everywhere as the most bombed hotel in Europe. But after suffering 28 explosions during the Troubles, the Europa has now had a multi-million pound facelift, and as the people of Northern Ireland are themselves looking forward it would be churlish of me to use the 'most bombed' thing as the BT fact. Besides, Belfast was also the birthplace of George Best, the pneumatic tyre, the *Titanic* and who knows what else – if I can't get some decent info out of that lot I shouldn't be in charge of this project to start with.

Before Belfast, however, there is an engagement to fulfil in London. Harry at the BPMA has very kindly arranged for me to go on a private 'Gems of the Archive' tour. The initial reason for this was the stamp he mentioned, the one commemorating a 1970s event which might theoretically have happened but in reality was never going to. But this will only be one of the gems – plenty more lie in wait. I present myself at Harry's office, which is actually in another Royal Mail building on Almeida Street, a short distance from the archive itself. As we set off for the walk he points to a street sign fixed on one of the houses.

'Look at the postcode,' he says, indicating the 'N1' in the sign's corner. Then he indicates one on the other side of the street. It's older, a beautiful white enamel job with blue lettering. It too announces the street's name, but this time the code in the corner says simply 'N'. 'That has to be pre-World War One,' continues Harry. 'They added the numbers during the war, when all the postmen were away fighting and mail was delivered by women. They'd been trying to add numbers for a while, but the blokes saw it as an insult to their intelligence. "We know these rounds like the back of our hands, we don't need numbers to help us," blah blah blah. The women doing the job didn't have any of that baggage, so they didn't mind.'

As we walk, I fill Harry in on my latest research, some of it from a recent sneaky visit to the archive room to savour those bookshelves again. This time my fingers alighted on *Her Majesty's Mails* by W. Lewins, a red leather-bound volume from 1864. Its final chapter, 'Being Miscellaneous and Suggestive', told of the GPO employee who on one road, between houses numbered 15 and 16, noticed a brass plate bearing the number 95. 'He made inquiry, when the old lady who tenanted the house said that the number had belonged to a former residence, and, thinking it a pity that it should be thrown away, she had transferred it to her new home, supposing that it would do as well as any other number!'

Dramatic news, meanwhile, from Montrose, where a postbox suffered a 'singular accident'. Somehow gas from a street pipe got into the box, the top of which was chosen by a night-watchman to strike his match against in order to light his pipe. 'The top was blown off and the pillar-box hopelessly damaged, although the watchman and the letters escaped without injury.' (This reminds Harry about one particular model of Victorian postbox designed with wonderfully ornate detailing and decorations, the only trouble being that they forgot to include a hole for letters.) Lewins also records some of the more unusual items sent by mail: 'two canaries ... leeches in bladders, several of which having burst, many of the poor creatures were found crawling over the correspondence of the country ... a pistol loaded almost to the mouth with slugs and ball ... a live snake ... fish innumerable ... and last of all, and most extraordinary of all, a human heart and stomach.'

'You should have a look at the modern "restricted items" list,' says Harry as we make our way through Islington. 'There are all sorts of regulations about what you're allowed to post and how you're allowed to post them. Alcohol, for instance – anything up to 24 per cent ABV is OK as long as it's wrapped in polythene and marked "fragile". Over 70 per cent it's a complete no-no.' Later I'll consult the full list on the Royal Mail's website. Christmas crackers are only allowed in 'their original retail packaging'. No magnet whose field reaches more than 4.6 metres outside its packaging is permitted. Nor is frozen water, dry ice or human ashes. UK Lottery tickets are allowed, but not those for foreign lotteries. You have been warned.

I also report to Harry on the book *Live Wires*, a collection of notable and historic cables. The telegraph (which used to be the responsibility of the GPO, hence the book's presence in the archive) revolutionised communication in the nineteenth century. When the Prince of Wales fell ill in 1871, cables flashed the news around the country, prompting the future Poet Laureate Alfred Austin to pen the lines: 'Across the wires the electric message came: "He is no better, he is much the same."' Like all innovations, the telegraph prompted controversy. Messages were charged for by the word, and a backbench MP asked for place names like 'Charing Cross' and 'Bethnal Green' to be counted as one word rather than two. The Postmaster General refused. Well into the twentieth century word counts caused trouble. In 1942 Churchill sent a memo to his officials: 'Is it really necessary to describe Tirpitz as the Admiral Von Tirpitz in every signal? This must cause a considerable waste of time for signalmen, cipher staff and typists. Surely Tirpitz is good enough for the beast?'

But most people got the hang of brevity. One soldier writing home to his girlfriend used a single word, 'amo', the Latin for 'I love you'. Unfortunately the person transmitting it assumed he'd missed a letter out, so the bemused girlfriend got a message reading 'Ammo'. The future Queen Mother, Elizabeth Bowes-Lyon, telegraphed her stingy father at the age of seven to ask for more pocket money: 'SOS LSD RSVP'. The agent of the opera soprano Frances Alda decided that the repertoire she'd been performing for years really had to change, so sent her the message: 'Hebrews XIII. 8.' Looking up the Bible reference Alda found: 'Jesus Christ, the same yesterday, and today, and for ever.' Other people saw the opportunity for mischief.

Arthur Conan Doyle once sent 12 distinguished men cables reading 'All is discovered. Fly at once.' Every last one of them, he claimed, left the country within 24 hours.

By now Harry and I have crossed the boundary from N1 to WC1, and reached the Archive itself. Passing through to the office behind the public room, we meet Chris Taft and Vicky Parkinson. It's always a bit worrying when in the course of researching books like mine you find yourself meeting archivists. Their sense of humour can sometimes be in inverse proportion to their level of expertise. Thank God, then, that both Chris and Vicky are exactly the type of archivist you dream of. If at any point I need to know the date of the 17th reprint of the second design of the British Empire Exhibition stamp, they will have the knowledge at their fingertips, if not in their heads. But at no point will they force that information on me against my will.

Moving through to a huge storeroom lined with shelves and boxes, we start, as I suppose we have to, with some Penny Blacks. The world's first adhesive postage stamp, the Penny Black was only ever issued for a few months. Soon after its debut in 1840 it became clear that the red ink used to cancel it (the GPO obviously couldn't use black ink, as that wouldn't have showed up) was easily removed, meaning people could reuse the stamp. So the Penny Red took its place, and the cancelling ink was changed to black.[1] Chris shows me a complete sheet of 240 stamps, which is how the stamps were printed and sold. Or rather it's almost complete: the top right one is missing.

'That would have been George V,' explains Chris. ' "The Philatelist King", as he was known. He built up a huge stamp

---

[1] Though Victoria's portrait remained the same – she liked the image of herself so much she kept it on stamps for the rest of her reign.

collection, and normally when you see the top right one missing from a sheet it's because it was taken for him.' The current Queen has inherited her grandfather's collection, which often cost astronomical sums to assemble. A courtier once asked him if he had seen that 'some damned fool has paid £1,400 for one stamp'. 'Yes,' came the reply, 'I was that damned fool.' No monarch, incidentally, is ever portrayed on a stamp wearing their crown until after their coronation has taken place – until then their bare head is shown, together with a small drawing of a crown in one corner. Chris shows me some Edward VIII examples, these, of course, being the only type ever issued of him, as he abdicated before being crowned. Then we turn to some 1965 stamps without the monarch on at all. They are the result of Tony Benn's efforts (mentioned by Harry at our first meeting) to de-royalise the nation's envelopes. He commissioned these samples, which commemorate the Battle of Britain. The 4d versions show silhouettes of planes and pilots, while the 9d adds the dome of St Paul's and some anti-aircraft guns. They also include the words 'UK Postage', which would have marked an end to Britain being the only country in the world not to put its name on its stamps (a result simply of it being the first to have stamps at all).

'Benn visited Buckingham Palace to present them to the Queen personally,' says Harry. 'She smiled politely, nodded in all the right places, then as soon as Benn left the room she got on the phone. You can see what happened here.' He points to the information panel's final sentence: 'Submitted to the Palace on 29 June, but subsequently withdrawn.'

The rules about who can appear on a stamp have, like those governing much of Britain's pomp and pageantry, been far less rigid and timeless than some might believe. The general headline for decades was that the only identifiable living people allowed were members of the Royal Family or those about to marry into it. If there's anything the Brits love more than their monarchy, however, it's pedantry, so that word 'identifiable' came in for some scrutiny. In 1967 stamps were issued to commemorate Francis Chichester's circumnavigation of the globe. They showed his yacht, *Gipsy Moth IV*, including a tiny blob that had to be a person. He'd been the only person on board, therefore it had to be him. Cue uproar. Cue more uproar when Freddie Mercury died, and a commemorative stamp showed not only the singer but also (*just* visible behind the drum kit) Roger Taylor. The rule was finally ditched in 2005, when England won the Ashes – Michael Vaughan, Andrew Flintoff and several other players were clearly depicted. Since then it's been a virtual free-for-all. Stamps have featured The Beatles, David Tennant as Hamlet, all the Dr Who actors (giving Tennant a second outing) and, during the 2012 Olympics, every British gold medal winner. The Queen is always there on each stamp as well, though, a tiny silhouette in the corner.

The archive is more than a huge stamp collection, of course. Next Chris fetches out a medal housed in a clear plastic case, a modestly sized cross attached to a scarlet ribbon. It's only as I peer closer and read the inscription – 'FOR VALOUR' – that I realise what this is: a Victoria Cross. It's the first one I've ever seen up close. 'It was awarded to Sergeant Alfred Knight,' explains Chris. 'He was a member of the Post Office Rifles, the unit in the British Army specifically for Post Office employees. He won his VC for charging an enemy position at Ypres in September 1917. He captured it single-handedly, didn't show any concern for his own safety.' After the war, Knight recalled being fascinated 'by the pattern made all the way round me in the mud by German bullets'. Not that the mud took all the punishment. 'Bullets rattled on my steel helmet – there were several significant dents and one hole in it, I found later.' A book in Knight's pocket was also hit, as was a photograph case and a cigarette case. The latter 'probably saved my life from one bullet, which must have passed just under my arm-pit – quite close enough to be comfortable!'

As we've already seen on the street signs outside Harry's office, the First World War affected the way the Post Office operated. But then again the Post Office affected the way the First World War operated. The Royal Engineers (Postal Section) was an army unit nominally under command of the military, but in effect operated by the GPO. The authorities knew how important it was for morale that troops on the front line should be able to send letters home, and indeed receive replies. So several acres of Regent's Park in London were covered with a huge wooden hut where 2,500 staff (mostly women) sorted the mail. At its peak the operation delivered 12 million letters and one million parcels a week. Every morning those in charge of the war told the Home Depot (as the sorting office was known) where battalions and ships had moved to, so that mail could be sorted accordingly. Trains delivered the post to points a little way back from the front line, where the final, detailed sorting took place before carts were wheeled out and letters delivered to individual soldiers. They were normally handed out with the evening meal. It was said that it didn't matter how hungry the troops were – they always read the letter before eating the food.

One man on the Western Front wrote to a London news-paper in 1915 saying he was lonely and would love some mail. Within three weeks he'd received 3,000 letters, 98 large parcels and three mailbags' worth of smaller packages. Reading the letters of those who *did* have families to correspond with, you're struck by the fact that for all its drama and importance in the grand sweep of history, war is, in the end, just one big lottery. 'My own beloved wife,' wrote Sergeant Major James Milne, '...We are going over the top this afternoon and only

God in Heaven knows who will come out of it alive ... If I am called my regret is that I leave you and my bairns ...' Lance Corporal Frank Earley, 19 years old, wrote: 'My dear father ... every letter now that I write home to you or to the little sisters may be the last that I shall write or you read ... Pray for me. Your son, Frank.' Milne survived the war and returned to his wife and bairns. Earley was killed the day after writing his letter.

The VC safely locked away again, Chris leads us to a heavy steel door, several inches thick and requiring several code numbers and keys before it swings open. Inside the strongroom he opens up a filing cabinet to reveal some guns. 'These date from around the 1750s,' he says. 'They were issued to the guards on mail coaches, to help defend the coaches against attack.' Whatever you think of the use guns are put to, these items are things of beauty: curved handles made of highly polished dark wood, ornately engraved mechanisms in brass and silver. The barrel of the one Chris lets me handle (not sure I could have lifted it to eye level, never mind taken any sort of aim) is inscribed 'For His Majesty's Mail Coaches', the tiny letters appearing around its circumference at the business end so that they would have been the last thing any highwayman ever saw. No mail coach was ever successfully robbed.

Chris has to leave us at this point, so Vicky takes over as we descend in a lift to another vast storeroom lined with shelf after shelf of postal goodies. First up she shows me an original top hat worn by the messengers who collected letters from your house in the days before pillar boxes. It is incredibly smart, a proper silk job with a wide gold ribbon around it. 'Some of the houses the messengers collected from were owned by very posh people,' explains Vicky. 'The Post Office didn't want their employees turning up looking scruffy.' There's also a colonial-style white hat once worn by workers in Mauritius, from the days when the Royal Mail[2] were helping to set up a postal system there, as they did in various Commonwealth countries. My favourite 'non-document' object, though, has to be the hessian mailbag addressed to 'Manager, Bank of Scotland, 30 Bishopsgate, London EC2' and marked with a red 'HVP' sticker. The initials stood for 'High Value Package' – the bag contained banknotes. The manager never received them, however, because they were intercepted in Buckinghamshire by the Great Train Robbers. The bag found its way into the archive after appearing as evidence during the robbers' trial.

Then Vicky produces an original of the map without which I wouldn't be here – the very first postcode map, dated 1838 and showing which of the ten London areas each sorting office would belong to. (As we've seen, the system itself didn't start until 1857 – good to know the Victorians weren't always that dynamic.) Actually it isn't a map of the capital at all, rather a circle split evenly into the eight compass points, with WC and EC in the middle. But a map doesn't have to be geographically accurate to count as eye candy for cartophiles (look at the Tube map). In fact, it's because this one *isn't* accurate that it's so interesting – it gives you a new way of looking at a very familiar city. I can't help looking at the slices of the pizza labelled 'North Eastern' and 'Southern', the two areas swiftly culled by Anthony Trollope, the Pete Best and Stu Sutcliffe of the postcode system. The S slice extends down through Clapham and Brixton all the way to Sutton and Croydon. NE reaches out as far as Chigwell, territory that was soon bequeathed to E. These days it belongs to IG, but E does

---

[2] I've been wondering if there's a difference between 'the Post Office', 'the GPO' and 'the Royal Mail' – Vicky explains that they've always been used pretty much interchangeably.

come out quite a way into Essex. If you live in Sewardstone, the small village north of Chingford and therefore part of E4, rejoice in your uniqueness: yours is the only place with a London postcode that lies outside Greater London.

Vicky tells me about the seventeenth and eighteenth centuries, when all mail went via London so the monarch could spy on his subjects. 'It didn't matter if you were posting something from Crewe to Hull, it still went via the capital. The king employed master forgers who could open letters without disturbing the seals, so the recipient would never know his mail had been read.' We also see a horse's sick note. 'The Post Office took good care of its animals,' explains Vicky as she hands over the form dated 29 October 1898. It reads: 'I certify that Mr J. G. Poppleton's horse of the Post Office is suffering from sore shoulders and unable to perform his official duties. He is to resume duty on or before the 7th of November or obtain a renewal of this Certificate.' Cats were on the payroll, too, catching mice right up to the 1980s. The longest serving was Tibs the Great. He did fourteen years. 'They all got pensions when they retired,' says Harry.

The Belgians went one stage further: using cats to deliver mail. Or rather trying to use them. Other countries have employed horses, dogs, pigeons, camels, even reindeer, but Belgium is the only country ever to take the feline route. They trialled 37 of the animals in 1879. The experiment – and this may come as a surprise to you, in view of how famously obedient and biddable cats are as a breed – was a total failure.

Half an hour later I'm back outside. My mind is buzzing, not just from the contents of the archive but also because on the way out Harry mentioned there are plans to open up the 'Mail Rail', the Post Office's underground train system running from Whitechapel to Paddington, which from 1927 until its closure in 2003 carried millions of letters a day across the capital. Tourist trips won't be happening for another couple of years, but 'selected' members of the media might be allowed a sneak peek in the near future. He doesn't say how that selection will take place, but promises to keep me informed. I'm beginning to view Harry as a drug-pusher, tempting and leading me on to ever harder substances – a postage stamp here, an underground tunnel there...

As I climb Mount Pleasant, I happen to do that thing none of us does often enough – look up. Painted in capital letters across the enormous sorting office are the names of British towns and cities: 'RUGBY, BATH, WIGAN, NEATH, LARNE, CREWE, PERTH, TRURO, YORK, DERBY, EXETER...' The message is clear: 'Look how far we'll take your letters, all for the price of a stamp.' Inspired by the list, I start ticking off some of the places:

BA (Bath): In the 1881 census, Isaac Pitman, inventor of the shorthand system that bears his name, spelled his Christian name 'Eisak'.

His memorial plaque in Bath Abbey prefers the conventional version, but Pitman spent his whole life campaigning for the reform of English spelling. He wanted to do away with all those confusing consistencies (why doesn't 'pint' rhyme with 'mint', for instance?), so that everything would be spelled phonetically, as it is in his shorthand system. 'Time saved,' went his motto, 'is life gained'. His brothers agreed. Jacob emigrated to Australia, where his grave reads: 'In luving memeri ov Jacob Pitman...' Benjamin went to live in America, using Pitman shorthand when he acted as stenographer in the trial of the conspirators behind Abraham Lincoln's assassination.

WN (Wigan): The music hall performer George Formby was born blind, only gaining his sight at the age of six months when a violent coughing fit dislodged a caul (piece of membrane).

Formby's song 'With My Little Stick of Blackpool Rock' was banned by the BBC because of its suggestive lyrics. You do wonder at Auntie's primness over the years. One of its censors once wrote about 'the need to buttress the forces of virtue against the unprincipled elements of the jungle'. All Formby had said was that 'it's nice to have a nibble at it now and again'.

PH (Perth): Strontian is the only place in Britain to have a chemical element named after it.

The village on Scotland's west coast lies in the shadow of the hills where a new element was discovered in 1790. They named it strontium in honour of the place. In America it's often the other way round: places are named after the elements found there. Hence Cobalt, Idaho, and Sulphur, Oklahoma.

When it comes to York there are several contenders. The street known as The Shambles got its name because there were once 25 butchers' shops on it, 'shambles' being an old word for a slaughterhouse (hence its modern meaning of a complete mess). Over in Scarborough the Grand Hotel was designed around the theme of time: 365 bedrooms, 52 chimneys and 12 floors. And Brompton Vale, between Scarborough and Pickering, was the venue for mankind's first ever flight in a heavier-than-air craft. Sir George Cayley designed himself a glider, though can't have been that confident in it because he got his coachman, John Appleby, to do the actual flying. Appleby steered it across the valley, crash-landed on the far

side and announced: 'Sir George, I wish to give notice. I was
hired to drive, not to fly!'

But in the end YO is snaffled by something that happened
much more recently, a satirical stunt pulled by a chain of
computer game stores founded in York in 1993:

**YO (York): On April Fool's Day 2010, Gamestation
inserted a clause in their online terms and conditions allowing them to claim their customers'
souls.**

The joke was aimed at highlighting the problem of 'click-
wrap' agreements, those boxes we all tick on websites to
confirm we've read the conditions when of course we've done
no such thing. 'By placing an order via this Web site,' ran the
Gamestation clause, 'on the first day of the fourth month of
the year 2010 Anno Domini, you agree to grant Us a non
transferable option to claim, for now and for ever more, your
immortal soul.'

Walking away from Mount Pleasant, I think back on the
various gems the archive yielded up. They all shone like
diamonds, but my favourite has to be the one that inspired
the tour in the first place, the 1970s stamp Harry mentioned
the first time we met. Chris showed it to me after the Penny
Blacks, as he explained that the Queen still has to approve
every stamp design personally. She has been known to refuse,
not so much because a subject matter is controversial, but
simply because she doesn't like the look of the thing. This is
one of the reasons stamps have to be prepared well in advance
of an event, whether or not that event is definitely going to
happen, and even when it almost certainly isn't. You have to
be ready just in case. So it was that I found myself examining
a stamp from 1978, showing a group of footballers in blue

shirts, all drawn generically so that they can't be identified as specific players, jumping up with their arms held aloft in triumph. The player at the front of the group is holding the most famous trophy the game has to offer. In the stamp's top right corner is the silhouette of the Queen's head and the price (9p). At the bottom the words read:

Scotland – World Cup Winners 1978

It's March now, and as I walk across the car park towards Stansted Airport a wind whips round my shoulders, one of winter's dying gasps. Friday's early morning sun is glinting off the terminal's mammoth panes of glass, and I remember how much I like this airport. Being so modestly sized it's much quicker to navigate than the behemoth of Heathrow. Not that Britain's biggest airport doesn't have facts to offer:

TW (Twickenham): Heathrow's Terminal 4 was built with gates 12 and 14 at opposite ends of the building, so that superstitious travellers wouldn't notice the absence of a gate 13.

Otherwise they'd have seen 14 as the 'new' 13 and refused to fly from that. The gates have since been renumbered, so perhaps reason is conquering Britain after all.

Another area can be filed under the same subject:

L (Liverpool): Paul McCartney once called Ringo Starr and said: 'Guess where I am? John Lennon Airport.'

McCartney, by the way, was in the running for TN, which eventually went to that inept German spy. Macca's country home is a farmhouse in Peasmarsh, the Sussex village in which Maria Ann Sherwood was born in 1799. She grew up to marry a man called Smith and emigrate to Australia, where she grew a new variety of apple. It was named in her honour as the Granny Smith – and just happens to be the variety pictured on The Beatles' Apple record label.

My plane takes off, and before we've reached more than a couple of thousand feet we're over the border from CM into SG. Until recently Rudyard Kipling's daughter had this area pretty well in the bag. Elsie Bambridge, as she'd become by marriage, lived at Wimpole Hall, the largest house in Cambridgeshire (it's now owned by the National Trust). So irritated was she by some sightseers having a picnic on her lawn that she traced their car registration number, ordered her chauffeur to drive her to their tiny suburban house and duly ate her own picnic in their front garden. But I'm afraid, Elsie, that as I gaze down on the countryside this morning your fact has to make way for one related to someone flying across these very fields:

SG (Stevenage): In May 1940 an RAF crew sent to bomb a German airfield in Holland mistakenly bombed a Fighter Command base in Cambridgeshire.

Now that sort of wrong turning needs a damn good explanation, so it's just as well that Captain Warren and his colleagues had one. Taking off from Yorkshire at 8.30 p.m. to approach Holland under cover of dark, they hit an electrical thunderstorm over the North Sea. Unbeknownst to them, lightning threw their plane's magnetic compass out of true. At about the time they were expecting to reach the Dutch coast they saw an estuary, and believing it to be the Rhine (it was actually the Thames), they followed it all the way to a nearby airfield. Here they dropped their bombs and headed, as they thought, for home. Later, as first light showed, they dropped through the clouds and saw a city. In horror Warren realised it was Liverpool. Working backwards he concluded that 'we can only have bombed somewhere in England. Christ, what are we to do?' Get back to base, Captain, that's what, and pray your attack on Bassingbourn hasn't killed anyone. Thankfully it hadn't. But that didn't stop Warren being demoted. From then he was known to colleagues as Baron von Warren.

Halfway through my hour-long flight I look down to see an expanse of water, followed by some land, followed by some more water. 'Aha,' goes my finely tuned navigational instinct, 'an island'. If you were reading a Thomas the Tank engine book you might expect it to be the fictional island of Sodor, home to Thomas and his friends and lying between England and the Isle of Man. As you're not, you know it has to be the Isle of Man itself:

IM (Isle of Man): The summit of Snaefell mountain is the only place on Earth from which you can see all four countries of the United Kingdom (England, Scotland, Wales and Northern Ireland).

Shortly afterwards we land in the last of these four countries, and I progress to the centre of its capital city. Except, as even the most cursory scoot around shows, Belfast is a large town rather than a city. Looking west down its streets (many of which are on a grid system), you feel you could reach out and touch the hills. In fact they're so close they inspired *Gulliver's Travels* – Jonathan Swift thought they looked like a sleeping giant keeping guard over Belfast. At the centre of the centre is Donegall Square, dominated by City Hall. And I do mean dominated. As if to symbolise the over-importance of politics in this part of the world, the council's grand Victorian home (Portland stone, lots of columns) takes up too much of the square, rather like a Lego feature that has been mixed up with a set of the next size down. I feel guilty having this thought so soon into my time here. But if you grew up in Britain in the 1970s and 1980s, Northern Ireland meant only one thing. It was the reason the Northern Ireland Secretary had more protection than any other Cabinet member apart from the Prime Minister, and it went by the shorthand of 'the Troubles'. Only if you were a Unionist, though – Republicans always called it 'the war' or 'the struggle'. Language, as ever, was a huge part of it. Still is: the BBC now refer to this country's second-largest city as 'Derry-Londonderry' (though not in their local bulletins here, I'll notice – it remains 'London-derry'). The language of IRA code words (used to confirm that a bomb warning was genuine) was chillingly mundane: a political journalist I know saw a list of them while covering the Good Friday Agreement, and was amazed at how everyday they were. A typical example was 'milk bottle'.

Those days are all gone, though, aren't they? I was going to come here and find a new Belfast, maybe not one totally free of trouble but one where *the* troubles weren't the major item on the agenda. Seems I was wrong, though. Yes, it looks a peaceful enough place, and the Ten Square Hotel opposite the hall is smartly boutique, its bar the venue for my first pint of Guinness.[3] The pump handle is shaped like a mini rugby ball, reminding me of Thomas Gordon who played for Ireland in the nineteenth century, the only one-handed rugby international ever (his right one having succumbed to a shooting accident). This is next to the stuff in my notes about

[3] It's called research, OK?

George Best (rejected as a youngster by local team Glentoran for being 'too small and light') and, also improbably in the sports section, the television personality Roy Walker, who in the days before he hosted *Catchphrase* was twice Northern Ireland hammer-throwing champion. Then I look up and notice the news on the TV, the captions telling me they're discussing an ongoing row over 'amnesty' letters for Republican terrorists. I glance at the paper being read by the guy next to me: a double-page spread on mail bombs intercepted at Belfast sorting offices. The flippant thought enters my mind that at least both these stories fit the project. It's replaced by the depressing thought that Northern Ireland still seems to be reading from its old script. As if to confirm this, on my walk from the Ten Square to the Europa Hotel I pass a police Land Rover. There are grilles over every part that could conceivably get broken, including small cages over the headlights and the spotlight on the roof, and a folding wire mesh over the windscreen. I'm no expert on armour plating, but even I can see that to make any sort of dent in that thing you'd need a *lot* of metal travelling *very* fast.

Round at the Europa, however, there's finally a feeling of a city that's moving on. It's a tall building, its frontage fanning out in two angled sections like a Vegas hotel, and though the upper part of the original structure still looks 1970s, a modern two-storey extension at the front brings everything nicely into the new millennium. All very different from the days when the 'most bombed hotel in Europe' title was being earned. One ITN reporter remembers a bomb warning coming while he was in the hotel barber's shop getting a shave – he had to stand out in the street with one half of his face bearded and the other bare. The bomb disposal squad displayed what you might term gallows humour: their jumpers had embroidered badges of Felix the Cat, in the hope that they too might get nine lives.

On the wall behind the reception desk a blue plaque com-memorates Bill Clinton's stay here in November 1995. This was the same month, incidentally, that he started 'relations' with Monica Lewinsky, although none of the 110 rooms taken up by his entourage were for her. (Even he wasn't that brazen.[4]) I mention the plaque to the woman behind the desk.

'Sure enough he was here two days ago as well,' she replies.

'Really?'

'He didn't stay, he just used a room to freshen up for an hour or two.' No disrespect to Alison's B&B in Kent, but the project's accommodation levels have definitely lifted a couple of notches.

Having dumped my bag in my room, I check out the hotel bar. Being mid-afternoon there aren't many drinkers in yet, though I do overhear the first of what will be many accents from Yorkshire and Lancashire – it seems Belfast is a popular destination among northerners. The local newspaper contains evidence of the legendary Ulster puritanism (the sort that in the 1950s saw playground swings locked up on Sundays) – a taxi driver has thrown two gay men out of his cab for kissing, even though his firm is one of the sponsors of Belfast's annual Gay Pride march. In fairness it's only a story at all because the prejudice stands out these days (despite it having been 1982 before Northern Ireland followed England's 1967 lead and decriminalised homosexual acts), and everyone seems to be condemning the driver. The next page reveals that life over the border in Dublin is more colourful: 'Blaming a pub owner,' it begins, 'for the alleged injuries of a woman during a rush

---

[4] Despite its many repetitions of the line 'a little bit of Monica in my life', 'Mambo No. 5' by Lou Bega was still selected as the theme song of the 2000 Democratic National Party Convention. Very annoyingly someone spotted the error in time.

to grab a spot prize at an Ann Summers sex toy party would fly in the face of common sense, a court has been told.' Well, quite. The 46-year-old is suing the bar 'after claiming she was shoved into a speaker when "a ring that goes around a certain part of a man" was thrown in the air'. Later sentences refer, in uncomfortably close proximity, to the 'Hunks of Desire male stripper troupe' and 'the onus of proof'.

Out on the streets again, I witness Friday's shopping gradually giving way to weekend drinking. A Caribbean woman in the pedestrianised Victoria Square uses an amplifier to preach her Christian message: 'God him love the *horl* world!' A man who's obviously been on it since lunchtime steams past in standard 'I'm not hammered, honest' gait – head locked so he faces permanently forward, shoulders rotating with every step. The window of Oxfam Books displays signs declaring 'My female hero is . . .' Nominations include Mother Teresa, Maria Callas, Aung San Suu Kyi and, from one brave soul, Margaret Thatcher. I take in the Ulster Hall, venue in 1971 for Led Zeppelin's first ever public performance of 'Stairway to Heaven'. The band hadn't recorded it yet, so according to bassist John Paul Jones the crowd 'were all bored to tears waiting to hear something they knew'. Also the city's cathedral, which because it's built on clay can't support a conventional spire. Instead there's a splendid thin modern metal one, a 177-foot needle. Inside things are more traditional, though each of the red lampshades in the choir's pews looks exactly like a fez, conjuring up an image of 40 Tommy Coopers singing the hymns.[5] The

[5] On holiday in Morocco, where he'd gone to avoid being recognised, Cooper tried on a fez. The stallholder said: 'Just like that.' 'How the hell do you know who I am?' asked Cooper. The stallholder looked confused. 'I don't know who you are. But I heard you were English, and whenever English people put on a fez they always say "Just like that".'

list of vicars and deans includes Cuthbert I. Peacocke (he was in charge from 1956 to 1970). As unlikely a name as the one I saw earlier on a blue plaque to former Belfast Lord Mayor Sir Otto Jaffe.

As in all gridded cities the wind gets fiercely channelled here, so on this bright but chilly day the cathedral isn't the only building in which I seek refuge. There's the one Oscar Wilde called 'the only beautiful building in Belfast', a Venetian-influenced gem built in 1869 as a linen warehouse (the city thrived on the trade), but which today houses M&S. There is, briefly, a Tesco Metro whose checkout is so close to the open door that to keep warm the sales assistant wears a onesie. And there is the occasional pub. The Crown Liquor Saloon opposite the Europa is another Victorian delight, all glazed tiling and stained-glass windows. You can see through to the kitchen, where a note on the dumb waiter reads 'Entering the car is forbidden'. You'd need to be a very small contortionist to even consider it – do the staff get *that* bored? The sixty-something man next to me at the bar disproves the old saying about first impressions. My instant judgement is 'golf club stalwart': only as the minutes pass do I notice the tiny unmended tear in the seam of his blazer, the almost-invisible speckling of dandruff on the shoulders, the faintest shake of his hand as he checks the racing pages.

A plaque at the Customs House out near the River Lagan reveals that our old friend Anthony Trollope worked part of his time for the GPO here. Street signs display the numerical parts of postcodes (Wellington Place 1, Franklin Street Place 2 and so on), and the map reveals, outside the city centre, a Friendly Street. Some of the alleyways are known as 'entries' – they include 'Joy's Entry', which did well to get past the city's puritan streak. It's a streak that never entirely leaves my mind. Somehow there's a thinness to Belfast, a feeling in the air that life here is restrained, curtailed, that letting go just isn't an option. This has some good side effects – not once in my time here do I see a seriously overweight person – but overall, despite everyone's friendliness, it's faintly oppressive. It recalls Graham Greene's impressions of his visit here in 1941. The dockyard cranes, he wrote, were like 'skeleton foliage in a steely winter'. After much trouble he found somewhere for Catholic confession, a 'dreadful parlour with pious pictures ... in the same street the pious repository selling Woodbines from under the counter to old women'.

You definitely can't forget in Belfast that you're in a different country. There's the accent of course, which reminds me of the Ulster girl I once heard in London saying she'd been to see 'a fillum in Fulham'. There are the colloquialisms ('I'll take a pint of lager' rather than 'I'll have ...') Also the banknotes, which instead of famous people depict the Old Bushmills Distillery in County Antrim. (If in future decades they go for the human approach there'll be more to choose from than George Best and Van Morrison. Kenneth Branagh, it turns out, was born in Belfast, as was Chaim Herzog, the sixth President of Israel.) But this other country in which you find yourself feels like a very small country. Both Liverpool FC and Glasgow Rangers FC have shops here, obviously doing a good trade in kits and memorabilia – what does it say when you have to import your football allegiances?

And all the time there's that question of whether or not Belfast is moving on from the Troubles. Certainly the city is changing: I can't imagine that previous decades would have seen the Deanes Deli Bistro and Vin Café offering its celeriac and poached pear tarte fine, or patrons of the Malmaison hotel relaxing over a Spicy Paloma cocktail. Sitting in Caffè Nero I hear a couple's dyed-in-the-linen Belfast accents. Turning I see that yes, she is pale with red hair, but he looks exactly like the

Sri Lankan cricketer Muttiah Muralitharan. Even the famous
end-of-terrace murals are changing. The most famous one is
round the corner from the Europa. Or rather it was: the Ulster
Freedom Fighters message ('You are now entering loyalist
Sandy Row . . .', next to a balaclava-clad man brandishing a
gun) has been replaced by a huge picture of King William
III, the Prince of Orange, and a message celebrating his 1690
victory at the Battle of the Boyne. 'This new artwork,' reads
a small panel on the adjoining wall, 'indicates a community
moving forward.' But another wall nearby bears foot-high
letters: 'They may have stole our banner but they will never
steal our culture.' And a couple of weeks from now a bomb
in Dublin will remind residents there that the troubles haven't
entirely ceased. The inept bomber, mind you, injures no one
but himself. When the timed device fails to explode he goes
back to investigate. The bomb promptly blows up in his face:
he has forgotten about the clocks going forward the previous
night. What would William Willett say?

In the end, as I finish off Friday night with a final Guinness
in the Europa's bar, the memory that stays with me most
strongly is of the old guy in the Royal Ulster Rifles museum
this afternoon. I'd stumbled across the place, which is housed
in a village hall-like room behind a 1970s office building. Not
being a war junkie, I was planning to give it a quick 90 seconds
for the sake of research and then depart. However the old guy
in attendance – ex of the regiment himself, a little unkempt
and fond of a chat – wasn't going to let the opportunity slip
by. Following me round the trestle tables and wall displays,
he pointed out items of particular interest. His soft voice,
carrying well in the high-ceilinged room, was hypnotic, facts
and dates and stories emerging like so many tracer bullets. I
heard about 3 April 1858, when members of the regiment
won three VCs before breakfast, storming the Indian city of

Jhansi. We read the text of Lieutenant Colonel Tim Collins's legendary address to his troops on the eve of the 2003 invasion of Iraq: 'The enemy should be in no doubt that we are his nemesis...' We examined an example of the folding pushbike issued to soldiers for the D-Day landings. 'They hated them,' explained the veteran. Easy to see why: even modern ones are weighty, but this beast (full-sized, plenty of metal) must have been a nightmare to carry. 'One section hid in a ditch from a passing German tank, dropping their bikes on the road as they scarpered, and when the tank ran over the bikes they all cheered. Another guy told me he jumped down from his boat into the sea, looked at the bike he was holding, thought "I can't eat it and I can't shoot it", and threw it away.'[6]

It was clear as we talked that the veteran was no Catholic-basher, no firebrand full of hate. He expressed regret rather than anger about 'inconsistencies' between the treatment of Loyalist and Republican terrorists over the amnesty letters. 'It's not a great peace,' he said of the years since the Good Friday Agreement, 'but it's better than no peace.' And yet towards the end of our tour of the museum, he said something I couldn't help feeling explained much of Northern Ireland's recent history. It was a reminder of how similar Northern Ireland is to the rest of the UK, how it's only an accident of history and geographical boundaries that has brought to life an instinct that everywhere else finds a home on football terraces or in pubs. We were examining a cabinet illustrating the Royal Ulster Rifles' service in Borneo during the 1960s.

'That was the type of gun I used,' said the veteran, indicating an archaic-looking rifle.

---

[6] Sixty years earlier John Boyd Dunlop had had the idea for the pneumatic tyre in Belfast, after his young son suffered terrible headaches while riding his tricycle.

'You fought there?'

'Oh yes, I was there.' He detailed one particular incident in the jungle. I didn't understand all the military terms, so couldn't follow every twist and turn, but it was clear that for several hours his life was in danger.

'That must have been terrifying,' I said.

'Not really. It's what you join up for, isn't it? You join up to see action, so you want to see some.'

He told me about his eagerness to join the cadets as a teenager, to sign up for the regiment proper as soon as he could. Then he took one last look at the cabinet that reminded him of his time in Borneo. 'Aye,' he said wistfully. 'They were the best days of my life.'

The next morning, I'm standing by the river watching three Geordie girls kiss a fish. It is blue, about thirty feet long and, if the girls' giggles as they take photos of each other are anything to go by, reports of its popularity are fully justified. Certainly the sculpture makes me smile. It has stood here since 1999. I can't immediately work out what it's trying to say, but as that's a question that bothers me less and less about art these days the smile is more than enough to be going on with.

Crossing the river I head for the docks area, where a little over a century ago the workers at the Harland and Wolff shipyard constructed a vessel whose working life was to last just five days, but which ended up as the most famous ship of all time. It has featured in the project already, and as I approach the spanking new £97-million visitor centre I remember Harry's pride in pointing out that the 'M' in RMS *Titanic* stood for 'Mail'. The ship itself now has 12,000 feet of Atlantic Ocean on top of it, but its memory – and the associated tourist trade – is thriving. Even if the young boy dragged here by his parents is unimpressed by the *Titanic*'s much smaller relative the *Nomadic*, now preserved in a dry dock. 'It's not even in the water!' he complains.

The shining silver visitor centre stands next to the site that once housed the gantry where the *Titanic* was built. It is 90 feet tall, exactly the same height as the ship itself from keel to deck. The gift shop offers branded T-shirts, baseball caps, scarfs and the like, even *Titanic* men's briefs, which I suppose count as a flattering gift. Dozens of visitors (mostly British, plus Americans, Europeans and Chinese) are queuing to see the various galleries. But at least one of those galleries, I've read, has Celine Dion's 'My Heart Will Go On' playing on a loop, so clearly there's no way I'm subjecting myself to that. Instead my money is spent on a walking tour of the area, taking in the disused drawing offices where the ship was designed, and passing the huge hall where its component parts were painted (now a film studio in which *Game of Thrones* is shot). The guy leading the group is in his thirties, a little over-exuberant (shades of the RSC guide in Stratford), but as a self-confessed 'Titanorak' perfectly placed to deliver us trivia aplenty. We hear that it took 20 horses to pull the ship's anchor, and 22 tons of soap to coat the slipway the first time the vessel was eased down into the water. Like all the White Star Line's ships, the *Titanic* was sent on its way without any formal ceremony – the company thought the traditional champagne-bottle routine was bad luck.

Passing the original gates to the yard, just a few feet wide, it's staggering to hear that they opened every morning at 6.30 for 15 minutes, in which time 15,000 men would surge through, desperate not to get locked out and suffer a day without work.[7] We stand in the very room (now derelict) where chief

---

[7] These days Harland and Wolff employ only a few hundred people, mainly making wind turbines.

designer Thomas Andrews argued with company chairman J. Bruce Ismay about the lifeboats. Ismay said too many would alarm passengers. His insistence on reducing the number cost hundreds of lives, including that of Andrews himself. William Pirie, Andrews's uncle, had been grooming his nephew to take over the Harland and Wolff business. For the rest of his life he never uttered the word 'Titanic' again.

Our guide illustrates the tour with several photos, including one of the ship under construction. It has a white mark in the foreground – one of the workmen, unnoticed by the photographer, had been taking a crafty pee at the time, so was scratched out of the negative. But interesting and educational as the walk is, I decide, heading back into town, that the BT fact will not be a *Titanic* one after all. The title goes instead to an incident from 1959, which shows – and in this of all postcode areas I feel it's something that needs to be shown – just how tolerant the people of the UK really are. Yes, they get in a tizzy (and sometimes things worse than a tizzy) about language and names and boundaries and affiliations. But deep down most people, most of the time, are pretty relaxed.

BT (Belfast): Ulster Television were responsible for one of UK broadcasting's earliest uses of the 'f'-word.

The occasion, six years before the much more famous Kenneth Tynan incident on the late-night satirical show *BBC3*, was a live interview on the teatime magazine show *Roundabout*. Presenter Ivor Mills was talking to a workman whose job it was to paint the railings on the embankment along the river in the middle of Belfast. These were so numerous that as soon as the task was finished the guy had to start all over again. Mills enquired if it was ever boring, constantly painting the same old railings. 'Of course it's fucking boring,' came the reply.

Back in the studio the channel's managing director froze in horror, then waited for the phone to start ringing. Surely this was it: his career was about to shudder to a premature end, buried beneath an avalanche of outrage at the obscenity. His name would live on in television circles forever as a reminder of the perils of live broadcasting.

In the event not a single person complained.

4

A TALE OF TWO CITIES

Early April now, and I'm standing in front of the map again. The far-flungedness of the Belfast trip was good, but the destination itself only netted a single fact. It's time to up the productivity level a bit – there are 124 of these areas to do, and I'm still down in the mid-thirties. What I need is a part of the country where postcodes cluster together like bees in a hive, so I can nip around and steal their nectar. Examining the country, I notice not just one place that fits the bill but two: Manchester and London. There's also transport to be considered: I've only done two-thirds of the 'planes, trains and automobiles' trinity, so that needs rectifying. A railway journey up north via the capital will give me an information-per-mile ratio to die for. Coincidentally, several of the facts themselves will relate to trains. It is clearly meant to be.

The map also brings home that there are some places I won't get round to visiting. Sad that even this early in the project possibilities are closing down as well as opening up, but one of the keys to a happy life is surely an acceptance of one's limitations. Ideas for future field trips are forming in my head, and some places, God love them and bless them, just don't fit. It makes sense, therefore, to deal with them now. The Channel Islands, for instance:

GY (Guernsey): Footballer Matthew Le Tissier once put a spread bet on his own team to concede an early throw-in, but was so nervous as he tried to 'accidentally' kick the ball out that he passed it too well.

The Southampton legend stood to make 'well into four figures'. The mistake (against Wimbledon in 1995) saw a team-mate keep the ball in play, and so cost Le Tissier his payout. Because of Guernsey's status (technically not part of the United Kingdom, merely a possession of the British Crown), it's a convention that its sportsmen can choose which of the four UK nations to play for. Thankfully for England fans, Le Tissier resisted the charms of Scotland, Wales and Northern Ireland.

JE (Jersey): The island in the Status Quo song 'Living on an Island' is Jersey.

Rick Parfitt was living there for a year due to tax reasons, and wrote the song because he was so bored. Hardly surprising that a rock star famed for his love of sports cars should struggle in a place with a blanket 40 mph speed limit.

I also deal with a hat-trick of language facts. One concerns the family whose country seat is Hatfield House in Hertfordshire ...

AL (St Albans): The phrase 'Bob's your uncle' was inspired by nineteenth-century Prime Minister Lord Salisbury giving his own nephew Arthur Balfour a job in the Cabinet.

... one concerns a place-name derivation you really wouldn't expect ...

CR (Croydon): The name Croydon means 'valley of the crocuses'.

...and one concerns a superhero...

NG (Nottingham): Batman's home city of Gotham is named after a village in Nottinghamshire.

An old story about Gotham (pronounced Goat-am) has its residents pretending to be mad in order to stop a road being built through their village. As Batman's Gotham was built to house the criminally insane, the story's writers copied the name. The superhero even owes his real first name to Britain – his creators chose 'Bruce Wayne' in tribute to Robert the Bruce.

And so, bag packed and train tickets in hand, I set off for London. My home area of CO has already been covered, meaning the first virgin territory is Chelmsford. The map revealed a village called Bocking Churchstreet, which from now on will be my favourite non-swearing swearing option (very handy when small children are around – Billy Connolly opts for 'gettifer yerbassa'). A recent news story from Braintree gave CM a shot at the award for best opening sentence ever: 'A motorist caught driving at 130 mph with a cup of tea between his legs told magistrates he was surprised to find his Mercedes-Benz E-Class didn't have a cup holder.' But in the end the fact is a political one. Not about Melford Stevenson, the barrister who contested Maldon for the Conservatives in the 1945 general election. The sitting Labour MP Tom Driberg was rumoured (correctly) to be gay. Stevenson said in a speech that he refused to believe these rumours: 'I can assure you there is no truth in them whatsoever. I say that with confidence as I happened to be appearing at the Old Bailey on the very day Mr Driberg was found not guilty.'[1] No, the fact concerns a Tory who did get elected: Norman St John-Stevas. Impossibly grand (when accused of name-dropping he replied 'The Queen said exactly the same to me yesterday'), St John-Stevas was said by opponents to be spending too little time in his Chelmsford constituency. This sort of thing can cost votes, so . . .

CM (Chelmsford): Norman St John-Stevas rented a flat above Chelmsford railway station so he could be seen returning to it before slipping out again and catching the last train to London.

Next we're into Romford. Tilbury Docks was where both Gandhi and Cliff Richard had their first sight of Britain (though Cliff was still Harry Webb, the name he'd been given at birth in India), but we're more concerned with St Laurence Church in Upminster:

RM (Romford): The first accurate estimate of the speed of sound was made by a vicar timing the gap between a shotgun being fired and the noise reaching him.

William Derham was our hero, rector at Upminster between 1689 and 1735. From the top of the church tower he used a telescope to watch an assistant firing the weapon several miles away. As soon as he saw the gunsmoke he started measuring

---

[1] In 1969 Stevenson was the High Court judge who sentenced the Kray twins to life. He said later they'd only told the truth twice during the trial – when Reggie called a barrister a 'fat slob', and when Ronnie said the judge was biased.

time with his half-second pendulum. The experiment was repeated again and again to average out any inaccuracy in the pendulum, and Derham arrived at the figure of 1,116 feet per second. The accepted answer today is 1,115.

Then it's Ilford:

IG (Ilford): Alan Sugar once signed a birthday card to his wife 'Best wishes, Sir Alan Sugar'.

He blamed a 'busy day in the office', but admitted that back home in Chigwell Lady S was 'not a happy bunny'.

Finally we're into the capital itself, eastern division. We could go for the first business founded by Whitechapel's Marcus Samuel – it sold painted seashells, which is why he called his later oil industry concern (founded 1897) Shell. But instead let's go back a few years further still:

E (London East): The tin opener was invented 40 years after the tin can.

Actually that's a conservative figure – tinned food was around in the late 1700s, though it was 1812 before the first patent was taken out, by Bryan Donkin of Bermondsey. Not until 1855, however, did Robert Yeates of 233 Hackney Road give us a dedicated tool for opening the tins. Before that the instructions had read: 'Cut around the top near the outer edge with a chisel and hammer.'

For the final few seconds of its journey, after it passes under Shoreditch High Street and curves round into Liverpool Street station, my train is in the land of EC. Here we find another invention that revolutionised daily life:

EC (London East Central): The toothbrush was invented in London's most notorious prison.

The site now occupied by the Old Bailey once housed the legendary Newgate gaol. In the 1770s William Addis was serving time there for causing a riot. Brushing his teeth the same way as everyone else – in other words using a rag to rub them with soot and salt – he decided that there had to be a better way. Inspired by the sight of a broom, he took a small animal bone left over from his dinner and drilled tiny holes into it. Persuading a guard to get him some bristles, Addis threaded them through the holes and glued them into place. On his release the invention made him a fortune. His most expensive brushes used badger hair, while the lower end of the range featured pig and boar hair. His company, now known as Wisdom Toothbrushes, survives to this day.

Over at Euston, my train to Manchester awaits. Even the conversations of fellow passengers seem destined to fit the railway theme at the moment – a besuited businessman says into his mobile: 'I'm sorry but your assurance isn't good enough ... After this morning it's obvious HS2 can't organise a breakfast meeting, never mind a train line.' Soon the metropolis has given way to fields and canals and the odd motorway, and at one point I realise all three have come together and we're passing just a few yards west of Watford Gap service station. I gaze across at the hotel that was home on the first field trip: always nice when a project starts tying up with itself. A little while later we speed through Lichfield Trent Valley station, meaning we're in WS territory:

WS (Walsall): The Queen keeps a suction-operated plastic hook in her handbag so she always has something on which to hang it.

The bags in question are made by Launer of Walsall, who also supplied Margaret Thatcher. Some of the royal contents are what you'd expect: glasses, mints, crosswords, a fountain pen. Contrary to rumours Her Majesty does carry cash, though only a folded £5 note in readiness for the weekly church collection. There's also a mirror and lipstick, which she often reapplies at the table after meals, even grand state banquets. But a plastic hook? Perhaps we shouldn't be surprised at such practicality – after all, she has those lead weights sewn into her dresses. One guest at a dinner in Berkshire witnessed the monarch remove the hook, 'discreetly spit' into the suction pad, then attach it to the underside of the table and hang her bag on it.

As we near Manchester the station names remind me of train journeys in the late Eighties and early Nineties, when I was at university up here. Next to Macclesfield stands a swish furniture store called Arighi Bianchi. You'd assume that's a sign of how the North-West has changed in recent years, but no, the firm's been here since 1854, founded by two immigrants escaping the Italian civil war. At a little before 1 p.m. we reach our destination, and I'm instantly greeted by a change to the Manchester landscape – a massive ferris wheel in Piccadilly Gardens. It's the same colour and much the same design as the London Eye, though not as big.

'Is that permanent?' I ask a passing policeman.

'Yeah.'

I happen to know that the more famous wheel has 32 pods (one for each London borough). A quick count reveals that this one has 42. 'You beat London in that respect,' I say.

'We beat London in every respect,' replies the copper. He leaves a gap between the last two words for a non-existent swear word, giving his comment just the right balance of humour and defiance. Manchester's swagger has always been of the relaxed variety. It's an attractive quality, unlike down the road in Liverpool, where they surely do protest too much. The difference is perfectly summed up in the old joke about which should be England's second city: 80 per cent of people from Leeds think it should be Leeds, 90 per cent of people from Manchester think it should be Manchester, but 100 per cent of people from Liverpool think it should be London.

Round the corner there's another big change since my college days: Manchester's tram system. It opened the month I left university, and has since expanded into the perfect tool for today's task – one branch goes out to Rochdale (OL postcode area), another to Bury (BL) and a third to Altrincham (WA). The yellow electric trains run along tramlines in the urban streets but use traditional train lines in between. The ticket machine shows me exactly which one-day pass I need, a bargain at £6.70. Including Manchester itself, that's £1.67 (and a half) per fact. Britain can still do great transport infrastructure when it wants to.

A Rochdale train comes along within minutes, and I sit near the front. The driver's cab is clear, letting you see through to the track ahead and so giving you more sense of your journey. (Why can't London Underground trains do this? Most of the network is above ground.) One of the stations we call at is in the Newton Heath area, where in 1878 workers on the Lancashire and Yorkshire Railway formed a football team. These days it plays a few miles down the road and is called Manchester United. Posters all over the network give information on improvements at one of the city centre stops: 'Please bear with us while we make Victoria posh.' The first station with an Oldham postcode is Hollinwood, whose eighteenth-century resident Hannah Beswick was so scared of premature burial that she had herself embalmed and kept above ground. Once a year, in the presence of two witnesses, the veil had to be lifted and her body checked for signs of life. She was finally buried in 1868, a mere 110 years after her death.

Through Oldham itself, where a sign advertises the 'Rainy City Roller Girls – All-Female Full-Contact Roller Derby' (do we suspect that not all the spectators will be there for entirely the right reasons?) Oldham was also the birthplace of Louise Brown, the world's first test-tube baby.[2] On the outskirts of Rochdale there's a shop called Reptacular, and then, after a 50-minute journey, it's the town itself. An elderly train enthusiast is on the platform to video our arrival. Note how I avoided the loaded term 'spotter' there. You couldn't call this man an anorak – instead he sports a rather natty red-spotted neckerchief. Rochdale is small but, like its bigger cousin at the other end of the line, has a great spirit. Sections of the ride out here were lined with derelict Victorian mills, but even these reminders of faded glory can't bring the people down. A statue of sheep in the town centre (unveiled in 1978 by local girl Gracie Fields) makes you smile, and the café where I have lunch is buzzing. The guy after me orders a latte, pronouncing the first syllable to rhyme with 'hat' rather than 'cart'. It strikes me that this is how the Italians themselves say it, only poncey English southerners insisting on the change.

I might be here because of Rochdale's Town Hall, photos of which reputedly impressed Adolf Hitler so much that he wanted to take it back to Germany brick-by-brick (it's thought he could have been told about it by local boy William Joyce, aka Lord Haw-Haw). I might be here because of Lord Byron, whose full title was Baron Byron of Rochdale (his ancestor bought the manor). But I'm actually here to visit a small building dating from the days when the street on which it lies, Toad

---

[2] Though if you want to be precise, the conception actually took place in a petri dish.

Lane, was still 'the old' ('t'owd') lane. Originally a warehouse, the three-storey brick building found itself marching into the history books in 1844:

OL (Oldham): The Rochdale Society of Equitable Pioneers was Britain's first successful co-operative movement.

Earlier movements had existed, but it's generally acknowledged that the modern Co-op has its foundation in the Rochdale Principles laid down by the group who opened their shop here. They're spelled out on a blackboard in the two-room museum which now occupies the building: payment of a dividend, political and religious neutrality, promotion of education and so on. Next to it, as an example of the goods that would have been sold here, is a sugar-loaf. It's never occurred to me, hearing the name of the Brazilian mountain, to wonder what a sugar-loaf is, but here I discover that it's a pointed column, about 18 inches tall, of packed-together sugar. Easier to transport that way, apparently. Shopkeepers sold it by taking slices off, much in the manner of modern kebabs.

The museum has achieved an ideal mix of new and old – enough exhibits to give you something to look at, but not so many that they get in the way of the best exhibit of all, the building itself. The stone floor, wooden beams and brickwork are all original, making it easy to imagine the Pioneers and their customers standing here. Unable to afford shop counters they used planks laid across barrels, displaying the goods (butter, flour, oatmeal and the like), which they had to buy in Manchester because local wholesalers refused to supply them. Similarly the local gas company refused to connect the shop. Undaunted, the Pioneers lit it with candles. They persevered with their bizarre new practices, such as one member one vote, even for women – this in a time when female workers weren't allowed to join trade unions, and a married woman's property automatically belonged to her husband. They encouraged poorer people to take part in politics by organising public-speaking competitions. Fittingly Rochdale was also the birthplace of the radical nineteenth-century MP John Bright. He coined the phrases 'mother of parliaments' and (while trying to rouse his fellow members from apathy on the subject of extending the vote) 'flogging a dead horse'.

I walk round the information panels, reading about the spread of the movement that started in these rooms. In 1896 the Co-operative Wholesale Society bought its own farm in Shropshire. Within six years it owned a tea plantation in Ceylon (now Sri Lanka). When 1930s radio manufacturers refused to supply sets (arguing that the dividend was a form of price cutting), the Co-operative bought equipment from Sweden, fitted it in their own cabinets and sold the sets under the brand name 'Defiant Radios'. Today the movement is so renowned in Japan that Kobe boasts a replica of the Rochdale building. Many of the old posters sound like twenty-first-century campaigns: one announces that 'there is no sweating in the manufacture of CWS furniture'. Meanwhile back at 31 Toad Lane more mundane problems had to be dealt with. A library had opened above the shop, and readers were so annoyed by the librarian's noisy clogs that they bought him a pair of slippers.

Books and DVDs are for sale, as well as (a nice touch in many museums these days) a selection of retro-toys. I buy a wooden yo-yo for Barney. As the young woman on the till rings it through, I attempt to operate it, and as usual with yo-yos I fail. She offers to coach me: the trick is flicking your hand up just before the string unravels completely. We get talking about the museum, and when she learns why I'm here says: 'Oh, you'll have noticed the postbox outside, then?'

Er . . .

'It's quite famous, apparently. We get people coming here specially to look at it.' So renowned is it in postbox circles that she's even ordered a book containing details of it. Opening it at the relevant page, we read that the box is a 'converted First National Standard pillar box of 1859'. It's the nature of the conversion that makes it so noteworthy. This, you see, is one of only two postboxes in the world to be incorporated into a lamp post. Outside, it's easy to see how I missed it on the way in: the thing is only about, oh, 12 feet tall. Philosophers could argue about whether it's a lamp post incorporating a pillar box or a pillar box incorporating a lamp post. The postal element is on the smallish side and in regulation red, a gorgeous enamel plate giving collection times, together with details of a later collection at 'Esplanade Rochdale' (now there's a name for a band). Stuck on top of it is an equally beautiful black Victorian lamp post, its bulb protected by an ornate six-sided glass case.

Only two in the world, the book said. This one in Rochdale, the other – and here's a juxtaposition reminiscent of Del Boy's van – in Paris.

If you imagine Manchester at the centre of a clock face, Rochdale is at one o'clock and Bury at eleven. It's silly to go all the way back into Manchester and then out again, certainly when the 471 bus is waiting to whisk me straight over to Bury. Fellow passengers are mostly schoolkids on their cheery way home, though there's also the woman on the back seat wearing a purple velour tracksuit which must have many 'X's before its 'L'. She treats her companion, and indeed the rest of us, to a monologue about everyone she's ever argued with and why they were wrong. One male acquaintance has 'only ever given me some dodgy bloody laptop what I never use', while another group are 'all Billy Bullshitters'. The bus heads through the town of Heywood, named after the family who lorded it round here in centuries past (Peter Heywood being the man who arrested Guy Fawkes). The Horse and Jockey boasts of being 'the Warmest Pub in Heywood' (large heating bills?), and stands on Wham Lane. The street sign's an old one, so whatever the explanation it can't be George and Andrew.

After half an hour we're over the border into the BL postcode area, and soon after that into Bury. The town is bigger than Rochdale, with a shopping centre/Vue cinema/bowling alley set-up, several magnificent lumps of Victorian architecture (one now reinvented as an arts venue) and a statue of John Kay, inventor of the flying shuttle which revolutionised weaving and helped this area build its fortune. Kay, the plaque tells us, somehow 'died in exile and poverty in France, where he lies in an unknown grave'. It's actually another inventor I've come here to honour, and to do so in an appropriate pub means asking around. People are very helpful, and soon I'm entering the Old White Lion via its revolving door (it used to be a hotel). The pub, you see, has a dartboard:

BL (Bolton): The numbering arrangement of the modern dartboard was invented in Bury.

Brian Gamlin was a carpenter in the town. In 1896 he worked out the sequence of numbers that would most heavily penalise inaccurate throws. The mighty 20, for instance, is sandwiched between minnows 5 and 1. The left-hand half of the board is known as the 'married man's side', because it has a higher proportion of large numbers ('married men always play safe' goes the explanation, though there does seem to be some evidence to the contrary on that). Ordering a pint,

I ask the landlady if the pub has a set of darts. 'Sorry love,' comes the reply. Oh well, it's probably for the best: I'd only get annoyed at how useless I am. That's the thing about darts – even more than in most sports, the pros make it look easy. This explains the unfair snobbery about it. Well, that and the shirts and the hairstyles and the audience members.

Examining the board (which is in a separate room with the pool table), I reflect on the minuscule distances between glory and disaster. In 1908 a pub owner in Leeds called 'Foot' Anakin[3] was prosecuted for allowing darts in his pub, on the grounds that it was a game of chance. To prove it was a game of skill he had a board brought into the courtroom, then threw three darts into the 20 and challenged anyone to do the same. A court clerk tried and failed, at which point the judge dismissed the case. The game had a strong claim to be part of England's tradition anyway – it evolved from archers in the Middle Ages using sliced tree trunks for target practice, the age rings and the developing cracks dividing the 'board' into areas. But the Leeds case really boosted the game's popularity. By 1938 a *News of the World* competition was entered by 280,000 players, the final in London being contested by Jim Pike and (if you thought Foot Anakin was an unlikely name I'd steel yourself) Marmaduke Brecon.

You can tell a game has found its way into a nation's heart when it develops its own lingo. 'Trebles for show, arrows for dough,' the professionals tell us. The author T. H. White, playing in a Wiltshire pub in the 1930s, heard a score of 81 called 'snowstorm', as southern England had suffered a heavy one in 1881. But for the very finest darting dialogue we turn of course to the late, lamented commentator Sid Waddell. The infuriating double 1 was always described in his Northumberland tones

---

[3] He had very large ones.

as 'madhouse'. One player had 'more checkouts than Tesco', while another's eyes were 'bulging like the belly of a hungry chaffinch'. Waddell once said during an especially tense match that 'if Elvis walked in with a portion of chips, you could hear the vinegar sizzling on them'.

Things are rather more relaxed in the White Lion this afternoon. Four blazered ex-serviceman discuss the lunch they've attended (a mural over the door celebrates the Lancashire Fusiliers). A younger crowd at the bar discuss plans for tonight. I love the accent here, the way 'all right' comes out as 'or rate'. A poster advertises the forthcoming appearance of a 'Top Male Vocalist', the photos depicting him as a crooner (bow tie), a Blues Brother (shades, pork-pie hat) and Bob Marley (yellow, red and green striped woollen hat – could have been worse). Another wall displays signed celebrity photos: Michael Caine, Des O'Connor, Frank Bruno, that pair from *Birds of a Feather*. In less lively regions this can be a desperate touch, but here the signatures are personalised in gratitude for the pub's contributions to various charities.

Time to rejoin the tram now, heading all the way back into Manchester and out the other side to Altrincham (which lies at seven on that imaginary clock face). One of the mills in the early part of the journey is so derelict that only the frontage remains: you feel you could blow it over. Passengers include two lads chatting happily away, one perhaps 16 in school uniform, the other 18 in suit and tie. They have to be brothers – friendships rarely cross that particular divide. In the city centre we pass a Co-operative supermarket, which I now see in a new light. Then, heading through south-west Manchester, we stop at the station whose name is famous all over the world: Old Trafford. The sporting ground right next to it is actually the cricket one, host in 1963 to Britain's first ever one-day match: it took two days to complete. The 'Theatre of

Dreams' is a few hundred yards up the road, reminding us of the best football chant of the last 20 years, when United's star defender Rio Ferdinand was banned for missing a drugs test – 'his name is Rio and he watches from the stand'. Back in 1970, when the ground hosted the FA Cup Final replay, David Webb, scorer of Chelsea's winning goal, was prevented from collecting his medal because he'd swapped shirts with a member of the opposition, leading officials to think he was a Leeds player.

Finally, it's Altrincham itself, which according to my friend Emma, who lives locally, was once pronounced 'Altrinsham' by one unwitting Radio 2 presenter. Emma isn't around this evening so we can't meet up, but she has been emailing me plenty of facts about the place. Bonnie Prince Charlie once drove through here ... local girl Angela Cartwright played one of the von Trapp children in *The Sound of Music* ... ex-Man Utd player Nicky Butt buys his pasties in the Co-op, *Corrie*'s Sally Webster her cotton buds in Waitrose. These last two are personal sightings by Emma, but even she has to acknowledge that their inclusion so high up the list gives a hint that Altrincham will perhaps prove a harder hunting ground than most. Widening the net slightly to Timperley (the penultimate tram stop, and the only other one in WA territory) we find some 'amazing rhubarb' being grown. Hmm. Never mind: on-the-ground research will no doubt produce something.

Altrincham turns out to be much more chichi than its satellite neighbours to the north of Manchester. Two expensively coiffed ladies are having their nails done at the Oxford One Spa, though as it's now well past six o'clock trading has finished at the Fab Patisserie. A good plaque, that's what I need. A classy circular one gets the hopes up, but it's only a spoof one advertising the estate agent underneath. A proper blue one commemorates 'Basil Morrison, 1915–2012', but he turns out to be nothing more than a pillar of the local community. A well-respected one, no doubt, and also at one point believed to be the oldest Morgan driver in the UK, but this still falls some way short of the mark. A text message arrives from my friend James, confessing that his database holds nothing of interest about Altrincham. When you bear in mind that the database in question is that of the programme *QI*, on which James is chief researcher, this really is the final nail. We must turn elsewhere. This could be the suburb of St Helens called Clock Face (there was once a large one on its pub), which would fit in with today's geographical analogy. But instead, fitting in with the railway theme, we choose Widnes:

WA (Warrington): The Simon and Garfunkel song 'Homeward Bound' was written on Widnes railway station.

The duo are so famously and resolutely American that it's amazing to learn of any connection between them and Britain, never mind one involving the backwaters of WA8. But apparently Paul Simon played plenty of British folk clubs in his early years, and 1965 found him heading back from a gig in the Lancashire town. 'If you know Widnes,' he said later, 'then you'll understand how I was desperately trying to get back to London as quickly as possible.' The love who 'lies waiting silently for me' was Kathy Chitty, whom Simon had met in equally exotic Brentwood the year before, when she sold tickets for his gig at the (amazing how a theme keeps itself going sometimes) Railway Inn. She's also the subject of 'Kathy's Song', and crops up in the lyrics of 'America'.

Back in Manchester city centre we find another American musician forging links with the North-West. My hotel for the night is the Radisson Blu Edwardian, which used to be the Free Trade Hall. This was a venue not just for political speeches (Disraeli gave his famous 'One Nation' address here in 1872) but also concerts. Home to the Hallé Orchestra, in more recent decades the hall hosted rock and pop acts. So it was that on 17 May 1966 Bob Dylan found himself here swapping his acoustic guitar for an electric one, at which point a folk purist in the audience emitted the legendary cry 'Judas!' I'd always thought this happened in America.[4] The Free Trade Hall closed for musical business in 1996, reopening eight years later as a hotel. The redesign preserved its sandstone façade and replaced the back half of the building with an impressive glass tower. The concierge, who himself attended Hallé concerts here as a schoolboy half a century ago, tells me that Bob would have been standing pretty well where the lifts are now.

By the time I'm gazing out from my eleventh-floor room Manchester has lived up to a reputation it's been ignoring all day: the raindrops have started. The intermittent drizzle matches my mood, which is eager anticipation at a stroll into misery. In their book *The Meaning of Liff*, a collection of spoof definitions for British place names, Douglas Adams and John Lloyd list Aberystwyth as 'a nostalgic yearning which is in itself more pleasant than the thing being yearned for'. My feelings go even further as I walk the couple of miles south through the university campus and on to my old halls of residence: I'm positively revelling in the memories of how unhappy I was for whole chunks of my time here. It's not masochism, rather a reminder of how life is a process of measuring yourself against different backgrounds until you can make out your true colours. Retracing these steps, the ones I took every day to and

[4] Just as I'd always assumed the famous 'Subterranean Homesick Blues' video, in which Dylan discards cue cards bearing the lyrics, was shot in New York. Not so – it was filmed behind The Savoy in London.

from lectures, I recall, re*feel*, the intensity of my thoughts and emotions in those days. It's an intensity you can only – should only – experience in your early twenties, so strong that tonight it's a nuclear glow from which I instinctively recoil. The old me is so different that he's almost literally a different person. I feel that if I stand still then sooner or later he's bound to pass by. I could have a conversation with him, explain things, tell him to stop worrying. But what good would that do? If you tell someone it's 93 million miles to the sun they believe you. If you put up a sign saying 'wet paint' they have to touch it to be sure. Quite right too.

All this damp introspection underlines an aspect of the project that's been fascinating me more and more – the personal memories contained in every postcode area. The other day, talking to a friend, I mentioned a particular alleyway near the Bank of England. Andrew said he can never walk down it without thinking of the day he saw a spanner, dropped by a workman high up on some scaffolding, go clean through the petrol tank of a parked motorbike. We all have these recollections of places, from the trivial to the momentous. It was in SW, for example, that I once saw a woman so horrified at absent-mindedly saying 'fuck' in front of a vicar that she said it again. Looking at the postcode map before setting out, knowing I'd be coming to this place from my past, I had the idea of a huge pile of maps, each filled in by a different person with what the various areas mean to them. Hardly anyone would have an entry for every area, but with enough people the whole country would get covered. Drilling down the pile in a particular area you could mine the story of how the same area had seen people being born, meeting their first love, narrowly avoiding a car smash, achieving a hole-in-one, trying oysters for the first time, committing a robbery, getting divorced, a whole cross-section of human experiences. Alternatively you could take a single map from the pile, see how one person had filled their life and where it had taken them. For instance every time I hear the word 'Rochdale' now, I'm going to think of yo-yos.

The blocks pass by as I trudge southwards. The one that once housed the BBC has become a car park, while one that was waste ground is filled by a leisure centre. The Jag dealership has turned into a bike shop, and a new building accommodating parents of patients at the Royal Manchester Children's Hospital is called Ronald McDonald House. Not a single one of the several dozen curry houses in Rusholme has kept the same name since my university days, so I plump for one at random, knowing that (as ever) they'll all be fantastic. Mango chutney is still slightly thinner in Manchester than elsewhere, and the chopped onions are still dyed red. I ask the waiter which mixture of spices achieves this. 'Tomato ketchup,' comes the reply.

Then it's on to my old hall of residence, my room number scored in the memory as securely as any postcode. I go and stand outside its door for a few seconds, though only a few – don't want anyone emerging into the corridor and wondering what this weirdo is up to. What has become of the twenty-odd people who have occupied this room since I left? You could play the same trick as with the postcode map: so many different stories united by the same location. Then I wander back out to the main road, passing groups of students. They all look so *young*. Not even the late-teens I know they must be – mid-teens at most. Surely these people belong in school, not university? I think of the occasions I've been back to this city. Most have been to watch Test matches. Then a thought occurs that has never entered my head in Manchester before: when will I find myself here for the *final* time? I suppose you could call this one of life's tipping points – the first time you consider a last.

Opposite the hall a strong contender for 'longest bus shelter in the world' has been built, fifty yards if it's an inch. I wait there for a bus back into town. Also in the shelter are two female students. One says to the other: 'My mum is *so* hormonal at the moment.'

It might have been a Frenchman who did it, but it was an English railway company that helped him out.

Next morning, over breakfast, I'm deciding which of the contenders for the 'M' fact will get the nod. If we were sticking to postcodes themselves there would be only one show in town, the show that would have been called *Florizel Street* but for a Granada TV tea lady pointing out that Florizel sounded like a disinfectant.[5] So *Coronation Street* it was, the residents of fictional Weatherfield enjoying M10 postcodes (the real M10 was re-coded as M40 in 1993). But in keeping with the railway theme of this trip, it's Louis Paulhan who wins out:

M (Manchester): The first man ever to fly from London to Manchester did so by following the whitewashed sleepers of the London and North Western Railway.

In 1906, the *Daily Mail* offered £10,000 (all but a million quid today) for the first person to fly the 185 miles from the capital city to Manchester within 24 hours, stopping no more than twice. It seemed impossible then – planes could only stay airborne for a few yards. But within four years French aviator Louis Paulhan was ready to make his attempt. He spent

---

[5] Actually he's a character in *The Winter's Tale*.

4 hours 12 minutes in the air, resting overnight in Lichfield. Not only did the L&NWR help out with navigation, they also ran a train carrying his wife and support team beneath him all the way. Paulhan was nearly defeated by turbulence: 'My machine rose viciously and then dropped so quickly that I was almost torn from my seat.' But at dawn on 28 April the Farman plane landed in Burnage, earning Paulhan the *Mail*'s money. The field in question is now covered by a road named after him.

The reverse journey takes me a shade over two hours this Friday morning. The train follows a slightly different route from yesterday, going via Wilmslow and Crewe, which means we pass the huge satellite dish (or more properly 'radio tele-scope') at Jodrell Bank. I didn't know that the tracks run within a few yards of it, so the looming white hulk standing in its field comes as a surprise. A 250-feet-in-diameter, still-the-third-largest-telescope-dish-in-the-world surprise. This is SK territory, on which research has been proving tricky, so it's very pleasant to read not only that the dish is steered by gun turret bearings taken from two ex-Second World War battle-ships, but also that:

SK (Stockport): The support towers of the Lovell Telescope contain a breeding pair of peregrine falcons, whose job it is to keep pigeons away and so prevent their droppings interfering with the telescope's working.

Sometimes even the highest of hi-tech needs a helping hand from Mother Nature.

There's more train info at the other end of the journey, when we reach the land of Harrow postcodes. Dangerous territory, it seems. In 1911 W. S. Gilbert (as in '. . . and Sullivan') died in the grounds of his house here, suffering a heart attack as he saved a girl from drowning in the lake. He was overseen in his final moments by the statue of Charles II that now stands in Soho Square – it was perching on an island in the lake while the square was remodelled. There's also the plaque in Harrow on the Hill reading: 'Take Heed – the first recorded motor accident in Great Britain involving the death of the driver occurred on Grove Hill on 25th February 1899.' But it's a death on the train tracks near here that concerns us. Reading about it the first time I assumed I must have misunderstood, so unbelievable was the cause of death. But no, further checking reveals it is indeed the case that:

HA (Harrow): In the early days of the London and Birmingham Railway conductors travelled outside the train, leaning in through the open windows to check tickets.

The first carriages were based on stagecoaches, in which the guard sat outside at roof level. Boards were fitted, along which the train guard could walk during the journey, reaching in to take passengers' tickets and make sure that no second-class passengers were travelling first class. The unfortunate Thomas Port was thus engaged on 7 August 1838. His train was travelling at its top speed of 30 mph when, stepping from one carriage to the next, he slipped. His legs were pulled under the wheels, which 'as they successively passed over, dragged his legs in, crushing them inch by inch up to one of his knees and above the other'. The train was stopped, and two doctors who happened to be on board administered emergency first aid. Port was then taken to Harrow where the doctors fully amputated both legs. But it was no use: he died from loss of blood, leaving a wife and two children. Within a few years trains were achieving much higher speeds, and guards were allowed the luxury of travelling inside (this was when British bosses really started to go soft). We only have Port's grave-stone to remind us of an incredible period in railway history. It seizes the chance with quite shocking directness: 'Ere noon arrived his mangled form they bore, With pain distorted and o'erwhelmed with gore, When evening came to close the fatal day, A mutilated corpse the sufferer lay.'

Arriving at Euston, I cross the capital to Waterloo, where the next fact awaits:

SE (London South East): Winston Churchill's coffin left London from Waterloo station purely to annoy General de Gaulle.

Relations between the wartime leaders hadn't always been cordial, so towards the end of his life Churchill ordered that if de Gaulle outlived him, the train carrying his coffin should travel to Oxfordshire (Churchill's final resting place) not from the logical station of Paddington, but from the much more awkward Waterloo. I'm leaving the station today to visit the final resting place of another British legend, this one in Kingston-upon-Thames. KT could have commemorated syl-labub: the Druid's Head in the town (still open today) was one of the first taverns to make the famous 'milk curdled by alco-hol' dessert, supposedly by a farmhand milking a cow directly into a jug of cider. Or it could have commemorated golf – a proposed new course near here has been in the news recently, protestors complaining that it would be Surrey's 142nd. Over the postcode border in TW, Richmond Golf Club's temporary rules from 1940 show just how much pluck there was round here: 'During gunfire or while bombs are falling, players may take cover without penalty for ceasing play ... The positions of known delayed action bombs are marked by red flags at a reasonably, but not guaranteed, safe distance therefrom ... A player whose stroke is affected by the simultaneous explosion of a bomb may play another ball from the same place. Penalty one stroke.'

Instead, however, it's the Kingston branch of Lloyds Bank that I've come to see. A plaque inside, next to a row of cash-points, honours the chap who is buried at the rear of the bank, though when he was interred the plot was merely a small park. Nipper was his name, on account of the fact that he used to bite people's legs: in a throwback to the project's very first fact, Nipper was a Jack Russell terrier. His owner Francis Barraud possessed an early phonograph (we're talking the 1890s here), and the dog used to sit with his head on one side, puzzled as to where the voices were coming from. Barraud was so taken with this that he did a painting of it, which he then offered to the Edison-Bell company. 'Dogs don't listen to phonographs,' came the abrupt reply. The Gramophone Company, however, had rather more imagination. Paying Barraud £50 for the painting, and another £50 for its copyright, they christened the image 'His Master's Voice'. And so it is that:

KT (Kingston-upon-Thames): Buried beneath the Kingston branch of Lloyds bank is Nipper, the dog in the HMV logo.

The tributes don't stop at the plaque. A small passageway round the corner has been renamed Nipper Alley. It runs down the side of a large pub frequented by some of the town's more seasoned drinkers, several of whom congregate at its entrance to smoke. At the far end the alley opens into a small yard, where an old public lavatory has been turned into the Toilet Gallery. This in turn has closed, though press cuttings visible through the padlocked doors tell of its opening by artists

Gilbert and George: they marked the occasion by cutting a length of loo roll. At first I feel disappointed on Nipper's behalf that his name should grace a stretch of ground filled with fag ends, discarded rubbish and an old toilet. Then I realise it's exactly what he would have wanted.

Surveying the rest of Kingston town centre I find a wonderful sculpture comprising 12 red phone boxes falling on to each other like dominoes (it's entitled 'Out of Order'), but not much else of interest. The place isn't as posh as I remembered. Well, I say 'remembered' – I'm struggling now to work out if I've ever actually been here before. I retire to Pret, where I order a coffee. The man who has looked up from tapping at the till screen continues to stare at me for a moment, before uttering a snooty, 'I don't work here.' I look down at the screen, then back at him. 'I'm here to fix the till,' he adds. On very close examination I can *just* make out that his shirt is a slightly different shade from everyone else's behind the counter. Silly me. Having eventually scored some caffeine, I sit down and decide that in fact I haven't been to Kingston before: I have been subliminally mixing it up for years with Kew, a mistake grounded on nothing more than them both beginning with the same letter. The lesson is useful not only in itself, but as a reminder that there are almost certainly some mistakes you *never* become aware of, ones that will influence your thinking for the rest of your days. The intimation of our human frailty is comforting.

Next destination is Southall, west of central London and north of here. There are no equivalents of the Rochdale to Bury bus, though, so it's all the way back into town and up to Paddington. Boarding the train there, I find the section between two halves of a carriage completely filled by an up-ended bike. It is *huge*, freakishly over-sized, wheels the size of a lorry's and a bright orange frame that could double as part of a suspension bridge. It makes the train itself look like a Hornby model. Feeling pleasantly Lilliputian, I turn to the bike's owner, a black guy in his late twenties. If his muscles are anything to go by the contraption certainly keeps you fit.

'Why so big?' I ask.

'Why not?' he replies, with a winning smile. He tells me about the bike: no gears, only one brake, cost not far short of a grand. Later, when he gets off at the same station as me, I'll see him ride away, looking for all the world like Dennis Hopper on a Harley. This station will be Hayes, the one after Southall. Why have I gone too far? Because I'm looking, in connection with my UB fact,[6] for something which stands right next to the track between the two stations. Something which, until the research for this project, I had assumed was an urban myth. In fact I've been scared to check it, so sure was I that this long-cherished mental image would fail to appear. But no, all the signs seem to point to it genuinely being there. Which is a fitting way to put it, really . . .

UB (Southall): There is a gasholder in Southall with the letters 'LH' and a large arrow painted on it to guide pilots towards Heathrow airport.

In the days before autopilot technology, when those in charge of planes actually had to do something beyond deciding which stewardess to chat up that night, visual markers on the ground were a crucial part of finding the airport you were heading for. The Southall gasholder was directly underneath the flight path into Heathrow. Unfortunately a very similar gasholder was directly underneath the flight path into nearby RAF Northolt. Several planes made the perfectly understandable error, and

---

[6] Although the area is centred on Southall, it takes its initials from Uxbridge.

had to be alerted by air traffic control that they were about to land at the wrong place. One American Boeing 707 did indeed go that final step, touching down at Northolt. Embarrassing enough in itself, but a further problem was that planes need a longer runway to take off than they do to land. Northolt, the pilot discovered, was too small for his 707 to get back into the air. They had to strip everything short of the joystick out of it before he could take off again, and even then the plane only just managed to clear the surrounding buildings.

After this it was decided it might be a good idea to differentiate the two gasholders. Hence the painted initials. On my first pass today, heading west from Southall to Hayes and looking out of the right-hand window, I locate the holder (a tall circular structure in blue metal), but not the initials. Getting off at Hayes and swapping platforms, I take the next train back, boarding in the first carriage. The driver, a friendly Australian woman, tells me exactly where to look: high up, on the far side of the holder as it curves away out of view. And sure enough there are the letters – a huge 'LH', with a long thin arrow underneath them. Flitting around here on this mode of transport reminds me of Alan Blumlein, the local chap who first had the idea for stereo sound. His early experiments in 1935 included footage of trains leaving Hayes station, recorded so that the sound followed the vehicle.

Then it's a leisurely walk round Southall itself. For years I've been meaning to come here. The area often crops up in reports about immigration, being almost entirely Indian. Much of *Bend It Like Beckham* was shot here, and one of its pubs was the first in the UK to accept rupees. The reports always show Southall as vibrant, a sea of colourful saris and nostril-teasing restaurants, so I've been looking forward to experiencing the place in person. There are some points of interest: the stalls on the High Street selling Bollywood DVDs, the fabric stall in the indoor market where two middle-aged men nimbly operate sewing machines, the marriage bureau whose window signs include two swastikas (the symbol belonged to the Hindus long before Adolf showed up – 'swastika' is a Sanskrit word meaning 'it is good'). But overall it's disappointing to find a lack of energy, a torpor overlaying the general scruffiness. I once read a piece by a doctor who practised predominantly in Muslim communities, and regularly heard complaints from hard-working parents that their children had integrated only too well into the British way of life, becoming lazy and slobbish. This seems to have happened here. Ladbrokes is full of Asian men staring listlessly at screens showing the horses from Sedgefield and the dogs from Swindon. The figures emerging from the pound shops shuffle and dawdle, and for every excited toddler there are three morose teenagers.

A big Edwardian pub on a major crossroads has a sign on the door warning 'No drinks beyound this point!!!', with another advising that toilets are for customers only – anyone else will be charged 40 pence. I love places like this, and leap at the chance to encounter a bit of life. But inside there are only two customers, both male (one Asian, one white), whose advanced drunkenness is soporific rather than inspiring, a horrible lesson in the damage alcohol can do. The place is borderline derelict, foul-smelling and threadbare. It's run by a middle-aged white couple, themselves far from sober. He wears slippers, she power-punches out of time to Queen's 'Don't Stop Me Now', though even this is done without much enthusiasm. I force myself to order a Coke, but can't bring myself to finish it. Five minutes later I'm back outside and heading for the train station. Oh well, at least Southall has been another discovery for the project. No one said they were all going to be good.

Into central London again, where the trip has one final port of call. It's a very large building on High Holborn, a few doors along from the Jockey Club. In fact for a while the club's rules on how you can and cannot name a racehorse in Britain were on the list of possibles for the WC fact. You are, for instance, limited to 18 characters, including spaces and punctuation. Names consisting entirely of numbers are forbidden, though you can include numbers above 30 as long as they're spelled out. (Sorry – 'thirty'.) Rudeness is a no-no, though silliness apparently isn't: the footballers Steve McManaman and Robbie Fowler named their beasts 'Some Horse' and 'Another Horse', purely to enjoy the race commentaries that would result. In the end, however, the nags have been leapfrogged by a recent change just up the road at number 252.

This vast stone building was placed on High Holborn in 1914 by the Pearl Assurance Company, who occupied it as their headquarters until 1989. After that it was converted into a luxury hotel, now run by the Rosewood Group. It has everything you'd expect of such an establishment, but also has one extra thing that no other hotel in the world can boast, something the Rosewood's Director of Communications Anna Nash has kindly agreed to show me. We ascend the main marble staircase, then walk along a corridor running parallel to the street outside. Eventually we reach a door and go through it. The room in which we find ourselves contains, among much else, a sofa with 11 cushions, a 52-inch mirror which at the press of a remote by Anna becomes a 52-inch TV, and a huge bowl of apples so highly polished they could take the place of the mirror. Passing through to a bathroom that is a marvel of marble (Italian), we find the bath itself, a steam shower stall, more than one hand basin (sorry, I lost track) and a Toto Neorest combined toilet-and-bidet whose settings, Anna helpfully reads out as I note them down, include 'heated seat', 'massage', 'dryer' and 'power deodoriser'.

Moving through a succession of rooms and corridors (please see earlier apology about losing track), we see walls clad in horsehair tiles, shelves bearing Geneva sound systems, kitchens with immense fridges and Nespresso coffee machines, walk-in closets and beds whose side tables contain specially selected books. Jean-Paul Sartre's *Being and Nothingness* sticks in my mind for some reason. One section of one room is dedicated to British icons – black-and-white photos of Keith Richards and Freddie Mercury (Wembley 1986 incarnation) stare down at us. Anna runs me through the different ways the suite can be configured, depending on how many of the six bedrooms, six bathrooms, three living rooms, one library and one dining room are required. Even within a bedroom there are options available: 'Our Middle Eastern guests often prefer separate beds.'

While we're chatting Anna's phone rings. It's Tom, the hotel's chief butler. As he's nearby (a relative term in a place like this) Anna gets him to call in. Like the doormen downstairs Tom[7] is nattily dressed in a Nicholas Oakwell outfit of dark jacket, grey checked trousers and blue tartan waistcoat. The light-tan Grenson shoes are a nice addition, as is the woollen bow tie.

'Real or pre-knotted?' I ask.

'Real,' says Tom. 'We have pre-knotted ones for especially busy days, but there was time to do the necessary this morning. You have to be able to tie one for guests anyway.' Apparently the best way to learn how to do it for someone else (that is, in reverse) is by practising on your own leg. Tom, it's clear, is exactly what a hotel wants a butler to be – in other words he can be different sorts of butler depending on what the *guest* wants him to be. If I were spending the £25,000 which

---

[7] Early thirties, tops. Forget policemen, when butlers start looking young you're really clocking up the summers.

one night in this suite sets you back, I'd chat with Tom as we're chatting now, possibly moving on to discuss football and cricket results and the merits of various Martin Scorsese films. With another guest, though, you just know he'd be able to give it the full Jeeves. Tom's is a nose that knows when to keep out.

It's also one that knows how to find things. 'One guest asked me to get a new case for her Yves St Laurent sunglasses.' Rest assured, by the way, should you happen to be the 'female pop star' in question, that those three words were the only clue Tom would give me to your identity. I asked more than once. 'You wouldn't believe it, but getting a YSL case in London is trickier than it sounds. The store wouldn't sell us one. None of my contacts anywhere else could help out. It was getting to be a real problem. But eventually, after *lots* of phone calls, I managed to track one down. I got it, brought it up to the suite, went in . . . and the guest was sitting there with half a dozen of them, all lined up. She'd had them all along. It's a test she sets any hotel she stays in, to see if they're up to scratch.'

Impressive as Tom is, however, he's not the reason I'm here. That's something quite different:

WC (London West Central): The Manor House suite at London's Rosewood Hotel is the only hotel suite in the world with its own postcode.

Letters to the rest of the Rosewood, you might wish to note for future correspondence purposes, should have 'WC1V 7EN' at the bottom of their envelopes. If you're writing to a guest in the Manor House suite, however, then you'll need 'WC1V 7DZ'. From what I've seen of Tom he'll be more than happy to do the necessary if you stupidly deploy the wrong option. But it's as well to get these things right in the first place.

The Royal Mail, it should be said, don't go throwing post-codes around like sweets at a pantomime. You need a very good reason for requesting a new one, and as we've seen with the residents of Ilford, Windsor and elsewhere, the Mail are loathe to mess around with their carefully constructed system just because you feel like it. But the Rosewood had a crucial fact on their side when it came to deciding the Manor House's code. Not merely that the suite is vast, but that it has its own entrance from the street. Instead of coming up through the hotel's main gated arch, across its courtyard and through reception as I did today, you can simply slip through a discreet black door at the building's eastern end, which leads directly up to the suite.

Not, Anna explains, that celebrity guests take this route. 'They tend to use the main entrance, because then we can close the gates across the archway and stop the paparazzi following them in.' I guess when you buy your own postcode for the night, you buy the right not to use the door which gave rise to that postcode.

5

QUARRYING FOR FACTS

It isn't often these days, I tend to find, that one gets the chance to conquer a country. Yet that's exactly the opportunity presented to me now. Surveying the map, and letting my gaze drift towards the left, I notice Wales. Only ever been there a couple of times. In fact, thinking about it, it might just be the once. This has to be rectified. Trying not to feel like a dictator surveying possible candidates for invasion, I count how many postcode areas there are in Wales. The answer is six.[1] I could do that in a couple of days. A warm feeling of anticipation spreads over me, which you couldn't say was *entirely* free of dictatorial tendencies, however benevolent they might be. 'How many divisions has the Pope?' asked Stalin. Not that different from 'How many postcodes has Wales?'

Getting across from Suffolk to the Principality will also allow the ticking off of several other areas, though not (unless my navigation goes completely to pot) anything west of Bristol, so I decide to deal with those now. Starting with:

TR (Truro): The Isles of Scilly have the fewest cars per household of any postcode district in the UK.

[1] There are tiny places where a couple of others seep in from England, but essentially it's six.

That's 'district', you'll note, not 'area'. We're talking the sub-divisions here, and TR24 (the Scilly Isles) has only one car for every ten households. Being a rural bunny myself I'm surprised by this: you *need* a car in the sticks. But no, apparently even the biggest island, St Mary's, has very few vehicles – people tend to use golf carts or walk. If you're wondering which district has the most cars, by the way, it's WR7 in Worcester: two per household.

Next comes Plymouth. This could be given to the Royal Citadel, constructed in 1665, with cannons facing both out to sea and into the town as a reminder from Charles II that none of the English should try on him what they did to his father. But instead it goes to a more recent ruler:

PL (Plymouth): Travelling to his holiday home, Harold Wilson replied to a Plymouth newspaper vendor's cry of '*Evening Herald*!' with 'Good evening, my man.'

EX has been done (in fact it was the project's very first fact), so next across it's TQ. Torquay, to a whole generation of sitcom viewers, can mean only one thing. The town was home not only to a certain fictitious hotel, but also to the real-life establishment on which that hotel was based:

TQ (Torquay): It was while staying at the Gleneagles Hotel in Torquay that John Cleese had the idea for *Fawlty Towers*.

The year was 1971. Filming on location in nearby Paignton, the Pythons holed up in the Gleneagles, where the owner, Donald Sinclair, treated them in exactly the same manner as he did all his guests: monstrously. When Terry Gilliam ate his steak in the usual American manner (cut it up, transfer the fork to your right hand, spear the pieces with it), Sinclair spluttered: 'You can't eat like that in *this* country!' Another guest, asking when the next bus into town would arrive, had a timetable thrown at him. Most of the Pythons left in protest after the first night, but John Cleese stayed on, eager to make notes. Eric Idle returned for a briefcase he'd forgotten, only to be told by Sinclair that it was at the bottom of the garden, hidden behind a wall in case it was a bomb. 'We've had some problems with the staff,' he added.[2]

The final area that needs mopping up in this neck of the postal woods is DT, which like Torquay offers us fiction inspired by reality, though in a far more sombre vein. On 9 August 1856, outside Dorchester Prison, Martha Brown became the last woman to be hanged in Dorset. A 16-year-old boy in the crowd remembered the incident years later:

DT (Dorchester): The hanging of Tess in *Tess of the d'Urbevilles* was based on an execution Thomas Hardy witnessed decades before writing the novel.

The writer said he was ashamed to have been there that rainy day. 'I saw – they had put a cloth over the face – how, as the cloth got wet, her features came through it.' He also recalled 'what a fine figure she showed against the sky as she hung in the misty rain, and how the tight black silk gown set off her shape as she wheeled half-round and back.' Hardy's death in 1928 had its own macabre element. He and his family both wanted him buried in Stinsford (near Dorchester), but

---

[2] Latest extract from the Improbable Files: Siegfried Farnon in *All Creatures Great and Small* was based on a different Donald Sinclair.

his executor insisted on Poets' Corner in Westminster Abbey. They compromised: Hardy's heart was buried in Stinsford, his ashes in the Abbey.

As I go about planning my Welsh trip – which will finish with me doing something astonishing in a quarry – there's also time to keep an eye on the news. A story about Birmingham gang violence shows how postcodes can sometimes inspire evil (the warring factions in this case being B6 and B21), so I determine that the city's fact should be a happy one:

B (Birmingham): The name of the 1970s children's TV series *TISWAS*, transmitted from Birmingham, stood for 'This Is Saturday, Watch And Smile'.

Then a newspaper article appears on how embarrassing street names affect property prices. Slag Lane in Wigan, Cock-a-Dobby in Sandhurst, that sort of thing. One of the examples given is a house in Upton-on-Severn, worth £70,000 less than comparable houses simply because it's on Minge Lane. Again, this sort of thing can't be allowed to bring a place down, so I single-handedly rescue the postcode area in question with the cheery little nugget that:

WR (Worcester): The village of Bricklehampton has the longest place name in Britain not to repeat any of its letters.

Fourteen of them. That's a majority of the alphabet. I would pay £70k *over* the odds to live in a place like that.[3]

---

[3] The 'majority' element applies to me too – that was my 62nd fact, and as there are 124 areas in total, from now on I will be nearer the project's end than its beginning.

Beyond the news, normal research continues apace, and often throws up wonderful 'strings' of facts tying several areas together. A football string, for example, starting at Burnley's ground on 12 December 1891. The visitors were local rivals Blackburn Rovers (whose town name would one day give Turf Moor the first two letters of its postcode). The match took place in a snowstorm so severe that by the second half the Rovers players had had enough and walked off, leaving only their goalkeeper:

BB (Blackburn): Abandoned by his team-mates during a match, goalkeeper Herby Arthur simply waited for a member of the opposition to touch the ball and then appealed for offside.

Eventually the referee did what he should have done before the match started: he abandoned it. If this had happened after 1963 the result would have been decided by the Pools Panel. The first week the Panel went into operation a player heard that his team had 'won', and asked his manager for a win bonus. The manager replied that he had been dropped that day. But the Panel wasn't the only thing inspired by snow-affected football:

NE (Newcastle): The windscreen wiper was invented by a Newcastle United fan driving home from London in a blizzard.

Gladstone Adams was even more justified in his misery than the 1891 Blackburn players. At least they suffered the white stuff in December – Adams was driving on 26 April 1908, one day after seeing his team lose the FA Cup Final to Wolves. His journey was punctuated by repeated stops to clear snow from the windscreen. At one point he tried folding the screen down completely, but that led to him getting frozen. Adams vowed that when he got back home he'd do something to solve the problem. And so he did. It's been a while since we encountered a serial inventor, so let us further note that Gladstone Adams also (with the help of his brother) gave us the trafficator, an early version of the indicator.

Hereford United versus Newcastle United in 1972 holds the record as the most weather-disrupted fixture in FA Cup history. The first match was postponed (waterlogged pitch), and then again (snow), before going ahead and resulting in a 2–2 draw. The replay at Hereford's ground was postponed three times (frost), before the non-league home team scored a famous victory over their top-flight visitors on what can only be called a quagmire. But this in itself isn't the fact. Another chapter in Herefordshire's footballing history provides that. In August 1980, a referee's decisions so annoyed the crowd at a Ledbury Town match that one of them ran on to the pitch and confronted the referee. It isn't recorded exactly what happened – the only detail I can find is that the referee's shirt was damaged 'beyond repair'. Now clearly hooliganism can never be condoned, but I do feel that our view of this particular hooligan has to be coloured somewhat by one specific detail about him:

HR (Hereford): Sam Phillips, the Ledbury Town spectator who confronted the referee during a match in August 1980, was, at the time of the incident, 82 years old.

Herefordshire FA, however, saw no reason to treat Mr Phillips any more leniently than they would a younger man, and banned him from attending matches for the rest of the season. As the season had only just started, Ledbury Town viewed this as an unnecessarily harsh sanction. They proposed a compromise in which Mr Phillips would be allowed into the social club, from where he could watch matches through a window. But Herefordshire FA stood firm, threatening to close the club if this happened. In the end Mr Phillips got round the ban by watching matches through a hole in the hedge.

Normally when you hear the words 'motorway' and 'tied up' in the same sentence you cringe. But this sunny April morning, as I head towards Wales, the M40 does me proud. Admittedly I'm only using a short section of it because the M25 is tied up in the conventional sense, but stopping at Beaconsfield services I notice the name 'Hope and Champion'. Rings a bell ... oh yes, it's the country's first motorway service station pub, opened shortly after I visited Watford Gap. Like my train journey to Manchester, this road journey is tying things back to the project's start. Needless to say the dire warnings of pissed motorists have failed to come true: not a single customer is on the booze. Huge fry-ups seem to be the order of the day. And as if to pay tribute to the project, the pub also boasts a sculpture made of horns from old mail coaches.

There's an alarming scene at one of the massive roundabouts on my way towards the M4: somehow a pensioner riding his shopmobility has ended up on it. Whichever exit he takes it's going to be a major road, and if he gets it completely wrong he'll be on the motorway itself. A lorry driver has parked up to shield him from the traffic while they try and work out what to do. You hear about these incidents on the news, but it's the first time I've ever seen it for real. Regularly these days I struggle to remember whether or not I've put sugar in a cup of tea. Is this how I'll end up? To reassure myself that the little grey cells aren't completely frazzled I mentally note the virgin areas I've covered so far this morning:

**EN (Enfield): Labour's victory at the 1997 General
Election was so enormous that Michael Portillo got
through his early television interviews without
anyone guessing he had lost his Enfield Southgate
seat.**

At 10 p.m. Portillo was interviewed down the line from
his constituency by Jeremy Paxman. Although the freshly
published exit poll showed a swingometer-busting victory for
Labour, no one had really got it into their head yet *how* seismic
the win would be. So despite Portillo's on-the-ground information telling him he'd lost, the possibility simply never occurred
to Paxman. He asked Portillo about the national picture, but
to the soon-to-be-ex-minister's relief the question of his own
seat never arose.

**WD (Watford): The lead actress in Britain's first
'talkie' film had to mime her words to another
woman speaking off-camera.**

It was at Elstree Studios in 1929 that Alfred Hitchcock directed *Blackmail*. Anny Ondra, his leading lady from Prague,
had the star quality that Hitchcock wanted, but she also had
a heavy Czech accent that he didn't. In later decades it would
have been simple for another actress to redub her voice. This
is what happened to Ursula Andress in *Dr. No*, for instance.
And while filming *2001: A Space Odyssey*, Keir Dullea, the
actor playing the astronaut Dave, was forced to react not to
the finished voice of the computer HAL (dubbed on later by
a Canadian actor), but to a crew member crouching behind
the set reading out HAL's lines, meaning Dullea heard, 'I'm
sorry, Dave, I'm afraid I can't do that' in broad Cockney.
Back in the 1920s, however, the technology for dubbing didn't

exist. So another actress, Joan Barry, stood on the set reciting the lines, with Ondra having to lip-sync to them in real time. Unsurprisingly this made for a somewhat stilted performance, parts of which you can still enjoy on YouTube.

We could keep the movie link going in the next area, with the fact that the famous Pinewood Studios gong 'hit' at the beginning of every Rank Film was made of papier mâché. Or we could instead cover SL with some information about Eton – perhaps that its old boys include Marwood (the 'I' in *Withnail and I*) and Captain Hook (his final words are '*Floreat Etona*', the school's motto), perhaps that it says 'Establishment' so loudly that plans to attack it were found on the body of a senior al-Qaeda leader killed in Somalia in 2011. But in the end some good old-fashioned silliness gets the vote:

SL (Slough): In 2008, a lorry driver trying to deliver 12 barrels of lager to a pub called the Windsor Castle accidentally delivered them to Windsor Castle.

Or rather he tried to. Staff at the residence knew the beer wasn't for them, and helped the confused driver correct his mistake. 'We have received mail for the royal household here before,' said the pub owner later, 'but I think this is the first time they have received anything meant for us.'

Soon the M4 carries me into RG territory. In keeping with my mode of transport I should probably make this fact the appearance in November 1919, on the Bath Road near Aldermaston, of Britain's first petrol station. Before this you had to buy fuel in cans from chemists. But I can't resist choosing another first instead, because it says something very important about us as a nation:

RG (Reading): The world's first ever text message, sent by a software engineer to the director of Vodafone, read 'Merry Christmas'.

Neil Papworth was the 22-year-old whizzkid. He sent the message on 3 December 1992, from the Reading office of the telecoms firm employed by Vodafone. Richard Jarvis, the recipient, was at his Christmas party at the time, so Papworth decided to make the first ever greeting a seasonal one. And what does this tell us about Britain? Well, compare it with the first ever mobile phone call, which was made by an American. Marty Cooper was vice-president of Motorola, who in 1973 were racing AT&T to develop a workable cell phone. Motorola got there first, a point Cooper proved by going out on to the New York sidewalk and using his new invention to call Joel Engel, his opposite number at AT&T. 'Joel,' he said, the Fifth Avenue traffic audible in the background, 'I'm calling you from a real cellular telephone.' We're pleasant to a colleague, the Americans are unpleasant to a rival. And you thought *you'd* been annoyed by an unwanted phone call.

After this it's SN, and bypassing Swindon itself I leave the motorway and head north for a few minutes to Cowage Farm, near the village of Bremilham. One of the farm's outbuildings now houses Perfection Health and Beauty, though unlike the owner of a breathtakingly pink Mazda MX5 I haven't come to avail myself of their services. Instead I'm interested in a stone structure standing on a raised patch of ground opposite the farmhouse:

SN (Swindon): Bremilham Church is, at 13 feet 1 inch by 11 feet 1 inch, the smallest church in Britain.

It's a peach of a construction, several centuries old and made from blocks of light-coloured sandstone. The roof slopes, and there's a small pointy bit at the front end, about five feet tall, which is obviously meant to pass for a steeple. So it does look churchy – it's just that it's a very small church. After I've walked a lap of it, and am standing back to admire it, I hear a voice from across the yard: 'You can go in if you like – it's open.'

The farmer is an amiable-looking guy in his fifties. When I've put my head round the old wooden door and surveyed the contents – a single pew flat against one wall, a stone font in the corner, a 1970s Bontempi-style electric organ – I walk over to thank him. 'Lovely building, isn't it?'

'Yeah,' he replies. 'We only have the one service a year in it.' This makes sense. 'The villagers gather on the grass outside, the organist sits inside and the vicar stands in the doorway facing out. It's a rogation service, one you hold after you've planted the crops so you can pray for rain.' He pauses. 'It seems to work – it's always pissing down when we have the service.'

The family have a strong bond with the church. 'I was christened there,' says the farmer, 'and so was my sister. My dad is buried there.' He indicates a grave a few yards from the building. 'We've buried loads of pets there over the years, too. Jack Russells, Labradors – even goldfish.'

After this I veer south-west. Before heading into Wales I'm visiting the Somerset village of Mark – a couple of years ago we stumbled across a Barney in Norfolk, and having taken a photograph of my son next to its sign I want the matching one to go with it. This diversion will have the added bonus of ticking off a couple more areas. Before leaving SN, though, I make a point of driving through the nearby hamlet of Tiddleywink. In fairness to the many map companies who omitted it until a 2003 campaign by residents, Tiddleywink doesn't even deserve the name 'hamlet' – it's nothing more than a row of eight cottages on the B4039. One of them was where cattle drovers used to stop for a drink (hence the rhyming-slang name). But if we can't celebrate a bit of nonsense once in a while then what has the world of road atlases come to?

Soon I'm into the next area:

TA (Taunton): When William Wordsworth visited his friend Samuel Taylor Coleridge in Somerset, locals found the two writers' accents so unusual they assumed them to be French spies.

Someone even wrote to the government to report their suspicions, and an agent was dispatched to keep an eye on the pair. He bought into the paranoia wholeheartedly, even mishearing the name Spinoza (Wordsworth and Coleridge were discussing the philosopher) as 'Spy Nosey'. Thankfully the residents of Somerset are more laid-back these days. At least none of those in Mark come out to make notes as I take a photo of myself by their village sign. Turning north again I pass a cottage being renovated with scaffolding from a firm in a nearby cathedral city: they rejoice in the name Tubular Wells. Then there's a hitchhiker whose acoustic guitar, peaked cap and bum fluff reassure you that some clichés will never die. His cardboard sign says 'Bristol', a reminder that there's another fact to be recorded:

BS (Bristol): The village of Rodney Stoke is a 'Thankful Village', denoting that none of its residents were killed in the First World War.

Such was the carnage that there are just 53 Thankful Villages in England and Wales, and none in Scotland or Ireland.

Of these, 14 are Doubly Thankful, meaning they lost no one in the Second World War either. It so happens that one of those 14 is the Gloucestershire village of Upper Slaughter. In France, meanwhile, the distinction is even rarer: only one village in the entire country – Thierville, not far from Rouen – got through the First World War with all its residents intact.

Finally I rejoin the M4, which rises high and proud to become the Severn Bridge. This carries you over the estuary of the same name into the only country in the world (other than Bhutan) with a dragon on its flag. One of the first things you pass in Wales is Celtic Manor, the golf resort which hosted the 2010 Ryder Cup. Vexillology pedants will be pleased to note that its flag is being flown correctly – in other words the dragon is facing the flagpole. This, the first of the Welsh post-code areas, is NP, for Newport. It's home to the Pot Noodle (155 million pots produced near Crumlin every year), a street in Caerleon which shows how militant the Welsh can be in their dislike of consonants – spelled Ffwrrwm, it's pronounced 'furrum' – and the Blorenge, a large hill which disproves the old 'fact' about nothing rhyming with 'orange'. In 1912 NP, in the form of Blackwood near Caerphilly, was home to Artie Moore, an early Welsh radio enthusiast. During the small hours of 15 April he picked up a faint Morse code message from a ship calling for help. 'Come at once,' it read. 'We have struck an iceberg.' He reported it to local police, who refused to believe him, despite the authentic detail that the message used the recently introduced 'SOS' rather than the traditional 'CQD'.[4] Only when newspapers reported the sinking of the *Titanic* a couple of days later was Moore vindicated.

But the fact that takes the title relates to a resident of The Hendre, a large country house near Monmouth:

[4] The first two letters short for 'sécurité', the last for 'distress'.

NP (Newport): Charles Rolls, the partner of Henry Royce, was the first British person killed in an aeroplane accident.

Rolls was, of course, a keen motorist. In 1896, at the age of 18, he travelled to Paris to buy a Peugeot Phaeton, this being only the third car ever in Wales. When the Duke of York visited The Hendre in 1900 Rolls took him for a drive, probably the first time the future George V had ever been in a car. But it was his love of flying that did for him. In July 1910 his plane crashed during a display at Bournemouth, earning Rolls his unhappy distinction.

A little further along the motorway is my first actual stop in Wales, the place I'll be spending the night: Cardiff. The dragons are out in force here too, Welsh flags cracking along the length of St Mary Street, where my hotel (the Royal) is to be found and which, like many of the city centre streets, is pedestrianised. The first big surprise is how bang-in-the-middle-of-things the Millennium Stadium is, only a couple of streets away from the hotel. The second is how international Cardiff feels. The girl on reception at the Royal is French, the waitress in the Italian restaurant where I eat is Polish, and with all the tourists and students milling about a native accent is relatively rare. You do hear them, of course, but – to quote an Australian assistant I'll encounter in Waterstone's tomorrow morning – 'even the Welsh people here don't sound that Welsh'. As ever the untruths can be so easily believed. Nationalists hog the headlines, and a Welsh comedian I once heard used the line that 'in my country it doesn't matter if a person is young or old, male or female – we're all... cousins'. Yet on the ground Cardiff, whose centre is much the same size as Belfast, feels a million times more cosmopolitan.

Its statues of homegrown heroes are being shown some

disrespect. John Batchelor, the nineteenth-century politician, has the lower part of his plinth used as an obstacle by skateboarders, though as his nickname was 'the Friend of Freedom' he probably wouldn't mind. Aneurin Bevan, meanwhile, has been dissed by many hundreds of pigeons in the way they know best. Poor chap. Perhaps the birds are channelling the ghost of Bevan's great Labour party rival Ernest Bevin – when someone opined that Bevan was 'his own worst enemy', Bevin replied: 'Not while I'm around he ain't.'

Repairing to the Duke of Wellington, I sample the local stout, disconcertingly named so that you drink a pint of Brains (the taste more than makes up for that). In the corner a Chinese man in his fifties and a local woman at least 20 years younger engage in a tense and (on her part) frequently tearful discussion. There is much holding of hands, and faces are rarely more than a few inches apart. My guess would be tutor and student. He manages to talk her down from a full-on monsoon, and they leave hand in hand. I, for what it's worth, wouldn't trust him as far as a gnat could throw him.

Walking back to the hotel I pass an enormous seagull attacking a hunk of bread with quite terrifying force. Turning in for the night I put my pocketful of change on the bedside table, and reflect that the coins have come home. Llantristant, north of here in the inland part of CF, is where the Royal Mint is located. It makes not only Britain's non-note currency but that of many other countries too: one in seven coins around the world started life here. If that isn't an international postcode area I don't know what is.

You can't help wondering what Captain Scott would have thought of the bees.

The Royal's breakfast room has a small display at one end, commemorating the fact that the room was the venue for Scott's farewell dinner before heading south to what would ultimately be his snowy demise. A society recreates the dinner every year, says a note, 'but has cut down the number of courses from eleven to seven'. Wimps. Up on the roof, meanwhile, a recently installed hive is continuing the trend, popular in several British cities, for urban beekeeping. The hotel's reservations manager, whose first rather than last name is Scott, kindly shows me the creatures. There are getting on for 20,000 of them, and if all goes to plan they will by the summer be producing honey for the hotel's tables. Scott tells me about the 'waggle dance', the coded signal given by returning bees to their colleagues to indicate the direction and distance of nearby flowers. Then he closes up the hive again. It has the room number 6B (geddit?).

Down at street level, avoiding the busker whose 'Stairway to Heaven' fares even worse than Led Zep managed in Belfast, I head for Cardiff Bay. A mile or so south of the city centre, this is a throbbing, multi-caféd leisure destination. A wall has been set aside as a shrine to Ianto Jones, a character in the Doctor Who spin-off *Torchwood*, which was both set and filmed in Cardiff. Notes, drawings and poems have been pinned here by fans distraught at Jones's death, many of them directing their ire at the show's writer Russell T. Davies. 'According to RTD,' writes one, '"just 9 hysterical women" are campaigning to save Ianto Jones ... Don't some of those "women" look rather large in the trouser department?' Ianto, who was gay, has become an icon. 'You say People should accept the homosexuality as such as normal thing,' runs another note, 'but how can we ... when you don't give us the chance to see it?'

A thirty-something couple are reading the messages. He stands back to take a photo. 'Do you want to get in the shot?'

'No,' comes her reply. 'I can cope with not being in the shot.' Something tells me their relationship might not have the most straightforward of futures.

The Welsh Assembly and Wales Millennium Centre both overlook the bay, and are fantastic modern buildings, but for Cardiff's fact we head back into town to a much older building:

CF (Cardiff): Britain's first ever mosque, founded by Yemeni and Somali sailors, was registered as a place of worship in 1860.

It's still there today, now known as the Al-Manar Islamic and Cultural Centre, the final couple of houses in Glynrhondda Street, a Victorian terrace a few minutes' walk from the city centre. Made of the same dark stone and slate as the rest of the dwellings, these two have a banner across their front asking 'Have you discovered Islam?' It's quiet this Thursday morning, no one entering or leaving the building. Those sailors, establishing the mosque for use on their trips between Aden and Cardiff Docks, would surely be amazed to learn that a century and a half later it would be inviting people to 'come inside and speak to us ... ask a question, express a thought or request literature'. Walking back to the city centre I see a young Muslim woman selling the *Big Issue*. The cover asks 'Is Britain really a Christian nation?' Handing over my money I notice that several of the woman's fingers are missing. 'Thank you, sir,' she says. 'Have a happy Easter.' The article inside mentions that whenever he left 10 Downing Street, Tony Blair packed a Bible in his luggage.

I continue reading the piece as I take one last tour of the city centre, the tour that includes Waterstone's and the revelation from their signs that the Welsh for 'Popular Science' is 'Gwyddoniaeth Boblogaidd', while that for 'Self Help' is 'Hunangymorth'. I don't know which country that woman came from, or how she lost her fingers, but Blair's Bible and those sailors in the 1860s and the frisson of ambivalence set off in me when she said 'Happy Easter' all combine together, and I know which way I'm leaning on the *Big Issue*'s question.

I do hope the residents of Port Talbot will forgive me, but the overriding thought that hits you as the M4 carries you past their town – comprising, it would appear, about seven houses and a billion factories, chimneys, yards and smoke-emitting pipes – is that you can totally understand why Anthony Hopkins lives in California.

Mind you, to be fair to both 'Puttulbutt' and the boy who left here as soon he could, you have to say that this whole region has struggled with the effects of industry. Swansea and its surrounding areas were known in the nineteenth century as 'Copperopolis' – they supplied 60 per cent of the planet's requirements for the metal, landing themselves with some of the worst air and soil pollution *on* that planet. Dylan Thomas said his birthplace of Swansea was an 'ugly lovely town'. Based on my brief visit today I'd say he was half right. If Cardiff is a city people come to, Swansea feels like one they depart from. Not just Thomas himself, not just Catherine Zeta-Jones,[5] but anyone, it seems, with any spark of life. The Welsh accents are thicker than in the capital, so thick they feel like a trap holding residents in place. I don't see many smiles in Swansea. A couple enter Tesco, the woman walking behind her man, talking to his back: 'She enjoys spending time with him? But she doesn't feel as though she's in love with him? There's a difference?' He carries on walking. I can see now why a recent local news story earned the column inches it did: 'Llwchwr Town Council is considering getting a colour photocopier...'

[5] Born here on the very day her future husband was celebrating his twenty-fifth birthday.

Local newspaper desperation, admittedly, can strike anywhere. Within the last couple of months Hertfordshire's Woolmer Green has had 'Village hall cooker to be cleaned more often', while north of here there was 'Thieves broke into a Mid Wales football club's refreshments hut and stole two packets of crisps. The incident happened at Newtown Football Club's Latham Park ground between 7 p.m. on February 26th and 10 a.m. the following day. Dyfed-Powys Police said anybody with information should call 101.'

Swansea's cityscape provides as little inspiration as its people. A statue of industrialist Sir Henry Vivian records that he chose the title Baron Swansea of Singleton. A huge wall overlooking a car park is adorned with the slogan 'More poetry is needed', conceptual artist Jeremy Deller's contribution to Swansea's 'Art Across the City' programme. If this is how he feels, he could just have put up a poem. Deciding it's time to move on, I head for Llanelli. Early signs as the town centre looms aren't encouraging. There's 'Dolled Up – Beauty by Catherine, Hair by Heather', then a pub offering 'Mobility Parking Valet Service'. The same establishment has a hand-written sign in the window announcing that 'As from today this premise is now open from 10 a.m. every morning.' To aid the explanation a clock has been drawn underneath: its hands point to 11 a.m. A nearby business offers 'Dog, Cat and Small Furies Grooming'. They specialise in 'Anal Glands'. It's at this point that I abort the town centre plan.

I head instead for the Millennium Coastal Park. This is to the west of Llanelli, one of whose sons never gets the recognition he deserves:

SA (Swansea): Boxing's Marquess of Queensberry Rules weren't written by the Marquess of Queensberry.

The rules are one of the two things for which the aristocrat is famous. The other was Oscar Wilde's downfall – the Marquess's son, Lord Alfred Douglas, was 'Bosie', the playwright's boyfriend, a state of affairs with which the Marquess was far from happy. The card he left at Wilde's club, over which Wilde foolishly sued for libel, showed Llanelli-like levels of spelling: 'For Oscar Wilde, posing as somdomite'.[6] But the Marquess didn't write the boxing rules, he only endorsed them. In reality they were the work of John Graham Chambers. Getting a tea from the Millennium Coastal Park's café, I retire to the beach overlooking the Loughor estuary and consult my notes about Chambers. Born in 1843 into an eminent local family, after Eton he went up to Cambridge, where a lifetime of sporting associations began. He competed in the 1862 and 1863 Boat Races, losing both times, then coached the crews in 1865 and 1866, again failing to win. Undaunted, he returned to coach Cambridge from 1871 to 1874, this time putting together four straight victories. They included, in 1873, one of those ideas that seem so obvious you wonder why it took so long: sliding seats.

Chambers was also a founder of the Amateur Athletic Association, helped stage the FA Cup Final and the Thames Regatta, rowed alongside the first man to swim the English Channel (Matthew Webb, 1875), established championships in billiards, cycling and wrestling, and was at one point English champion walker. But it's his contribution to the 'sweet science' that fascinates me. He drafted the rules which, with a few alterations, still define modern boxing, yet merely because someone with a higher social ranking endorsed them,

---

[6] Wilde's own epistolary habits were lazy – after writing a letter and putting a stamp on the envelope, he would throw it out of the window on to the pavement, knowing someone would assume it had been dropped and so pick it up and post it for him.

Chambers's name has been written out of the annals. His code introduced gloves (rule 8), three-minute rounds with a minute between them (rule 3), and the ten-second count (rule 4). Indeed that rule is my favourite, because of its contribution to the English language. The floored contestant didn't just have to 'get up unassisted' within the ten seconds, he also had to 'come to the scratch', a mark in the middle of the ring. This is where the phrase 'up to scratch' originated.

A look at the map reveals that the scenery is going to improve from here on. Having followed the bottom of Wales, I'm now halting my westwards progress and heading north into the country's centre. The map also tells you that there are some serious hills up there, a few even earning the name 'mountain'. Before the terrain really opens out, though, I pass through the town of Gorseinon, where a van belongs to a tree-stump removal firm called Conifers From Hell. Then there's a golf club whose Welsh flag is at half-mast. I don't know who's moved on to the great fairway in the sky, but rather than having the flag halfway down the pole the original convention was to fly it one flag's height from the top, leaving 'room' above for death's flag.

After this the really wild stuff begins. The rock-strewn hills get ever higher, and some very sturdy mountain ponies work hard at their grazing. A shaggy black cow scratches its neck on a barbed-wire fence, and there are plenty of sheep that redefine the term 'hardy'. Given the slopes they have to deal with it's a miracle they're not all gathered in one huge woolly ball at the bottom of the valley. Surely if you switch off for a second gravity would catch you unawares? It'd be a long way down, too – at one point the climb causes my ears to pop.

A few miles before Brecon, below me and to the left, the Cray Reservoir appears, built at the beginning of the twentieth century to supply water to Swansea. It had to be sited this far north to avoid the pollution of 'Copperopolis'. Then, in the town of Brecon itself, I note that as well as a High Street there's a High Street Superior and a High Street Inferior. The town also has an estate agent's called James Dean. A tiny dot between the two names is your clue that the business was established by David James and Adam Dean – but still, you'd think they might have reversed the order.

The 'winding along a road halfway up a valley' journey keeps reminding me of the opening credits from *The Shining*.[7] The film stays in mind as I pull into the small spa town of Llandrindod Wells and find, overlooking the triangular green at its centre, the Metropole Hotel. Not that the establishment resembles its fictional counterpart the Overlook either in terms of remoteness (as I say, it's bang in the middle of town) or atmosphere: everyone is very welcoming, and not once do I see imaginary twin girls blocking the corridors or blood gushing out of the lifts. No, it's the size of the place: the Metropole is very big indeed for the size of town it's in, a five-storey Victorian job with several wings and more than one turret. Branching off reception are a large lounge area, the main restaurant and steps down to the gym, swimming pool and health spa. A corridor leads through to the rear section of the hotel, which contains the enormous breakfast room and several function rooms. As I check in (for this is where tonight will be spent) I notice a door marked 'BBC' with a lightbulb above it.

'Is that a studio?' I ask.

'Yes,' says the receptionist. 'The Beeb use it for down-the-line interviews with anyone near here. It's cheaper than them having their own building.'

---

[7] This in turn reminds me that the set assistant at Elstree whose job it was to polish Jack Nicholson's axe – not a euphemism – was a young Simon Cowell, a fact even more unsettling than the movie itself.

Talk about being the centre of the community. In fact the hotel's character and history are the reason I've picked it. Now run by the fifth generation of the same family, the Metropole is a fascinating reminder that history is never just a collection of facts, it's made up of people – the things they've done, the ways they've behaved. Until the hotel appeared on the project's radar, LD belonged to Henry de Winton. He was Rector of Llandrindod Wells in 1893, keen for his flock to attend the town's new church. But they stubbornly insisted on using the old one, as well as the church in nearby Cefnllys. De Winton, therefore, simply took the roofs off the other two churches. Stubbornness continued, and de Winton had to concede defeat: the roofs went back on. The rector has also been defeated in the fact stakes: LD now goes to Elizabeth Miles. It was she who bought this hotel in 1897. Originally founded in 1872, it was then known as the Bridge. The previous owners had levelled the lawns opposite so a circus could perform there every year. On one visit the circus's lioness escaped, making her way into the Bridge's bar before being recaptured.

Miles, widowed with two sons at just 24, expanded the business to cater for the ever-increasing number of tourists visiting Llandrindod in order to take the waters and enjoy the scenery. By 1923 the Bridge could sleep 250 guests, making it the largest hotel in Wales. Miles also changed the name, though not for any reason involving marketing experts or focus groups:

LD (Llandrindod Wells): The Metropole Hotel in Llandrindod Wells got its name because the owner bought a job lot of cutlery and china monogrammed with the initial 'M'.

The stuff came from Norfolk, where a hotel whose name began with 'M' was selling off its old stock. This proves that

Elizabeth wasn't averse to travelling long distances for a bargain, but when she got back home her sons pointed out the obvious problem. Brooking no nonsense, Miles replied that they would simply change the name of the hotel to match the china. Bedrooms were also sized to match the carpet she'd bought, rather than the other way round. This was an advantage a few generations down the line, when en-suite facilities had become de rigueur: the bedrooms were so large that it was no trouble at all to add bathrooms into the same space.

Stewardship of the hotel now resides with Justin Baird-Murray, Elizabeth's great-great-grandson. He joins me for a drink as I'm finishing dinner in the restaurant (Welsh lamb – I've tried not to think about all the cute ones I drove past this afternoon). Justin's in his late forties, tall and lean, well-spoken (English accent rather than Welsh) and with an enthusiasm for his job that, had it been shared by the owner of the Gleneagles in Torquay, would have deprived us of *Fawlty Towers*.

'I feel like I know you already,' I say, mentioning the photos of Justin included in the 'Timeline' display running along one of the ground-floor corridors, documenting the hotel's past.

'I know,' he says. 'I suppose it's strange having your life on public display, but I don't mind. Like that shot of me as a young boy in the old outdoor swimming pool: it's nice to be part of something that everyone in the town remembers. Most of them from the 1950s through to the 1970s learned to swim in that pool.' There's also a copy of *Caterer and Hotelkeeper* magazine, its front cover showing Justin holding his newborn daughter as he stands next to his father David. 'It looks like he's tiny in that photo. He wasn't, but for some reason they wanted me to stand on a box.'

Justin breaks off as the waiter comes across. 'I'll have a bottle of lager please, Vaughan,' he says.

'You must have to watch it in this job,' I say, 'what with all the socialising. I dare say it'd be easy to end up drinking too much.'

He nods his agreement. 'We named the bar after my great-uncle Spencer – let's say it was his favourite room in the hotel. Didn't make him the easiest person for my father to work with. But it did make for some interesting parties.'

The restaurant is very busy, so to ease pressure on tables Justin and I move through to the lounge area. Sitting down we notice a pound coin on the floor.

'If ever I need a bit of change I do a sweep of the sofas in here,' says Justin. 'You wouldn't believe how much money you find in them. It's a nice second wage packet for the cleaners.'

'I've heard that the cleaners at Studio 54 in New York used to get high from all the cocaine lying around when they did the hoovering.'

'Hmm. Not sure we can match them on that front.'

We talk about the hotel's history, much of it documented in the Timeline. There's the photo of Elizabeth Miles herself, wearing a hat which (to borrow from the project's theme) deserves its own postcode – I can see how she brought the force of her personality to bear on the hotel. There's the price list from the 'Hydro', an early spa specialising in hydro-electric baths: 'Special precautions have been adopted in order to prevent the slightest possibility of earth shocks, which previously constituted a grave objection to the use of these otherwise most efficient modes of Electrical treatment.' Justin also mentions the Monte Carlo Rally of 1958, which used the Metropole as its headquarters for an overnight stop (in those days the rally headed towards Monaco from different parts of Europe). 'The great Raymond Baxter of the BBC did his commentary from our Wedgewood Room. He started with "I'm reporting from the third coldest place in the world – there's the North Pole, the

South Pole and the Metropole in Llandrindod Wells." The days before central heating, of course. Once upon a time every one of the rooms had its own chimney. Incredible to think of that now.'

In 1971 the hotel's exterior colour was changed from white to green to match the ivy. 'By then it had completely covered the building, so the paint was chosen to blend in with it. That ivy was a nightmare. Bats used to live in it, and they'd get into the hotel . . . Horrendous. We still keep the outside green to this day. We've got rid of the bats, though, thank God.' Justin cites the most recent paint-job as the sort of thing which only happens because the hotel is family-run. 'It cost a lot of money, but we wanted to do it. If we were part of a chain head office would be saying "Really? Can we justify this money? Exactly how many extra guests are we going to get because of it?"'

The fact that the hotel is still in the family, it might be argued, is due to the Peugeot car company. 'It was 1988,' says Justin. 'I'd left home a couple of years earlier and gone to live in London. I was working for a wine merchant, hadn't got any grand plans or anything, and my father called. "Do you want to come back to the hotel? I'll give you a Peugeot 205 GTi 1.9." That was it – I was back here like a shot. It shows how little I'd thought about what I was going to do in life, whether or not I'd come back here – all it took to get my attention was that car.' He smiles at the memory. 'It was a great car, though. That 205 was *the* hot hatch of the year.'

Guests are constantly passing us, heading to and from the restaurant, and Justin exchanges the odd word with regulars. Running a hotel must be a great education in human nature, I say.

'You could say that. You do see the same patterns repeating themselves. Anniversaries, for instance – they're always the biggest cause of complaints. It's Special Occasionitis. There's such a huge pressure of expectation, but the truth is it's just another day, just another meal. That's why people can blow up. Plus of course there's the thing of "Am I annoyed about the hotel or am I annoyed because I've been married to this person for ten years?"'

The job also hones your diplomatic skills. 'We've had all sorts of scenarios,' says Justin. 'Wives turning up when their husband is upstairs with another woman, you name it. You learn what to say and what not to say, let's put it that way.' The pressure can be all the greater because Justin lives on-site, in a room at the top of the hotel. 'I go away regularly for a few days at a time, to get away from it all. You have to. Otherwise you'd go mad.'

You can tell that, at heart, Justin loves the task of carrying his family's legacy into the twenty-first century. 'There's always something going on. Like a while back someone got in touch and told us he'd found a voucher from thirty-five years ago for a weekend stay at the hotel. He'd won it in a competition or something. We thought it'd make a nice story, so we honoured it, and he turned the weekend into a big family gathering – it was lovely. When he left we gave him another voucher redeemable in another thirty-five years.'

As we finish our chat Justin drains his lager, which reminds him about great-uncle Spencer. 'The rep from the brewery came to see him once, around the time bottled lager was being introduced. He had a crate of it with him, which he left when he went off on his rounds so Spencer could try a bottle or two. When he got back he found Spencer had polished the lot off, the entire crate. Of course being him it hadn't had the slightest effect. "This stuff's like water," he said. "It'll never catch on, you know."'

The third day of the trip starts with the knowledge that it will contain a British record and a European one. What I don't know yet is that it will also contain two revelations.

A word on the records, before we start: I won't be setting them. Rather I'll be encountering them. But still, they'll feel pretty special, involving as they both do a spectacular descent. Before I get to them, however, there's more climbing to be done, as the road north from Llandrindod Wells leads ever upwards, winding through the mountains. And it really is 'winding' at points: the road markings repeatedly teach me that the Welsh for 'slow' is '*araf*'. Come to think of it, signwriters in Wales must be minted – *everything* is in both languages. A big Amazon warehouse near Swansea yesterday was announced as both 'Amazon Park' and '*Parc Amazon*'. The park-and-ride service came out as '*Parcio a Theithio*', prompting memories of the Spanish newsreaders on *The Fast Show*.

Within a few miles LD has given way to SY, the area which takes its name from a town over the national border: Shrewsbury. There are possible facts from both countries. Shrewsbury itself contains St Chad's Church, where you can find the gravestone of Ebenezer Scrooge. Don't get excited, though – it's a prop still in place from the Muppets' *A Christmas Carol*. The English bit of SY also gives us Ruyton-XI-Towns, the only place name in Britain containing a capital 'X' – it's pronounced 'Eleven', Ruyton having once been the major town of that many – and the village of Knockin, whose store is called The Knockin Shop.[8] The Welsh sector offers Borth, inspiration for Morrissey's 'Everyday Is Like Sunday', and Aberystwyth, home to the underground tunnel where the contents of the National Library of Wales were stored during the Second World War. The same tunnel, if rumours are to be believed, also housed the Crown Jewels, though the authorities

---

[8] Both places came to my attention via the excellent blog of Rob Ainsley, who undertakes rhyming cycle tours – Barmouth to Yarmouth, Barrow to Jarrow, Poole to Goole and so on.

have never confirmed it. They do confirm that the jewels were moved from the Tower of London, but won't say where. Seventy years after the event this seems to be taking secrecy a tad far.

Unable in the end to adjudicate between the two countries, I sit on the fence. Or, more precisely, on the national border:

SY (Shrewsbury): A pub in the village of Lla-nymynech allowed Sunday drinking in its two English bars but not in its Welsh one.

The Lion sat right on the border, meaning that different licensing laws applied to different parts of the building. The Shropshire magistrates who oversaw the English section were happy for customers to make merry on the Lord's day. Their Montgomeryshire counterparts, however, insisted that Sundays remain dry. Sadly this beautiful anomaly has come to an end: the Lion has closed. The border still splits the village, though. Different councils collect the bins, and different police forces keep the peace.

The terrain gets more impressive by the mile now. Cloud shadows move slowly across the moss-covered mountainsides, and occasionally a rock-strewn river gurgles alongside the road. There's a village called Clatter. Further north, between Mallwyd and Dolgellau, the walkers appear, many in their fifties and sixties using those big long poles you can't believe do anything but which obviously must. Then, past Dolgellau, tall, straight pines tower over the road, and as I've now reached the Irish Sea, the water glistening in the sunshine on my left combines with the trees to give everything an almost Californian feel. That might sound silly, but this west coast really does feel like the West Coast. And that's the day's first revelation: this bit of the Principality is astoundingly beautiful. It must be an expectations thing. Heading to the very north of Scotland for the first time I looked forward to the incredible mountains everyone had raved about. Yet they were a disappointment. Impressive, yes, but not mind-blowing. It's the same when you finally get round to watching a classic film: it can't possibly live up to the decades of rave reviews. Here, on the other hand, in the geographically more modest of England's immediate neighbours – the one that emphasises its valleys rather than the mountains that form them – I've had a very pleasant surprise precisely because I had no expectations.

Soon I'm into Barmouth, a proper little seaside town popular with people from the West Midlands. One of its cafés is called the Carousel, though as they misspelled it and then the 'C' fell off you're confronted with the Arousal. After this the route heads due north along the coast, with nothing to protect it against the wind blowing in from the sea. Many of the trees accept the inevitable and grow at a 45-degree angle. There are plenty more tourists in the next town along, Harlech. They've got more peaceful intentions than the one who built Harlech's castle in 1286 (Edward I – he was invading at the time). The lie of the land has changed, too: originally next to the sea, the castle now sits half a mile from the shore, because this part of Britain is gradually rising again after being weighed down during the Ice Age.

I've made a point of coming through Harlech to encounter the first of the day's record breakers. One of the roads leading down from the centre of the town is the steepest in Britain, a brakepad-threatening 40 per cent. It isn't immediately clear which one, however – there's lots of steepness round here generally – so I park up and investigate on foot. Inquiries reveal that it's Ffordd pen Llech, a narrow lane starting next to an Indian restaurant and winding down past a few small houses to shore level. I don't know *why* you'd build a home on a slope like this, unless it was for the guarantee that the only passing traffic will be your neighbours and idiots like me. A sign at the top confirms the 40 per cent gradient (though as it's a standard red triangle one the black silhouetted slope looks hopefully inadequate), while the one underneath offers another Welsh lesson: '*Anaddas i fodur*' means 'unsuitable for motors'. However my informant, a resident of a nearby street that's a mere 25 per cent, has assured me that it is indeed legal to drive down it. In fact you used to be allowed to drive *up* it too. Having acquainted myself on foot with the lane's early stages, I retrieve the car. The 'I've run up Britain's steepest road' boast seems too good to resist, so for the last few yards I do just that. Even this is enough to put me out of breath, and a couple walking slightly ahead of me get completely the wrong idea. They step swiftly to one side. The 'drive' down the lane is, of course, nothing of the sort: the accelerator doesn't feature at all, the steering wheel sees plenty of service as the twists are negotiated, and the brakes only get lifted completely when I'm almost at the bottom. Still, I can now claim that I have successfully tackled a British record.

There's another record with links to LL (for Llandudno's is the postcode area in which we now find ourselves). It is, in its way, the opposite of my downhill exploit. Not far from here is Mount Snowdon, on which Edmund Hillary and his team practised for their 1953 ascent of Everest. (Overlooking Blaenau, which I drive through, are some massively intimidating slate-covered mountains. You couldn't be big-headed if you lived here.) Hillary's rehearsal could itself have been the LL fact. As could the gold nugget from which the current Queen's wedding ring was made, mined near Dolgellau. Or Edward II, born in the castle his dad built after the one at Harlech – Caernarfon – and who grew up to pay a 'tumbler' 20 shillings every time he fell off a horse purely for the King's amusement. Then there's the Menai suspension bridge, its U-shaped girders inspiring Samuel Fox to invent the collapsible umbrella. But in the end, LL goes to another fact, the day's second record and one with which I'm about to become intimately acquainted:

LL (Llandudno): A disused slate quarry near Bethesda houses the fastest zipwire in Europe.

The Penryhn quarry was a record-breaker even before Zipworld got their hands on it. Once the world's largest slate quarry – it's a mile long and 1,200 feet deep, meaning you could stand the Shard in it with 200 feet to spare – Penryhn also hosted the longest industrial dispute in British history, the workers downing tools on 22 November 1900 and not picking them up again for another three years. To show solidarity, a firm in Ashton-under-Lyme sent the strikers a Christmas pudding weighing two and a half tonnes.

Jo has referred to my adventure today as the 'deathslide'. She claims it was a slip, but that would surely be a Freudian one, so I'd rather believe she said it deliberately. You can see her point, mind you. When I first read about Zipworld at home I reported my findings.

'You go at a *hundred* miles an hour!'

'Don't be stupid,' said Jo. 'That can't be right.'

I returned to the website. 'No – look – a hundred miles an hour. The wire's a mile long.'

'Are you sure?'

And so on. Only now, as I leave the road to Bethesda and drive down a dirt track to the quarry entrance, does the scale of the place become clear. Getting out of my car, I hear a buzzing sound not unlike that of a light aircraft. Looking up I see the zipwires high above. There are two, side by side. Way in the distance, on the far side of the quarry, each of the wires has a red dot on it. The buzzing gets louder and the dots get bigger until you see that each is a person, jump-suited and suspended from the wire horizontally, face-down, head-first. They zoom overhead, getting smaller and quieter again until they reach the end of the wire way to our left. At least I assume they do – it's too far away to make out against the mountains rising behind the quarry. All of a sudden my stomach relocates slightly.

In the small reception hut are photos of previous visitors, including Ant and Dec. For once they're breaking their golden rule – Dec is standing on the left, Ant on the right. On TV and in publicity shots it's always the other way round. The rule even extends to their houses – they live on the same road, with Ant's house to the left of Dec's.[9] Once I'm suited up I join the dozen or so other people in my group, and we're led to the start of the Little Zipper. This is another pair of wires, which the curve of the quarry's side has hidden from us, and which provide a 'break you in gently' start to the experience. A humble third of a mile long, and running diagonally underneath the Big Zipper, this ride takes you down to the bottom of the quarry. The way it works is very simple: you lie face down on a platform, the staff attach the back of your suit to a metal bracket whose wheels run along the wire, then they simply let go. You don't have to do anything, just lie forward and think of Wales, in particular the part of it that's flying past 70 feet below you. No sooner have you had time to take on board that it's all going to be OK, and that the wire's 'dip in the middle' trajectory means you're now heading slightly upwards and therefore slowing down, than the staff member waiting on the platform at the other end is reaching up to

[9] This is not a joke. It might be a coincidence, but it's not a joke.

shake your hand. It's impossible not to say 'pleased to meet you'. Keeping hold of your hand they then pull you along to a part of the platform that rises up mechanically to meet you and take your weight. Unclip, stand up, job done.

We all say how enjoyable it was, what a breeze, literally. Then we climb into the back of an open-sided lorry ready to be driven right to the top of the quarry. Passing huge boulders and discarded pieces of slate, the vehicle grinds its way slowly up the twisting track. The ride, we have been warned, will take twenty minutes. For most of this the inside of the quarry itself isn't visible, only the mounds of earth surrounding it. We chat happily to each other, having almost forgotten what we're here for. Then the driver rounds yet another bend, slows down and comes to a halt. Looking out of the truck's right-hand side we finally see the quarry again. We're directly underneath the wires of the Big Zipper, still with a hundred feet or so to climb but high enough for the view to silence all conversation. After a few seconds someone finally says something. It begins with 'F'. The longer of the two rides, it now hits us, is an entirely different beast from its junior sibling. My stomach goes on further manoeuvres.

Up at the top banter resumes, but this time it's rather more forced. No one wants to watch the wires stretching a mile across the yawning chasm, or the figures queuing up to ride them, but somehow no one seems able *not* to watch them. Even though we know that in principle we're only going to repeat what we did on the first ride, the scale of it all makes it a very different prospect. For the first section of the ride we won't be too far above the ground, but then the quarry suddenly opens out. OK, the wires themselves have dipped by that point, but we'll still be 500 feet above the large lake which these days fills the bottom of the pit. The water is beautiful, a shimmering turquoisey-blue. It's just the height from which we'll be studying it that gives us pause for thought.

Soon, perhaps too soon for some of us, our group has made its way to the platform, and the first pair are trussed up. Before each duo is released the staff make walkie-talkie contact with their counterparts at the far end, checking that all is in order and we're good to go. Then with a '3 ... 2 ... 1' the safety cables are released and the ride begins. Awaiting my turn I chat to one of the staff.

'Do you ever get people backing out at this stage?'

She nods. 'One or two. But if I'm up here I *really* try not to let them. You know they'll always regret it.'

'How do you persuade them?'

'Talk to them calmly, remind them of all the safety features. Then if that doesn't work...' A mischievous smile plays on her lips. She doesn't say any more. Am I imagining it, or was that slight movement a mime of pushing someone towards the edge?

Eventually it's my turn. I lie on the platform, gazing out across the quarry as the clips go on and the walkie-talkies crackle. Then the numbers descend, the cable clicks and I'm away. The ground rushes by beneath, then after 20 seconds falls away leaving me high above the water...

...which is when the day's other revelation arrives. I'm waiting for the speed to pick up – timing the previous riders revealed that you complete the mile in about a minute, implying an average of 60 mph – but it doesn't feel as though I've reached even that speed yet, never mind the promised ton. The longer nature of this second ride, however, means you have time to think things through. Only now do you work out that with everything so far away – the sides of the quarry as well as its floor – you don't have anything to measure your speed against. Yes, it feels fast, but not like 100 mph on the motorway, where other cars and the crash barriers are only a few feet away. A phrase from the Zipworld website comes back to you, one you didn't really notice at the time: 'the nearest thing to flying'. Amid all the talk of speed and adrenaline and thrills and excitement, that bird-like element to the experience didn't register. Up here, though, it really does. *That's* what's beautiful about this experience – not that you're speeding, but that you're soaring. Rather than becoming a cannonball you've become a bird.

And with half the ride left, there's still time to savour the sensation. As I gaze down on the lake, then lift my eyes to take in the quarry wall and the sunset-tinged slopes beyond it, I very calmly and carefully note to myself that this is what the project is all about: making yourself do new things. Sometimes a normal life seems attractive, a life free from obsessiveness, from making lists and ticking off their items. But then without those lists I'd never end up having experiences like this. Another day would have slipped by when I thought 'must get round to that'. And then another week, another month…

Nearing the far end of the wire now. Just time to promise myself that when Barney's old enough I'll bring him here so we can fly across the quarry together. Simultaneously the place's original function comes back to me, and I think of the men who toiled here, the slate they gathered, the strike they endured. For a single instant the past and the future exist together in my mind, a magical thought of those workers standing at the bottom, gazing up at me and my son and wondering what the hell we're doing. There's a lesson about happiness in there somewhere: relish where you're going, remember where you've come from.

6

THE MOST NORTHERLY HOUSE
IN THE UNITED KINGDOM

Jo's doing her look. It's one I've got used to over the years. We're visiting friends in Sussex, and Andy has cooked a Thai curry. Being a considerate chap he's erred on the mild side, placing a bottle of Tabasco sauce on the table for those desiring more oomph. 'Did you know,' I say to him, as I pepper my dinner with a few drops of the Louisiana institution, 'that every bottle of Tabasco is...'

But already Andy is smiling back. 'I know – brilliant, isn't it?'

We both pause in silent tribute to the unspoken end of the sentence.[1] Jo, meanwhile, is doing the look, the one combining the message 'what the hell are you going on about?' with the message 'no, on second thoughts don't explain any further, I might actually lose the will to live'. Andy's partner Cheryl is doing the exact same look, meaning we get the treatment in stereo.

'Never mind your disapproval,' I counter. 'You'll be sneering on the other side of your face tomorrow, when my trivialist tendencies take us on a small detour on the way home.'

Jo looks suspicious. 'What have you got planned?'

I remain, however, undrawn. On Sunday evening, therefore, as we pull up in a quiet cul-de-sac off the main street in the village of Merstham, Jo is none the wiser. Nor is Barney. He sits patiently in the back.

---

[1] '...aged in barrels previously used to age Jack Daniel's whiskey.'

Jo fails to follow his lead. 'Come on,' she snaps. 'What are we doing here? If you faff around any longer we're going to hit tomorrow morning's rush hour.'

I reach for a carrier bag, but don't take out its contents. 'Did you notice the name of this street?'

Jo looks at the detached houses, some of them from the seventeenth and eighteenth centuries. But from where we've parked she can't see any of the street signs. 'No. I didn't, Mark. Just tell us, will you?'

Only now do I reveal what's in the bag. A box of chocolates. But not just any box of chocolates. 'You are about,' I announce, 'to eat Quality Street on Quality Street.'

RH (Redhill): Quality Street chocolates were named, like Quality Street in Merstham, after a play by J. M. Barrie.

The comedy, which Barrie penned in his pre-*Peter Pan* days, premiered on Broadway in 1901, then transferred to London. It became so popular that in 1936 confectionery maker John Mackintosh named his new line after it. The 'soldier and his lady friend' characters who for decades were pictured on the tins (Miss Sweetly and Major Quality) were based on the play's two main characters. And when the husband-and-wife team who portrayed them on stage moved to this cul-de-sac in Merstham, it was renamed in honour of the play. Jo digs around in the box until she locates the Brazil nut variety known universally as the Purple One. Thankfully there is more than one of these per box, so no scene ensues. Barney opts for a Green Triangle, and soon the car is filled with contented munching sounds, punctuated only by me reading out my research note about Quality Street chocolates being offered by Saddam Hussein to George Galloway when the MP visited him in 2002.

Several days later, Jo is doing the look again. I have returned from our local market town in Suffolk, proudly bearing on my phone pictures of a pillar box. It stands outside some not especially interesting houses on a not especially interesting street. Even the pillar box itself is not especially interesting: round, chest-high, standard-issue red, three or four characters' worth of illegible graffiti drawn in felt tip across its 'Last Collection Time' notice.

'Why am I looking at this?' asks Jo.

'This,' I reply, 'comes under the heading "Items of Generic Postal History".' I magnify the photo, zooming in on the monarch's initials at the bottom. 'Look – there.'

'E and R,' says Jo. 'So?'

'It's not Elizabeth. Look at the little numerals between the letters.' Jo has clearly misread them as 'II'. I magnify the picture even more to assist her. 'See? "VIII". This is an Edward the eighth postbox.'

'And?'

'There are hardly any of them left. Only about 130 in the whole country. Obviously not that many were installed in the first place, as he was only king for ten months.' I think about sidetracking into what Chris at the BPMA told me about 'crowned' stamps of Edward VIII never being needed, but decide against it. 'And then when he abdicated the public were so disgusted they went round vandalising them. People actually used to take files along and grind the initials off...'

I pause. The look is now firmly in place, and, to be honest, for once I'm on Jo's side. Yes, the tale of how Edward's subjects reacted to him trading the crown for an American divorcée is, I would maintain, an interesting slice of social history. But nevertheless it's hard not to sympathise with my partner.

Her eyes at this moment paint a picture of deep despair, the despair of a woman who has realised that her life has finally reached the point where she is sharing it with a man who takes pictures of postboxes.

Spring hands over the baton to summer, but the project's entering its autumn. The last couple of trips have seen off 21 and 22 areas respectively. This only leaves 45 to do. At the current rate my next trip will probably be the penultimate one. Distraction from my sorrow about this appears in the form of an email from Harry, inviting me on a press trip for that planned re-opening of the Mail Rail. If I'd care to present myself at Mount Pleasant on the nominated morning, the Post Office's underground railway will be mine for the viewing. Not many gift horses take the form of a tiny train riding subterranean tracks 70 feet below London, so I avoid looking this one in the mouth.

Arriving at the BPMA, the chosen scribblers are presented by Harry with hi-viz jackets. He then accompanies us a few yards further along the building. We descend a slight incline to an underground car park, resorting to single file as a Royal Mail van passes us on its way out. Here Harry introduces us to Ray, one of the three engineers whose job it is to maintain the Mail Rail, a legal obligation on the company even though the system is no longer used (and one that looks very sensible now it's going to be reopened). It's obvious from the first glance that Ray, who started his job when the Mail Rail was still carrying letters, is everything you want in an engineer – overalls, glasses, a general air that for all the system he's in charge of gives him headaches he still loves it like an owner loves a dog.

Ray takes us through a door and down several steps to the maintenance depot. This is the size of a very large commercial garage, and with the same appearance: bits of machinery, cables, wires, grey metal tool boxes, health and safety notices of various vintages. A set of drawers is labelled 'm20 castle nuts ... m6 x 16 cap head screws ... 10m hex half nuts ...' and so on. Embedded in the concrete floor are sets of two-foot-gauge tracks, one of which runs to the far end and disappears down a slope into a tunnel leading to the Mail Rail itself. We mooch around for a while, and Harry returns from a shelf in the corner. 'Look what I've found.' He's holding out an old bar of soap with the 'EIIR' logo cut into it. 'Standard Royal Mail issue.'

Ray then leads us back up the steps, across the huge sorting area I glimpsed on my first visit to the archive (as then it's nearly deserted by this time of day), and round to a lift. On the way we pass dozens of discarded red elastic bands.

'How many of these does the Royal Mail get through in a year?' I ask.

'God knows,' says Ray. 'I passed a room here once, it must have been at least fifteen foot square, and it was packed floor to ceiling with sack after sack after sack of rubber bands. I had a look at the label on one of them. It said "Contents: one hundred thousand".'

The lift deposits us into what is essentially a slightly-smaller-than-normal Tube station, with an eastbound and a westbound platform, and a map showing the layout of the system. Between here and Whitechapel the tracks run via stations underneath King Edward Street (near St Paul's, the GPO's old head-quarters) and Liverpool Street. The aim was to link up with mainline railway stations – west of here you travel underneath Oxford Street out to Paddington. 'The tunnel is really close to the Bakerloo Line tunnel at Oxford Circus,' says Ray. 'If you stand still you can hear passengers talking on the platform.'

The carriages on which mailbags were carried are dinky little affairs, about four feet high with one side left open for loading and unloading. In 1977, to celebrate the Mail Rail's fiftieth anniversary, a few carriages were joined together and converted into a 'VIP' train for distinguished visitors. It's on this that we'll be travelling today. Metal loops support a Perspex roof over the double seats into which the taller among us have a bit of difficulty squeezing, but once we're in it's perfectly cosy. The equally dinky engine in which Ray's going to drive us is painted yellow.

'It's this colour because of *Hudson Hawk*,' he tells us. 'They filmed the bit here which is set on the Vatican's underground railway, and they wanted the papal carriage painted yellow. Bruce Willis escapes from someone in one of the carriages, I think.' He points to the electric display board on the tunnel wall, which shows information about the system using words like 'shunt', 'loop' and 'car shed'. 'They got me to put something up on that in Latin.'

Before we pull away Ray explains that the Royal Mail used money from the *Hudson Hawk* shoot to fund Christmas trips for children. 'They used to do two each year – one for disadvantaged kids, one for the kids of Mail employees. We used to get the fattest postman each year and dress him up as Santa. Also you should look out for the twelve days of Christmas painted on the wall as we go along – they did that to give the kids something other than a tunnel to look at.'

We depart the westbound platform and head into the tunnel. The pace is stately rather than speedy, the wall near enough that you could reach out and touch it from the open side of the carriages. The tunnel is lit, so we can make out the Christmas drawings when they appear – the two turtle doves are particularly well drawn. Ray takes us on a looped journey, veering through a side tunnel on to the eastbound tracks. As we pass back through the station, I notice that the wall of the platform has a dartboard hanging on it. When we've changed direction a second time, and pulled back into the platform from which we started, I mention this to Ray.

'Well,' he replies, 'the guys had to have something to do in the gaps between trains.'

Heading back to the lift, I fall into step beside Harry. 'That was really relaxing,' I say. 'Trundling along through the tunnels.'

Harry nods. He's spent quite a bit of time down here recently, preparing for the press trip. 'Sometimes when I'm down here, I get them to stop the train in the middle of a tunnel. Just for a minute or two, so I can savour the peace.' He lifts up his phone. 'You know no one's going to bother you on this for a start.' I know what Harry means, but I also wonder if there isn't something more fundamental at play. Could being underground feel so comforting because it reminds us of being in the womb? Is it where we go when hiding under the duvet doesn't quite cut it any more?

Back above ground, as we collect our bags and jackets, Harry asks about my next field trip. I tell him I haven't decided on a destination yet. But within minutes, after our conversation has taken a chance turn towards postage stamps (we've been telling someone else in the group about the Scotland World Cup specimen), an idea has formed. We've mentioned that a first-class stamp costs 62 pence these days, but that for this sum the Royal Mail will deliver your letter anywhere in the UK. Not just to the next town, not even the next county – right to the other end of the kingdom. 'Where is that furthest address?' we find ourselves saying. 'How much value can you squeeze from those sixty-two pennies?'

Back at home in Suffolk, the answer appears. An initial glance at a map confirms we're talking the Shetland Islands. Further searching on the internet reveals that the most northerly house in the UK – and therefore the most distant address to which the Royal Mail will travel to earn my custom – is a cottage called The Haa, at the top of Unst, the northernmost of the islands that make up Shetland. A crow departing from the postbox at the centre of my village and heading straight for The Haa would clock up 611 miles, almost all of them over the North Sea. According to an online routefinder the journey by car would cover 918 miles. Or rather a little more – the site won't believe that the cottage can be reached by road, and keeps depositing me a couple of miles short. Then it emerges that the ferry to Shetland leaves from Aberdeen, meaning it takes you from AB to ZE – alphabetically the first and last of the UK's postcodes. When you stumble across a fact like this, you know that things are written in the stars.

Harry puts me in touch with someone from the Royal Mail's Scottish office, and soon everything is in place: I am going to post a letter to The Haa, then travel to Unst and accompany the local postwoman as she delivers it. Yes, I know that'll mean I could have saved myself the 62 pence. But you get the idea.

Before the trip commences, I consult the map to see which areas need ticking off. The ones that won't now be visited, I mean. England's south-east and south-west were pretty well covered by the Kent trip and the journey over to Wales, so it seems sensible to draw a line across from London and mop up the few remaining areas below it. Starting with a seismic cultural event on the south coast:

BN (Brighton): Portugal's entry in the 1974 Eurovision Song Contest was played over the radio as a coded signal to begin a military coup.

This was the contest won by a little-known Swedish band called Abba. Their rendition of 'Waterloo' only took place in Brighton because Luxembourg, who'd won on home turf in 1973, didn't fancy the expense of staging the event for a second consecutive year and so pulled out. Britain volunteered to take over hosting duties. But the departure from Eurovision norms didn't end there. For a start the new home country was represented by an Aussie, or at least someone we all now assume is an Aussie – Olivia Newton-John. Turns out she was born and lived the first six years of her life in Cambridge. (Her Welsh father had worked at Bletchley Park during the Second World War.) France withdrew at the last minute when its President Georges Pompidou died, and Italy refused to broadcast proceedings because it was feared its entry '*Sì*' could subliminally influence viewers in a forthcoming referendum on divorce. But the strangest sub-plot concerned Portugal's offering '*E Depois do Adeus*' ('And After the Farewell'), performed by Paulo de Carvalho. It only garnered three points and a joint last when crooned to the good burghers of Brighton, but a couple of weeks later it earned de Carvalho a place in political history. Shortly before 11 p.m. on 24 April it was played by a Portuguese radio station as a pre-arranged signal for left-wing army officers to begin their coup against the country's ruling dictatorship. The coup succeeded. When you consider the quality of music offered up by Eurovision over the decades it's incredible this is the only time it has led to actual violence.

Down the coast in PO we're spoiled for choice. The Isle of Wight falls within Portsmouth's postal range, and as well as its previously mentioned role as England's smallest county at certain times of day, the island also appeared in the news recently – 37-year-old Anna Wardley became only the fourth person ever to swim round it. (She's done several other islands, too, though had to abandon Tiree in the Inner Hebrides when the water temperature made her hallucinate.) A yacht called *America* won a race around the Isle of Wight in 1851, and the cup awarded to its owner ended up being named after the vessel, so giving the sport its most famous trophy. In 1937 the review of the navy's fleet at Spithead was commentated on by Lieutenant Commander Thomas Woodrooffe, who after a pre-programme session in the bar delivered a broadcast that is still enjoyed today. He keeps repeating the phrase 'the whole fleet is lit up!', referring to the lamps outlining the ships against the night sky. At one point he yells 'It's gone! ... It's disappeared!', not realising that a lurch by the ship he is standing on has left him looking out to sea.

But it's a humbler maritime pursuit that gets the title:

PO (Portsmouth): The windsurfer was invented after a 12-year-old boy noticed the weathervane of a church on Hayling Island.

One morning in 1958 Peter Chilvers was messing about on a stretch of water not far from the seafront, using a piece of plywood to which he'd attached a mast and sail. Facing the right way to catch the wind was tricky, even with the foot-operated rudder he had cleverly incorporated into the design. But seeing a weathervane blowing on a local church spire made him wonder – what would happen if he replaced the fixed mast with one that could rotate? Windsurfing, that was what.

Popping inland for a moment, we journey north to the Hampshire town of Alton:

GU (Guildford): The expression 'Sweet Fanny Adams' comes from a notorious child murder of the nineteenth century.

You assume, don't you, that the name is an invention to cover up a well-known phrase whose second word is 'all'? But no, Fanny Adams really existed. Aged eight, she was murdered in Alton in 1867 by a solicitor's clerk. He dismembered her body, leaving the various parts scattered around. When the Royal Navy introduced tins of mutton for its sailors in 1869, the rations proved so unpopular that the men joked (if that's the word) about them being the remains of Fanny Adams. Use of the expression later widened to cover anything tiny or worthless. Adams's gravestone in Alton's cemetery still has dolls and teddy bears left on it to this day.

Westwards to SO, where we find more tragedy, this time from the animal kingdom:

SO (Southampton): In 1977 a giraffe called Victor accidentally did the splits at a zoo in Hampshire and never managed to get back up.

No one knew for sure how Victor's legs ended up going in opposite directions. Some thought it may have involved his girlfriend Dribbles. Whatever the reason, he ended up with his back legs splayed out behind him, a muscle in one of them hopelessly torn. Messages of support came from all over the world, but actual physical support proved impossible, even when workers at Portsmouth Dockyard made a hoist. Victor never made it back on to his feet, and though he sat there contentedly chewing food, without exercise the end was never going to be far away. A few days later his heart gave up, Victor dying peacefully in his owner's arms. But to lift the mood, let us finish with this detail, which gives credence to the theory about how Victor met his end: a giraffe's gestation period is 15 months, and the following summer Dribbles gave birth to a calf. It was female. The zoo named her Victoria.

Two of the other areas concern royal building projects:

THE MOST NORTHERLY HOUSE IN THE UNITED KINGDOM

SM (Sutton): One of Henry VIII's palaces was called Nonsuch because no such building existed any-where else.

Henry commissioned the palace in 1538 to celebrate the birth of his son, as well as to outdo his great rival François I of France. The plot he wanted in Surrey was already occupied by the village of Cuddington. Simple solution: knock the village down. Nonsuch cost a fortune to build, some of it paid to the ironmonger who supplied the nails, all 250,000 of them. There were stucco reliefs of the Labours of Hercules and the Liberal Arts and Virtues, as well as one of Henry and his son Edward. Carved slate was set off with gold leaf, and all in all the palace really was fit for a king. But Henry only ever visited it three times. After his death it passed in and out of royal hands for over a century, until Charles II gave it to his mistress in 1670. She demolished it to sell off the parts and pay her gambling debts.

A later royal mistress took better care of her property:

BH (Bournemouth): The Langtry Manor Hotel in Bournemouth has a small peephole looking down on its restaurant, put there so Edward VII could decide whether he felt like joining his dinner guests.

The hotel was originally built by Edward (then still the Prince of Wales) as a house where he and his close friend Lillie Langtry could spend quality time together. Langtry designed much of the property herself. As well as the peephole she gave one room a lofty ceiling specially fashioned to disperse the Prince's cigar smoke. The hotel still has the window into which Langtry carved her initials with a diamond ring given to her by Edward. The couple used the house for entertaining guests formally as well as themselves informally, though as the peephole shows Edward sometimes bailed out at the last minute. The affair wasn't without its storms, and finally ended when Lillie came down for a fancy dress dinner party in the same outfit as the Prince. He ventured the opinion that this wasn't on. She put a chunk of ice down his back. By the time he became king Edward had collected so many mistresses that a special pew was reserved for them at his coronation: it was known as the 'Loose Box'. Before we leave BH, by the way, an honourable mention for this report from the *Bournemouth Evening Echo*: 'Mrs Irene Graham of Thorpe Avenue, Boscombe, delighted the audience with her reminiscence of the German prisoner of war who was sent each week to do her garden. He was repatriated at the end of 1945, she recalled. "He'd always seemed such a nice friendly chap, but when the crocuses came up in the middle of our lawn in February 1946, they spelt out Heil Hitler."'

There are now three areas left south of that line across from London. Only one is outside London itself: Southend-on-Sea, glorying in the code 'SS'. You'd think a way could have been found round this. Jaguar managed it, after all – they were originally named SS Cars (standing for Swallow Sidecars, that being their first product), but changed it after the Second World War for reasons that were obvious to them if not to the Post Office. Coincidentally the fact concerns a fictional character who drove a Jag himself:

SS (Southend-on-Sea): The *Inspector Morse* theme tune spells out 'Morse' in Morse code.

Composer Barrington Pheloung may have a name straight out of a murder mystery, but the venue in which he penned the music is very un-Morse-ish: the Southend suburb of Westcliff-on-Sea. Pheloung was living there when he wrote the music, later versions of which would sometimes spell out the name of the episode's killer, or (if Pheloung felt like toying with the viewer) that of a totally innocent character.

One of the other two areas is North London, which I'll be covering on the Shetland trip, so we're just left with the capital's western regions. Without wishing to offend W's higher numbers, the fact has to come from W1. You could do a whole book on this patch alone, from Fortnum and Mason being the first shop in the UK to sell baked beans, through Edward Elgar opening the first ever HMV store on Oxford Street in 1921, all the way to *Chariots of Fire* composer Vangelis trying to march past reception in EMI's Manchester Square. Surveying the flamboyant Greek star, all flowing locks and copious beard, the gruff commissionaire said: 'Oi, where do you think you're going?'

'I have an appointment,' came the reply.

'Wait there.' The commissionaire rang upstairs. 'You expecting anyone? There's a bloke here says he's got an appointment... Hang on, I'll ask him.' He turned back to the star. 'What's your name?'

'I am Vangelis.'

The commissionaire resumed the call. 'Says his name's Frank Ellis.'

But it's to Bruton Street in Mayfair that we turn for the fact. Number 17, to be precise, where in the early hours of 21 April 1926 a baby was born by Caesarean section. As well as all the people you'd expect to be there, a man called Sir William Joynson-Hicks was present. He was unrelated to the mother or the child, and had no medical expertise at all. His was a very different role:

W (West London): Queen Elizabeth II will be the last British monarch whose birth was attended by the Home Secretary.

The convention that the holder of this office witnessed royal births had its roots in the 'Warming Pan' scandal of 1688. A rumour went round that James II's son had been stillborn, and that a replacement baby had been smuggled into the room in a warming pan. To ensure everyone knew a possible future monarch really did have blue blood, it became a tradition for the Home Secretary to confirm that the baby in question had indeed emerged from the royal womb. The last time this ever happened was at the birth of Princess Alexandra in 1936. Home Secretary Sir John Simon must have been delighted – it was Christmas Day.

Still in 'tidying up' mode as I survey the route of my London-to-Aberdeen rail trip (that 900-odd-mile figure proved too daunting in the end – let's allow a train driver to do the work), I note not only the areas we'll pass through but also the ones we'll narrowly miss. The first is Cambridge, co-star with Oxford of a well-loved quiz question: 'Who, apart from Isaac Wolfson, is the only person to have a college named after them at both universities?'[2] We could take the sporting approach, either with cricket – Fenners was the first sporting ground to have its grass mown in patterned strips – or rugby: when it was first played at the university some passers-by thought a fight had broken out and ran on to the pitch to intervene. But the honours go to Thomas Hobson:

[2] No, it's not St John – the two colleges commemorate different ones. Nor the Earl of Pembroke – ditto. The answer is Jesus Christ.

CB (Cambridge): The expression 'Hobson's choice' comes from a horse owner who only let customers hire the animal nearest the door.

Thomas gets the nod because he fits in with the project: his horses were used to deliver mail between Cambridge and London. When they weren't needed for that, students and academics could hire them from Hobson's stables outside the gates of St Catharine's College. Most owners allowed customers to choose whichever beast they wanted, a policy which inevitably meant a tiring life for the best-looking horses. To prevent this, Hobson operated a strict rotation system – you had to choose the horse nearest the door. Hence the choice he offered you was no choice at all.

Next up is the city whose cathedral was, from 1311 to 1549, the tallest building in the world:

LN (Lincoln): Chad Varah was inspired to found the Samaritans after conducting the funeral service of a young girl who had committed suicide.

It's normally the London church of St Stephen Walbrook, round the corner from the Bank of England, that gets all the glory. And yes, this is where Varah actually started the Samaritans, when he was the rector there in 1953, operating with a single Bakelite telephone on the number MAN (Mansion House) 9000. The phone itself now sits in a glass case inside the church. But the idea first came to him years earlier, when as an assistant curate in Lincoln he led the funeral of a 14-year-old girl who, mistaking her first period for a sexually transmitted disease, took her own life. 'Little girl,' said Varah to himself, 'I didn't know you, but you have changed the rest of my life for good.' He vowed to start a service that would 'befriend the suicidal and despairing'.

Up in Yorkshire we meet someone who provided brave resistance to the growth of the state:

WF (Wakefield): Harry Willcock was the last person in Britain to be prosecuted for refusing to produce an identity card.

Willcock, who hailed from the village of Alverthorpe, was stopped by police while driving on 7 December 1950. The constable, Harry Muckle, demanded that Willcock produce his ID card, which was still a legal requirement even though the Second World War (during which the cards had been introduced) was long since over. 'I am a Liberal,' replied Willcock, 'and I am against this sort of thing.' He got a ten-shilling fine for his trouble, despite arguing at his trial that ID cards really weren't on in peacetime. His appeal was handled by some prominent Liberal lawyers, all waiving their usual hefty fees. They lost, but not before the Lord Chief Justice had shown considerable sympathy for their cause. 'To use Acts of Parliament passed for particular purposes during war,' he said, 'in times when the war is past ... tends to make the people resentful of the acts of the police.' Willcock's case attracted so much support that he founded the Freedom Defence Association, tearing up his ID card as a publicity stunt. Inspired by his example, members of the British Housewives' League did the same outside Parliament. Winston Churchill may have defeated Hitler and Mussolini, but knowing that British housewives were made of sterner stuff he vowed to repeal ID cards if he regained power. The promise was kept, too: on 21 February 1952 an announcement was made in the House of Commons that the cards were to be scrapped. Harry Willcock died a few months later. His last word was 'freedom'.

We stay in God's own county for the next fact:

LS (Leeds): The theme tune to *The Archers* is named after a village in Yorkshire.

The ditty's title is 'Barwick Green', honouring the village of Barwick-in-Elmet. Written in 1924 by the Yorkshire composer Arthur Wood, the tune had to wait for its fame until 1950 when the good folk of Ambridge first appeared. The version used on the programme until the 1990s was produced by a pre-Beatles George Martin. The theme has now escaped from *The Archers* on to other Radio 4 programmes: a round of 'One Song to the Tune of Another' on *I'm Sorry I Haven't A Clue* once paired it with the lyrics from 'Love Me Tender' (try it – they're a perfect match). It even saves lives: doctors are instructed that the tempo of 'Barwick Green' is the ideal rate for performing chest pumps when resuscitating someone.

Further north there's anagrammatical wizardry at play:

SR (Sunderland): The Stadium of Light contains a cunningly hidden reference to Sunderland FC's hated rivals Newcastle United.

When the club built the ground in the late 1990s, they offered fans the chance to take part. For 25 quid a go, you could have your name engraved on a brick in the 'Wall of Fame'. With 25,000 bricks available, this brought in a handy bit of cash. It also allowed pensioner Joe Ritchie the chance for some fun. 'I'm a Newcastle fan,' he explained, 'but I've lived in Sunderland for thirty years. You can imagine how much stick I get from my mates. So when the bricks came up for sale I thought it was time for a little pay-back.' He paid his money, telling the club that he was called Cwen Least. Only when the brick had been in place for several months did a Sunderland fan notice the unusual name. 'I can't believe it took them so long,' said Ritchie.

The rain is getting heavier now, each drop hitting the window and following a slightly different trajectory to the bottom. Down on the pavement pedestrians are splashing their way to work, umbrellas angled forwards to prevent them flipping up. I am loving every second. The rain is exactly what I wanted. There's no point staying in a hotel linked directly to a train station if you don't feel the benefit.

The Great Northern Hotel at King's Cross was London's first railway hotel (1854), and with a 10 a.m. train to catch I decided to avoid a rush-hour dash across the capital by spending last night here. The hotel was refurbished a year or so ago, part of the general gentrification of this area of London. Twenty years ago when I lived in King's Cross there were sights at bus stops that you really didn't want to examine too closely. Now the manor has been given a new postcode, or rather a new sub-division of its existing one: N1C. No one seems to know what the extra letter denotes: my assumption is that it's meant to imply 'NICE'. The Great Northern itself is certainly very nice. Not only does it allow me to step from reception on to the station concourse without a single raindrop getting anywhere near me, its breakfast tables also sport some rather nifty napkin rings. The item always puts me in mind of the Duke of Devonshire. Seeing some in Asprey's one day, he was mystified as to what they were.

'In some houses,' came the reply, 'napkins are rolled up at the end of a meal ready for re-use, instead of being laundered every time.'

'Good heavens,' said the Duke. 'I never knew there was such poverty in England.'

So to the train, whose departure marks the start of what will be three days spent almost entirely in motion. Seven hours from here to Aberdeen, overnight ferry to Shetland, meet Bruce Crossan (the Royal Mail's delivery manager there, who's going to drive me up to Unst), accompany the postie (Michelle) on her round, then repeat the train–ferry–car combination but in reverse order. I don't know how far I'll travel on Shetland itself, but the other elements of the journey total 1,527 miles – 547.5 each way on the train, and 216 on the ferry (216 land miles, that is. In nautical miles it's 188[3]). The first part of the trip is through the aforementioned N area. Knowing that more than one of the facts further on in this train journey will relate to football, I decide to set up a theme. We could go for Tottenham Hotspur deliberately setting Jimmy Greaves's 1961 transfer fee from AC Milan at £99,999 to avoid putting him under the pressure of being the first £100,000 player. But instead let's make it another fact about the same club:

N (North London): In 2001 a Spurs fan lost £10,000 by betting on his team to win when they were already 3–0 ahead.

The visitors at White Hart Lane that day were none other than the mighty Manchester United. By half-time the home team had established a three-goal lead, which understandably put their supporters in high spirits. One decided to add a pecuniary cherry to the cake, placing a bet that his team would

---

[3] One nautical mile per hour, of course, being one knot. It used to be measured by throwing a log off the back of the boat and seeing how many of the knots on a piece of rope tied to that log went past in a set time.

complete the victory. Not surprisingly the odds weren't that great – he could only get 16 to 1 on. So to ensure a return worthy of the name, he gambled £10,000. Settling down to watch the second half, and wondering how he would spend his £625 winnings, he saw United score a goal, then another, then another... Spurs eventually lost 5–3.

The countryside is positively gleaming after all the rain, and large swathes of Hertfordshire and Cambridgeshire and Nottinghamshire slide past the window. But it takes until Doncaster before we reach a virgin postcode area. What an area, though:

DN (Doncaster): Michael Jackson's 'Thriller' was written by a man from Cleethorpes called Rodney.

Mr Temperton not only composed the title track of the best-selling album of all time, he wrote two of the other songs on it as well, meaning he's now a man from Cleethorpes who owns houses in Los Angeles, the South of France, Switzerland and Kent, plus an island off Fiji. Not bad for someone whose musical training as a child involved setting up his drum kit near the telly and playing along to the test card. When the day came for Vincent Price to record his spoken part at the end of 'Thriller', Temperton hadn't finished it. Scribbling feverishly as his taxi approached the studio, he looked up to see Price getting out of his limousine. 'Go round the back,' Temperton told the driver. Eventually it was completed, and Price did his thing. Not that he made as much from it as Temperton: offered a choice between $20,000 and royalties, Price foolishly chose the former.

Just as Temperton went from DN to America, so four of my co-passengers have come from America to DN. 'Don-*cas*-ter,' reads one of the three fifty-something women when we pass through the station. The male of the group looks like Charles Bronson in an Adidas baseball cap, and it's hard to work out which, if any, of the women he belongs to. Meanwhile I'm childishly delighted by the lid of my coffee cup, with its sliding horizontal cover protecting the little hole through which you sip. These are the things that impress me these days. Digital devices and the internet have reached the point where you're only amazed if they *can't* do something, but an elegant solution to an age-old problem like spilt coffee is proper engineering.

My radio, however, fails to cope with the electrical interference from the train and so refuses to bring me the midday shipping forecast. I haven't been on a ferry since the Channel Tunnel came along, so as this is the first time in over 20 years that I've had a vested interest in what the sea will be doing, I wish to be prepared. Looking up the forecast on my smartphone, I realise that this device can also procure an explanation for what the figures actually mean. In essence it's 'wind, sea state, weather and visibility'. Cromarty and Fair Isle, through which I'll be travelling tonight, look as though they'll hold few terrors. You have to love the shipping forecast's sense of time: 'soon' is defined as 'within six to 12 hours', while if something's expected in under six hours that's 'imminent'. There's something very wistful about it, too: the phrase 'losing its identity' always makes me feel sad. In her Twitter biography Corrie Corfield, who as a Radio 4 announcer has read her fair share of shipping forecasts, describes herself as 'moderate, occasionally poor'.

At York we're joined by two grannies. They're not together but they sit together, both wearing spectacles, both eating sandwiches from Tupperware containers, both with scarves draped around their necks. After finishing lunch one of them sets to work on a book of Sudoku puzzles. The other starts reading the *Socialist Worker*. Soon we pass into DL

(Darlington) territory. The countryside is more rugged now, characterful rather than picturesque but no less attractive for that. A small brick building in the middle of a field has 'Coal Now And Future' painted on it – the socialist granny would surely approve, had she not nodded off. One of the firms keeping the area's engineering heritage alive these days is Cleveland Bridge Ltd. Its employees have a keen sense of humour:

DL (Darlington): The arch that spans Wembley Stadium is filled with Middlesbrough FC shirts and scarves.

There are also old season tickets, match programmes and various other items of memorabilia, placed in the arch by the steelworkers who made it.

The next area we reach is Durham. Although the train doesn't stop here there's time as we pass through to admire the city centre, dominated by the cathedral which doubled (with a digitally added spire) as Hogwarts in the first two *Harry Potter* films, and whose bishop stands at the monarch's right hand during coronations. When it comes to the area's fact, I could plead project relevance in noting that the train line beneath me is the demarcation line between DH2 and DH3, or that Chester-le-Street's post office, opened in 1936 during Edward VIII's brief reign, is one of very few in the country to feature that king's emblem. But the memories of the 'Jo/postbox' incident are still too fresh, so let's seek another fact. Perhaps the UK's heaviest badger (27.7kg, found in Durham)? Perhaps Australia's cricketers getting scared while staying at 'haunted' Lumley Castle in 2005, leading Darren Gough to creep up behind Shane Watson on the field the next day and do a ghost impression? No, let us commemorate instead one man's determination to take laziness to new heights:

DH (Durham): In 2010 a man was convicted of walking his dog through the window of his moving car.

Paul Railton was spotted by a cyclist driving his Nissan Navara near Consett at five miles an hour. The cyclist alerted the police, who then performed what must have been the simplest car chase in criminal history. They found Railton driving along holding a dog lead, on the other end of which was his lurcher. His defence in court included the claim that 'a lot of people exercise their dogs in that manner'. The magistrates disagreed, and fined him £124. They also gave him three penalty points, which along with the nine he already had meant he was banned from driving. Six of those points were for a speeding offence, which proved that at least Railton varied his crimes.

Britain's smorgasbord of place names offers another delight north of Durham: the village of Pity Me.[4] The Angel of the North appears over to the right, and then we're into Newcastle. I love multi-layered cities like this – the track winds past windows halfway up 15-storey buildings, reminding you of that 'sci-fi metropolis' BBC2 ident. After Morpeth there's a huge open-cast mine, a man padlocking an allotment shed watched by his sheepdog, our first teasing glimpse of the east coast, then a field full of pigsties, each with a red Calor gas bottle next to it and a pipe leading into the sty. Is this to keep the pigs warm, or to deliver the final blow in as gentle a manner as possible? Either way it seems considerate. Soon we're into TD, officially the Galashiels area but taking its letters from the Tweed, the river which historically formed the border between England and Scotland, and still defines quite

---

[4] No one knows for sure. Could be that it's a desolate place, or perhaps a corruption of an ironic reference to the arid land – '*petite mer*' ('small sea').

a bit of the border today. Near Cheswick there's a concrete pillbox mysteriously graffitied 'Come see my cat', then we reach Berwick-upon-Tweed, where foaming white waves crash angrily on to the beach. We stop at the station that came to a Prime Minister's aid:

TD (Galashiels): Sir Alec Douglas-Home once shot a bird that fell into a passing train, whose driver then left the bird for him at a subsequent station.

Not just any train, either. Sir Alec and his chums were shooting above a cutting on the line, 'when I shot a high woodcock which fell into the tender of the *Flying Scotsman*'. Displaying the sort of nous that took him to the very top, Douglas-Home managed to 'signal to the driver as he flashed past'. Exactly what the signal entailed isn't recorded, but it was clear enough for the driver to understand. He 'left the bird for me with his compliments with the station master at Berwick-upon-Tweed'. Birds weren't the only thing to get shot round here in the past, given the disputed nature of the territory (similar to the Debatable Lands we encountered over in Dumfries and Galloway). Coldstream, home of the Guards and also Sir Alec's final resting place, was where Edward I invaded Scotland in 1296. A century or so later 'The Ballad of Chevy Chase' was written, based on real border skirmishes and telling the story of the Earl of Northumberland leading a hunting party into the Cheviot Hills. The Earl of Douglas interpreted it as an invasion of Scotland and retaliated, leading to a huge battle. The American comedian born Cornelius Chase got his nickname Chevy from a grandmother because she, and therefore he, was descended from the Douglas clan.

These days Berwick, having flitted between the two countries several times, lies a couple of miles inside England. Shortly after leaving the station we pass a sign displaying the crosses of St George and St Andrew either side of the words 'Across the Border – British Railways'. Before Dunbar the train veers slightly inland, the hills to our right lined with huge, dense pine forests. Eventually they give way to the ugliness of an industrial plant, while back on the coast at Belhaven Bay two kite-surfers twirl and prance in the wind. It's gone two o'clock now, and the Great Northern's breakfast is finally wearing off. Heading to the buffet car I pass three hipsters. One (ginger hair and beard, massive headphones over a knitted bobble hat) edits something on his MacBook, while his two companions, one with an Irish accent that sounds almost American, discuss Banksy's autobiography in reverent tones.

Edinburgh offers more multi-level magic, as well as stops at two of its stations (Waverley and Haymarket), as if to show how important a city it is. A few minutes later we reach the Forth Rail Bridge. The far end is in the Kirkcaldy postcode area, so I consult my notes on the structure in readiness to tick off KY. Players of *Grand Theft Auto: San Andreas* will recognise the bridge from the game's fictional town of San Fierro: the designers included it as a nod to their native Edinburgh. The old chestnut about needing to start painting it again as soon as you've finished turns out to be a myth: the most recent application (finished in 2011) is expected to last at least a quarter of a century. Should think so too, at a cost of £130 million. As we travel across I admire the pleasing shade of red, as well as the reassuringly sturdy rivets, of which there are 6.5 million. The final one – gold-plated, don't you know – was driven in by the Prince of Wales (post-Lillie Langtry but pre-taking the throne) on 4 March 1890. The previous November, however, the very first rivets had presented problems:

KY (Kirkcaldy): A spell of unexpectedly cold weather meant the two halves of the Forth Rail Bridge didn't quite meet in the middle.

God knows how cold 'unexpectedly cold' it is in the Firth of Forth in November, but the north and south halves of the bridge, eight years in the making, remained separate entities. Only when things warmed up and the metal expanded could the rivets be driven home.

Scotland's palette works hard as we continue: the wheatfields may not have yellowed yet, but the oilseed rape certainly has. At Burntisland an optimistic funfair has opened up, but the weather isn't fair so there's not much fun. More unlikely place names – Leslie, Star, Windygates, Bottomcraig – lead us up to an equally unlikely coincidence in Dundee:

DD (Dundee): The two heaviest defeats in British football history happened a few miles apart on the same day.

It was the first round of the 1885–86 Scottish FA Cup. Minnows against giants are the nature of cup competitions, so hammerings are always on the card. But one particular minnow, Bon Accord, was in the wrong pond altogether – they'd only been invited to take part because the FA mistook them for another club. Bon Accord (named after the code word which started Robert the Bruce's storming of Aberdeen Castle in 1308) were in fact an offshoot of a cricket club. The draw pitted them against the (relatively) mighty Arbroath. The bigger club's goalkeeper didn't touch the ball once, and spent part of the match hiding from the rain under a spectator's umbrella. When the referee's whistle finally put Bon Accord out of their misery the score stood at a record-breaking 36–0.

It still holds the British crown, though surrendered the world title in 2002 to a 149–0 result in Madagascar. All 149 were own goals, scored by one of the teams as a protest against a penalty decision during a previous match.

But Arbroath's 36-goal triumph might never even have held the British record. On the same day, 18 miles away, Dundee Harp played at home to Aberdeen Rovers. When the final whistle went the referee noted the score as 37–0 to Harp. But Harp's secretary told him that by his reckoning there had only been 35 goals. As it had been so difficult to keep count while officiating, the ref accepted the secretary's lower figure and wired the result to the Scottish FA. Another telegram was sent by Harp full-back Tom O'Kane. He had once played for Arbroath, and in fact still lived in the town. Wanting to let his old team-mates know about the incredible event, he wired them saying his team had won 35–0. They replied straightaway saying, in effect, 'you won't believe this but we've won 36–0'. Of course O'Kane *didn't* believe it – he thought his Arbroath friends were winding him up. Only when he got the train home that Saturday evening did he discover Arbroath really had gone one better than Harp. Understandably this somewhat removed the wind from his sails, but not, in fairness, from his lungs: the next morning he ran those 18 miles to Dundee in order to share the bad news with everyone at Harp.

Arbroath, as it turns out, is the next stop after Dundee. While we're there a man emerges from the gym next to the station, wearing a tracksuit and carrying a heavy weight in each hand. He takes one step forward, bending his front leg as much as possible so that the knee of his straightened back leg almost touches the ground. Then he repeats this move with the other leg, and so on until he has travelled the entire length of the car park. In the grey Scottish drizzle of a Wednesday afternoon it forms one of the most bizarre sights I have ever seen. Finally, at bang on the appointed hour of five o'clock, we pull into Aberdeen. Emerging from the station, you find that the 'Granite City' nickname is more than justified. The entire place is a monochrome symphony, a whole new meaning to the phrase 'fifty shades of grey'. If the Londoners among you want to nail one of the shades think Waterloo Bridge: it's made from Aberdeen granite. There's hardly a building here that hasn't placed itself in the middle ground between black and white. But somehow Aberdeen feels wonderful, a vibrant and modern city full of attractive young people. The huge displays of architecture are impressive rather than oppressive.

Perhaps it helps that the weather has improved in the last hour, but you get the impression that Aberdeen has bounded into the twenty-first century with style. Yes, it displays its history (ornate lamp posts outside the Victorian library, a massive statue of William Wallace), but there's modernity too. Esslemont and Macintosh, a former department store with the founders' names mosaically tiled above the door, is now a Jamie's Italian.[5] The Korova Bar advertises a 'Husband Creche' ('is he moaning about shopping?... Drop him off... we'll take good care of him...'), the Cumin Tandoori offers 'Low Fat' Indian cuisine, and a yellow American school bus takes children home. Perhaps the finest mix of new and old is on School Hill, where L'Occitane En Provence and Ispiro Estetica Hair and Beauty stand either side of a Greggs.

There are modern contenders for Aberdeen's fact, too, such as Saddam Hussein's bedroom door now residing in the Gordon Highlanders Museum. Well, some wood panelling from the door to *one* of his bedrooms in *one* of his palaces. The regiment served in Basra, and have the wood as a memento,

[5] OK, they could have sold out to someone less annoying and with a correctly sized tongue, but let's not quibble.

along with the huge bronze head from a statue of the fallen leader. We could also mention Scotty in *Star Trek* being 'an old Aberdeen pub crawler' (his own description), the actor James Doohan having based the accent on an Aberdonian he met while serving in the Second World War. But the fact is historic in project terms – it's the one hundredth – so it should be historic in real terms:

AB (Aberdeen): William Wallace's left leg is buried in the wall of St Machar's Cathedral.

Once the English had executed the Scottish hero they quartered his body, sending the various parts to different towns and cities as a warning to potential rebels. His head was dipped in tar and impaled on a spike on London Bridge. His right arm went to Newcastle, his left to Berwick, his right leg to Perth and his left to Stirling. From here it eventually ended up at Aberdeen, where it received the sort of treatment sometimes meted out by London gangsters but for slightly different reasons.

Down at the harbour I search for my ferry. It must be hiding among the half-dozen or so larger vessels ... No, hang on – it *is* one of the larger vessels. I was expecting a dainty old-fashioned thing (how many people can there be wanting to visit the Shetland Isles?), but the ferry is huge, the size of a mid-league shopping mall. It has a restaurant, a bar, a shop, a cinema, a children's play area and several lounges. My cabin boasts an en-suite shower room. Adorning the side of the ship is a huge drawing of Magnus, the helmeted and bearded Viking who acts as NorthLink Ferries' logo. He's a reminder that the islands I'm visiting are a very long way out in the North Sea, with strong historical links to Scandinavia. In Norway, my Quality Street research revealed, the chocolates are known as

'Shetlandsgodt' ('Shetland Sweets') because fishermen visiting the isles used to take them home.

The cinema is showing *Noah*, which bodes well. The captain announces himself as Captain Scott, which doesn't, but soon his Scottish burr is wishing us 'every comfort and care during the journey', a solidly formal turn of phrase that brings reassurance. By now it's getting on for seven and I'm starving, so I head up to the restaurant. The Shetland poached salmon in a citrus chive and dill Hollandaise sauce might be more appropriate in view of our destination, but the rumbles from my stomach call out for the Orkney steak casserole with a herb dumpling.[6]

Only when I try to shift the position of my chair mid-meal do I notice that it's chained to the floor. Oh yes – we're on a ship, aren't we? On that thing called the sea, which can cut up rough once in a while. That's why there are all these piles of paper bags everywhere on board. It's so long since I've been on a ferry that I really can't remember whether or not I have decent sea legs. Certainly there were never any horror stories, though there might have been the odd queasy moment. Tonight, however, all seems fine. In fact I'm so much of a seadog that I don't even notice us setting off. The engines starting up, yes. You can't miss a noise like that. But lifting a forkful of casserole to my mouth I look up to find Aberdeen a hundred yards away: I hadn't even felt the movement. Finishing my main course I take a chocolate bar and coffee up on to the open deck for dessert. A few of the hundred or so other passengers are here to enjoy the view, including a father and his young son, the latter wearing a Ness United top (they're one of Shetland's football teams). A light coating of salt covers

---

[6] Some of the ferries call in at Orkney en route, but tonight we're heading straight to Shetland.

the handrails. A dolphin leaps happily behind us, while on the beach to our left (sorry – starboard) a black Labrador goes mental as its owner throws a ball. It takes a good ten minutes to clear the harbour wall, then we're out into open sea. This makes things a touch choppier, but nothing to worry about. Not for an old salt like me.

Heading back to the lounge, I pick up a copy of the *Shetland Times*. It's sad to read that the isles' oldest resident, 105-year-old Ruby Lindsay, has passed away in the capital Lerwick, but proving that life goes on there's a new skateboarding park in Knab. The '50 Years Ago This Week' section is auspicious in project terms – it relates the delivery to Unst of a new Post Office van, complete with a picture of the vehicle being loaded on to the ship. Things were more relaxed back then: they used basic rope slings and large cushions jammed into the wheel arches to protect the van from damage.

At half past seven I find myself thinking about going back to my cabin. All of a sudden I feel like a bit of a lie down. This is simply, you understand, because it's been a long day's travelling. In no way whatever is it related to the steady up and down movement of the ferry. There's absolutely no thought in my head that I might be starting to feel seasick. No thought at all.

You really don't want to know what happens between eight o'clock and eight-thirty.

By nine o'clock, calm has returned. I'm lying in bed, a trifle listless and I dare say rather pale, but no longer vowing to cancel the return half of my ticket and book a flight back from Shetland. In fact it's quite cosy here now, the vessel's undulation acting as gentle rocks on my cradle. I drift off to sleep, waking briefly at three, when a lifting of the blind reveals that dawn really is that bit earlier this far north: the eastern part of the sky is already pinkly lit, though it's a shade darker to the south. Dozing until five, I wake fully and realise that I can now listen to the shipping forecast in situ, as it were. Tuning the radio to roughly the right part of the dial, I find an English voice, obviously the World Service about to hand back to Radio 4. But after several minutes the handover still hasn't happened. A quick shimmy of the tuning button – turns out I've been listening to BBC Radio Scotland by mistake. The shipping forecast has been going on a millimetre to the right. I catch the final few words. 'Thanks, Chris,' says the Radio 4 announcer. 'I thought "thundery in Lundy" was particularly poetic.' Even the announcer's name gets in on the act: Neil Sleat.

By now land has appeared to our left, so I go up on deck. Lerwick is quite a way along Shetland's main isle rather than at its southern tip, meaning there's plenty to see before we arrive.[7] It looks like any other rugged, almost uninhabited stretch of coast you might encounter in Britain, but because of the distance we've travelled to get here it doesn't *feel* that it can be. There is a foreign aspect to all this, a sense of reaching someone else's home rather than your own. Adding to the strangeness is the appearance of the sea: a thirty-yard wake behind the ferry foams white, but either side the water is a dramatic stealth-bomber black, with an unreal CGI sheen to it. After a while another island appears to our right. Checking the map I find it's Bressay, and there's a village on it called Mail. Later this will inspire a search for other project-relevant

---

[7] The island is bigger than the Isle of Wight, even the Isle of Man – in fact it's the fifth largest of the 6,000-plus British Isles. Great Britain and Ireland are obviously one and two, followed by Lewis & Harris in the Outer Hebrides, then Skye in the Inner Hebrides.

places. There are settlements in Scotland and Northern Ireland called Letter, villages in Iran and Texas called Post, and an Arkansas town called Stamps.

We dock in Lerwick at seven. Bruce is waiting in the terminal building for me. He's about my age, tall and assured, so in control of things on Shetland that he's even arranged for weather as different from yesterday's as you could possibly imagine. As we walk to his car for the drive to Unst the sun comes out, turning the thermostat a notch or two upwards. The plan, Bruce explains, is to catch the ferry from the mainland to Yell, then one from Yell to Unst, getting us to Baltasound for mid-morning. The first bit of this confuses me, until Bruce explains that 'the mainland' is what Shetlanders call this, the main island of the group.

'What do you call the mainland, then?' I ask. 'The bigger mainland, if you see what I mean?'

Bruce has to think about it. 'I don't know, really. If you're going to Aberdeen you just say "Aberdeen".'

It raises the question of how much Shetland feels part of Scotland. As Bruce points out, allegiances are never easy to define – most football fans here support one of the big Scottish clubs (Celtic, Rangers or Aberdeen), but some islanders have asked during the referendum debate why, if Scotland can have its independence from the UK, Shetland can't have its independence from Scotland? 'They'd say "we've got oil here, after all".' But the one thing everyone agrees on, he adds, is that they hate being called 'the Shetlands'. 'It's definitely "Shetland".'

Lerwick's old buildings are concentrated around the harbour, the rest of the small town dating predominantly from the 1960s. I'll find that most of the buildings on Shetland as a whole are of the same vintage: that's when the oil was found, so that's when the place really started to grow. In as much as it has grown, that is. Settlements here are 'village' edging down towards 'hamlet', and usually not even that – most houses are in ones or twos, and very often you'll be able to see several miles to a horizon and not need a second hand to count the dwellings. Sheep, however ... Perhaps it's because they out-number people by eight to one that they're so confident, but the way they wander on to the road is positively suicidal. At one point a lamb severely tests Bruce's emergency stop skills. 'It's the salt,' he explains. 'When they put it on the road in the winter the sheep lick it off. It's a habit they can't get out of even in summer.' A cruel irony, considering the relationship the animal ultimately has with salt.

The ferries which island-hop us to Unst are much smaller than the overnight one, with room for just a few cars and no inclination to annoy my intestines. At a couple of points Bruce has to take work calls. The pace of life being what it is on Shetland his job isn't exactly stressful, though it's not without the occasional drama. 'A while back we intercepted eight grand's worth of heroin. Or rather the police did. They'd tipped us off about this particular address, so when we got a package for it we alerted them. The guy came in to the post office in Lerwick to collect it – he'd been really anxious about it, asking if it had arrived yet. As soon as he picked it up several plain-clothes cops jumped on him.'

We reach Baltasound, where a day of the UK's 'most norther-ly's begins. Every post office in the kingdom is south of this small single-storey building which doubles as a shop. There's a bungalow next to it, and another slightly larger shop 30 yards away, but other than that Baltasound is what you might term 'geographically dispersed' – in other words it doesn't really exist. We have reached a part of Britain where rural really does mean rural. Inside, Bruce introduces me to Michelle, who's sorting the post ready for her round. Including, she shows me, the envelope I posted in Suffolk several days ago. 'We've been holding it back for you,' she says. Bruce explains its journey: by van to my local town, then Chelmsford Mail Centre, then Stansted airport... plane to Edinburgh... road to Aberdeen Mail Centre, then Aberdeen airport... plane to Sumburgh (on Shetland's main island)... road to Lerwick... and finally the same road/ferry combination that brought me from Lerwick to Baltasound today.

As well as the letters there are plenty of packages, several bearing the name of a South American rainforest. 'Obviously Amazon deliveries are a huge part of the job now,' says Michelle. 'Them and eBay.'

'I suppose you could be delivering anything with eBay, couldn't you? There must be a maximum size of parcel you don't go beyond?'

'Aye, but that doesn't mean I haven't delivered some strange stuff. Car parts, a hen house – I even had to deliver a radiator once.' Nice to be trusted, I suppose. In 1905, when the Cullinan diamond (to this day the largest ever found) was transported from South Africa to Britain as a present for Edward VII, detectives travelled by ship carrying a decoy jewel – the real one was sent by ordinary post. Registered, mind you. Stones cut from the diamond ended up in the Crown Jewels. Though not the crown on the side of Michelle's van: Scotland has a separate crown, sceptre and sword (known as the Honours of Scotland), brought out when the Queen opens the Scottish Parliament. To reflect this the crown in the Royal Mail's Scottish logo is also different.

Once Michelle has finished her sorting we're on our way. It's soon clear that there's no rigid route to follow – having sorted the mail herself Michelle knows whether or not she has anything for a particular house or collection of houses, and so improvises accordingly. A lot of people on Shetland leave their front doors open, which lets her place oversized letters inside. As she walks back from one house she opens the door of a car parked outside and leaves a bundle of letters inside. 'That's the lady's daughter,' she explains. 'She's usually here seeing her mother this time of day, so I leave her mail in her car for her.'

Several times Michelle has parcels requiring a signature, and knows the recipient won't be at home until later. 'We'll leave that one now,' she'll say, weighing up her options at a T-junction. 'Catch them at the end of the round when they're in.' I'm reminded of the postman mentioned on Danny Baker's radio programme a few years ago. One street on his round was slightly uphill, so to avoid having to walk all the way back to his van he would put the automatic gearbox in 'Drive', allowing the vehicle to crawl along beside him as he delivered the mail. 'What,' as Baker himself said, 'could possibly go wrong?' Absolutely nothing. Until the day the van hit a large stone, mounted the pavement and took out several garden fences.

After an hour or so we deliver the mail to the salmon farm run by Michelle's husband, John. He invites me in to take a look. 'How many salmon do you have here?' I ask as we cross a large barn-like building to one of several round tanks that are waist-high and several feet across.

'Up to a million.'

'*What?*'

John indicates the contents of the tank. 'These ones are a few weeks old.' Tiny little creatures barely recognisable as fish are darting about in the water. There are tens of thousands in this tank, apparently – as they grow they're moved to larger tanks, reaching full size in about eleven months. Unlike Michelle, a Shetland native, John is originally from the mainland of Scotland. We talk about their sons, both in their twenties, one of whom has moved away to work in Edinburgh. Michelle herself lived in Gibraltar between the ages of five and eight, when her father was in the RAF. But then her parents returned to Unst, taking on the sheep farm they still run today. Michelle has always known she wanted to stay in Shetland. This talk reminds me of Justin in Llandrindod Wells, leaving for London only to be tempted back to the family hotel by a Peugeot 205. And of my brother – he still lives near to where we grew up, whereas I think I knew from an early age that I wouldn't stay. Which gene is it, which string of letters in your DNA that decides whether you'll travel, whether the home you knew as a child will be your home for life? Later on Michelle will mention the walking she and John like to do at weekends. A few years ago their son walked the whole coast of Unst with some friends. It took three days. Perhaps once you've circled your home you need a new one.

Gradually the deliveries take us northwards. We hand an envelope to a man in his sixties. 'Great,' he says, 'this'll be my eagle.' Then, seeing my confused face: 'The comic. I used to read it as a kid, but I was always cutting the pictures out of the sports pages. So now I'm using eBay to replace them all.'

'Are they expensive?' I ask.

'This one was 99p,' comes the reply, but only because his wife is within earshot.

'Funny,' she says. 'The bank statements never say that.'

Soon afterwards we reach the famous Unst bus shelter. I heard about this researching my local bus book, but as that journey finished at John O'Groats I never got to see it. The structure is sometimes known as Bobby's shelter, after the seven-year-old boy who cycled there to catch his school bus, leaving his bike in it for the return journey. The council took the shelter away, but after a pleading letter from Bobby they reinstated it. Then someone added a sofa – on a remote Shetland hillside you need every bit of comfort you can get. Over the last couple of decades further adornments have appeared, and a local woman now maintains the shelter, changing the theme of her displays annually. This year it's Nelson Mandela. There are posters and books about him, while a comfy chair is covered by a colourful throw and the desk and wooden chair have been painted with the South African flag. Everything is watched over by a toy giraffe. The visitors' book contains praise from natives of Australia, Nottingham, the West Midlands and (a sure sign you've succeeded) Yorkshire. I would say it's the strangest structure I've seen all day, but in the garden of a house we delivered to earlier there was a full-sized Tardis.

Eventually we reach Haroldswick. It was from this tiny settlement that my friend David telephoned through to *The Times* on General Election day in 1997 with his piece about getting as far away from Westminster as possible without leaving the United Kingdom. In fact it's David who has furnished my Shetland fact:

ZE (Shetland): If you live at the northernmost tip of the island of Unst, your nearest IKEA is in Norway.

Bergen, to be exact. Well over a hundred miles closer than your second-nearest option of Edinburgh. David's phone is still here and still working, but the post office over the road, in 1997 still the UK's most northerly, is now a private residence. Michelle and I had reached the UK's most northerly hotel back in Baltasound (it's the only one on Unst), but the other record-holders now appear more regularly. We pass the most northerly brewery (called Valhalla – one of its ales is 'Simmer Dim', after the local name for the summer nights up here when darkness never really descends), garage and shop (they inhabit the same building – I stock up on mini pork pies in case hunger returns, which it still hasn't after last night's 'incident'), and church. The last is, like so many of the other buildings in Shetland, a modern concrete affair. At only a single storey it keeps its bell outside. I can't resist pulling the rope.

As you'd expect Michelle is an important figure on the island, known to virtually everyone on her round. Talking to friends during the project I've realised that the much-loved postie exists all over the country, even in badass London, but somewhere like Unst they can be the only person you see all day. Michelle and I pause for brief chats with many of her deliverees. As well as those born on Unst there are plenty who weren't. A woman from Australia who married a Scotsman she met in Egypt: 'I love living on an island – though as I always remind him Australia is the biggest island of all.' (She didn't see rain until she was ten: 'Our teacher let us go outside just to stand in it.') A couple from Norfolk, who ask me to send their regards to East Anglia. A woman from Leicestershire whose Newfoundland dog is bigger than many of the Shetland ponies we've seen today. He's lovely, but as we walk back to the van I suggest to Michelle there must be others that aren't.

'You soon get to know which dogs you can trust,' she says. 'There was one that used to run out and bite the tyres on my van. Absolutely mad, it was. Eventually it'd wear itself out and run back through the gate. That was my cue to get out and deliver the post.'

Finally, in the early afternoon, we reach the building I've been waiting for: the most northerly house in the United Kingdom. The Haa is yet another modern bungalow, but whitewashed to fit in with the centuries-old drystone building to its left. A few other buildings of both vintages cluster round to make up a farm, and standing waiting for us is Alison, the woman who along with her husband owns that farm. Michelle has kindly arranged for Alison to be here – she actually lives a couple of miles to the south (The Haa these days is home only to some lambs). Alison takes us into the small kitchen to show us the cans of condensed milk with which she feeds them, and the cooker on which she heats the milk up. 'We've a new cooker going in soon,' she adds. These are some well-catered-for animals.

My letter simply explained what the book's about and why I wanted to visit, but even though Michelle has already forewarned Alison it still seems proper that the envelope is officially handed over. In return Alison shows us the second visitors' book of the day. People from all over Britain have been coming to see The Haa for decades – the book's earliest entries date from 1961. I'm honoured to add my name, before Alison takes us back outside to show us the building to the right of the main house. It's a drystone construction similar to the one on the other side, with the exception that its roof, when you look closely, is an upside-down rowing boat.

'That's another lambing shelter,' explains Alison. 'It was built after the war. The boat came from *Sea Venture*, a British ship that was going across to Norway in 1939. She was torpedoed by a U-boat. All the crew managed to get into the lifeboat and they came ashore here.' She indicates the small sandy beach on the other side of the field next to the farm. 'The Sinclair family were living here then – they welcomed the men ashore.' The men left but the boat stayed. Talk of world war leads to a discussion of the first one, when the messenger boys who delivered the telegram telling of a loved one's loss became known as 'angels of death'. They were forbidden from whistling.

Alison and Michelle and I are joined after a while by Bruce, who's going to take me back to Lerwick in time for this evening's ferry. We talk about nearby Out Stack and Muckle Flugga, the two uninhabited rocks which form the northernmost points of the UK. Muckle Flugga comes second by a few hundred yards, though wins in the 'amusing name' stakes. (It means 'large steep-sided island', and according to legend was a stone thrown by a giant fighting another giant who loved the same mermaid.) Shetland language as a whole is wonderfully rich, especially when it comes to wildlife. Puffins, I learn, are 'tammy nories', porpoises are 'neesiks', while a 'bonxie' is a bird none of my companions knows the proper name for but, says Bruce, 'it's a massive great thing that dives at you'.

Soon it's time to go. I depart with a subtly altered sense of what 'Britain' means to me. It has to change your picture of the country, knowing it includes somewhere that has bonxies and where the nearest place you can buy Scandinavian flat-pack furniture is Scandinavia. And yet still, as far as the Royal Mail are concerned, this place fits underneath a first-class stamp.

Michelle heads off to complete her round, and Bruce and I bid farewell to Alison. The last thing we see as we drive away is her disappearing into the main house, followed excitedly but obediently, their tails wagging, looking for all the world like new schoolchildren following their teacher into a classroom, by two tiny lambs.

7

THE LAST POST

And then there were 23.

I'm looking at them on the map now, with that feeling you always get near the end of a job you've enjoyed – half proud that soon you'll have achieved it, half sad that soon it'll be over. Only one more trip to make, one big sweep up and down the country to take in some of those remaining areas. I feel like a caretaker conducting his final tour of the night, checking the windows and locks on a building he cares for deeply.

An itinerary forms – up the west of England, into Scotland, turn right and right again then back down Britain's east. Before setting out I tick off the areas that definitely won't be visited, the first of them LU. Pretty sure that a story told by TV presenter Nick Owen happened at Luton Town's ground, I check with him. Just as well – it actually happened at Aston Villa's. We're talking 1979, the days before Owen graced breakfast sofas with Anne Diamond, back when he was still a football commentator. After years of radio he'd been given his first ever television match, and had 'calmed my nerves' before kick-off with a few pints of lager. The media gantry at Villa Park was reached via a ladder, which then had to be hauled up to allow the crowd in. It couldn't be lowered again until the crowd had left after the match. By half-time on this cold March evening Owen realised that the liquid intake had been a mistake. By the final whistle he was 'desperate'. But the crowd hung around, waiting for the night's other scores to be read over the tannoy. Trapped in his torment, Owen appealed to colleagues for help. They didn't fail him – no fewer than 13 empty polystyrene cups were collected. Owen filled every one.

Had Birmingham not already been taken this could have done duty for B, cueing up a side mention for the fact that during the Second World War Villa Park's home dressing room housed a rifle company from the Royal Warwickshire Regiment. But LU would still have been vacant. Have no fear, though – Nick steps into the breach with something that *did* happen at Kenilworth Road:

LU (Luton): Nick Owen was once refused entry to the Nick Owen Lounge at Luton Town FC's ground.

Wanting a drink before a match he was attending with his sons, Owen presented himself at the door. 'You can't go in,' said the steward, 'it's packed.' Not being the sort of celebrity to use the dreaded line 'don't you know who I am?', Owen accepted the situation and walked away. As he went he heard someone ask the doorman: 'Don't you know who that is?' 'Haven't got a clue,' said the doorman, only to be told that 'his name's in bloody great capitals above your head'.

Chester next, where we could use the plaque unveiled by Gyles Brandreth during his time as the city's Member of Parliament: 'This plague was unveiled by Gyles Brandreth MP...' But let us instead record a canine landmark:

CH (Chester): One of Britain's first guide dogs for the blind ate its owner's false teeth.

It should be noted that the owner wasn't wearing them at the time. The use of dogs to help blind people had been pioneered by a German doctor during the First World War. Walking in the grounds of his hospital with a patient who'd been blinded at the front, the doctor was called away for a few minutes. On his return he noticed how well his German Shepherd had behaved with the man, and decided to investigate. The guide dog programme that resulted came to the attention of two women in the Cheshire town of Wallasey, who in 1931 began training the first British guide dogs, four German Shepherds called Flash, Meta, Judy and Folly. The public initially thought the idea cruel, and even intervened physically to stop the training taking place. But then they saw the delight on the faces of the owners, four men who (as in Germany) had been blinded during the war. OK, there were some teething troubles, literally in Meta's case, but a new chapter in the relationship between man and his best friend had begun. Folly's owner, Thomas Ap Rhys, was soon 'walking at the fastest pace or even running with her'. He died in 1979 at the age of 82, while retraining with his sixth dog.

The Kilmarnock area covers a whole stretch of the west coast of Scotland below Glasgow, as well as the Isle of Arran lying off that coast. Cleat's Shore on the island is widely cited as the only official nudist beach in Scotland, but there seems to be some dispute about that so I can't use it as the fact. Given its location you won't be surprised that the beach is described in the guidebook *Bare Britain* as 'probably the least visited nudist beach in the known universe'. The country's first official beach of this kind opened in Brighton in 1980, despite the objections of Councillor John Blackman, who called it 'a flagrant exhibition of mammary glands ... What distresses me is that people naively believe what is good for the Continent is good for Britain.' If we can't have nudity on a beach as our fact, then, let us have a murder on one:

KA (Kilmarnock): Lawyers in an eighteenth-century murder case argued about whether it should be treated as a crime at sea, because the killing had taken place beyond the high-tide mark.

The 10th Earl of Eglinton was the man on the wrong end of the shotgun. He could have featured as the 'G' fact: the village of Eaglesham (now in the Glasgow postcode area) was laid out by the Earl, otherwise known as Alexander Montgomorie, in the shape of a capital 'A' to denote his Christian name.[1] But leaving geographical narcissism to one side, Eglinton came to his end in 1769 during a dispute with a supposed poacher who had been seen on his estate of Montfode, near the town of Ardrossan. By the time Eglinton reached the area the man, Mungo Campbell, was on the beach. Refusing to hand over his gun, Campbell first retreated, then shot Eglinton in the stomach, wounding him fatally. His trial was delayed because the incident had occurred between the high- and low-water marks, and murder at sea lay within the jurisdiction of the Lord High Admiral of Scotland. In the end the proceedings went ahead. Campbell was found guilty and sentenced to be hanged. But his friends smuggled a silk scarf into his cell, allowing him to do the job himself rather than suffer the indignity of a hangman taking charge. This didn't go down very well with the public, who had been looking forward to a good old-fashioned public execution. As recompense they dug up Campbell's body and abused it. His friends eventually rescued the corpse and buried it (where else?) at sea.

Yet more criminality – and indeed more sea – in the next fact:

---

[1] It was on a farm outside Eaglesham that Rudolph Hess landed during his secret 1941 attempt to negotiate a peace treaty with Britain.

**HS (Outer Hebrides): Men who stole whisky from a
shipwrecked vessel off the island of Eriskay wore
women's dresses to protect their clothes from
incriminating oil.**

In 1941 the SS *Politician* was on its way from Liverpool
to the USA with a cargo that included 28,000 cases of malt
whisky. It came to grief off the coast of Eriskay, and the islanders decided to help themselves. Eight years later the incident
would form the basis of the Ealing Comedy *Whisky Galore!*,
but customs officer Charles McColl didn't see anything at all
funny about the thefts. He insisted on prosecutions, and went
ballistic when fines of just a few pounds were handed out.
Eventually McColl blew the ship up with dynamite to prevent
further illegality. *Whisky Galore!* itself was filmed on nearby
Barra, home in *Dad's Army* to Private James 'We're Doomed!'
Frazer. He called it a 'wild and lonely place'. That may have
been his opinion, though I can't help warming to an island that
names its annual half-marathon the 'Barrathon'. And before we
leave the Outer Hebrides, how about a mention for Gerhard
Zucker, an exile from Nazi Germany who was brought to
my attention by Harry. The BPMA's files, it seems, record
Zucker's 'Mail Rocket', which would have conveyed letters and
parcels between the islands of Harris and Scarp. He persuaded
the Royal Mail to let him demonstrate the device in 1934.
'Unfortunately, but possibly predictably,' goes the account,
'the first flight ended in an explosion and the destruction of
most of the cargo of 1,200 letters. Having singularly failed to
impress in the UK, Zucker was deported to Germany where
he was promptly arrested on suspicion of co-operating with
the British.'

On to KW, covering not only the Orkney Islands (on which
the town of Kirkwall is to be found) but also the north-eastern

part of mainland Scotland itself, the bit that includes John O'Groats. It's a vast area with not many residents, meaning it contains fewer postcodes than any of the other 123 areas. The mainland residents frequently get annoyed. 'Every time we tell people our postcode,' says one, 'they think we live on Orkney.' As a result they get stung for 'exorbitant' delivery charges, and are campaigning for a separate code. Second place in the race to be KW's fact goes to the daily plane journey between the islands of Westray and Papa Westray, which with the wind in the right direction can take as little as 47 seconds, making it the shortest scheduled flight in the world. For sheer strangeness, however, the title goes to some cows:

KW (Kirkwall): The uninhabited island of Swona is home to Britain's only wild herd of beef cattle.

The last remaining humans on Swona, brother and sister James and Violet Rosie, left in 1974 when James was taken ill. Their herd of cows – eight females and one bull – had to be abandoned. The bull clearly set about having a good time, because four decades later the herd is still going strong. Every spring two calves are born (though they don't always survive), and the island's population averages 17. Because they've been separated from the mainland for so long the cattle are totally free of disease, and with the grass kept constantly short by their grazing Swona's flower count has gone off the scale. There are orchids, corn marigolds and so many other rare plants that the island now enjoys Site of Special Scientific Interest status.

Back over the border again, we reach the Cleveland postcode known as TS, for 'Teesside'. It was here, outside St Mary Magdalene Church in Trimdon, that Tony Blair (during a weekend in his constituency) made his famous 'people's princess' remark about Diana. This is now commemorated by a plaque which indulges modern Britain's love of the Unnecessary Capital Letter: 'On this spot The Prime Minister The RT Hon Tony Blair MP Announced the tragic death...' But we didn't make Gyles Brandreth's plaque a fact, so political neutrality dictates that we can't honour Tony Blair's either. Instead let us return to 1827, and the Stockton-on-Tees shop of chemist John Walker. Stirring a pot of chemicals one day, he saw that a lump of the mixture had formed on the end of the stick and dried. He tried to scrape it off. It burst into flames. Which means that:

TS (Cleveland): The match was accidentally invented by a chemist in Stockton-on-Tees.

Walker called his invention the 'friction light'. He started selling three-inch-long versions, packed together in boxes of 50. Each box came with a separate piece of sandpaper, which you folded in half before dragging the match through it. Despite friends telling him he should patent the idea Walker refused, not wanting to stop others benefiting from it. Improved designs soon reached the market, including one called the Lucifer (meaning 'light-bearer'). To this day the Dutch word for 'match' is 'lucifer'.

Further down the coast is Hull. The area includes Beverley, whose elections to Parliament were notoriously corrupt, even in an era when corruption was a way of political life. Anthony Trollope, not content with writing his novels and shaping the early postcode system, also fancied being an MP. Resigning from his job at the Post Office (civil servants weren't allowed to enter the Commons), he stood in Beverley. The campaign proved to be 'the most wretched fortnight of my manhood'. He threw £400 at it and still came last. Kingston-upon-Hull itself is the town where Philip Larkin lived most of his adult life, enjoying its position 'on the edge of things'. Not during the Second World War it wasn't: Hull was the most severely bombed British town or city other than London. 95 per cent of its houses were damaged. One resident remembered heading for the air-raid shelter: 'Mam dashed back into the house. "Where are you going, Mary?" said Dad. "Back for my false teeth," she replied. "Come back here," shouted Dad, "the Germans are dropping bombs not meat pies."' But the area's 'edgy' reputation certainly applies to its fact:

HU (Hull): The beach at Tunstall marks the Greenwich Meridian's last point on land before the North Pole.

You could say it's the line's most northerly land-bound point full stop. Not until researching this book (here comes an admission that might count as shameful for someone in his early forties) did I fully get my head round the fact that the North Pole doesn't really exist. Not in the sense that the South Pole does, a proper point on a proper land mass. The North Pole is in the middle of the Arctic Ocean, occupying a stretch of water almost perpetually covered with shifting pieces of ice. Thinking about the Greenwich Meridian, and learning that its ratification dates from 1884, you'd be forgiven for assuming it was an act of Victorian imperial arrogance, the country which owned most of the world telling the rest of the world that it was the centre of the world. But in fact the International Meridian Conference took place in Washington, DC, at the behest of then US President Chester A. Arthur. Delegates from 25 nations agreed that the meridian passing through the Royal Observatory in Greenwich, already the most popular for shipping purposes, should get the global nod. Only one country abstained from the vote, persisting for another few decades in using the meridian that passed through its own capital city. You may or may not be surprised to learn that this country was France.

Sadness over in HD, and specifically in the parliamentary constituency of Colne Valley:

HD (Huddersfield): The Reverend Charles Leach is the only person ever to be removed as an MP after being declared of unsound mind.

Leach had already lived a pretty full life even before he entered the Commons. Born in 1847, his work as a Non-conformist minister saw him deliver hundreds of Sunday afternoon lectures and write 20 books, among them *Old, Yet Ever New*, *Is My Bible True?* and *Ten Reasons Why I Believe the Bible Is the Word of God*. He spread that word – and sometimes built churches – in Birmingham, London and Manchester, also finding time to act as a tour guide in the Holy Land for an up-and-coming travel firm called Thomas Cook. At the age of 61 he was elected Liberal MP for Colne Valley, but this didn't reduce his work on behalf of the Lord. Preaching took him to Canada and the USA, and when the First World War broke out he became a chaplain to the armed forces. However the strain of visiting the wounded took its toll, and in 1915 it was reported that he had moved to a 'nursing home' in London. It was actually a lunatic asylum.

Not unknown for our elected representatives to part company with sanity, of course, then or now. 'Eccentricity', a trait we often admire in them, can occasionally develop into something darker. Soon after the 1992 General Election one Labour MP succumbed to Alzheimer's, and by 1997, when his party finally won, he was unable to understand what was happening.

But for those five years he was allowed to stay in the House. This is how it had always been done: keep it quiet, sort a successor, let them take over at the next election. This is how it would have been done for Charles Leach, but the war meant no one knew when the next election would be held. By 1916 it was decided that Leach had to be replaced. So for the first and only time ever, the 1886 Lunacy (Vacating of Seats) Act was invoked. Leach left the Commons, and entered history.

The customer in front of me at the petrol station knows the cashier, and not having seen him for a while she asks after a mutual acquaintance.

'I'm afraid he died,' replies the cashier.

'Oh no,' says the customer. 'How?'

'He got run over by ten police cars.' He hands the customer her receipt. No more is said of the matter by either of them.

It's a blazing morning in late July, and I'm on my way to the first appointment of the final trip. Six days of mopping up Britain's loose ends are going to start with a footpath. So bad luck, Ken Richardson. For a while your 32nd birthday celebrations had the HP (Hemel Hempstead) title tied up. You remember, that day in 1977 at the Oddfellow's Arms when you played pool with your wife Gill. As you took aim your dentures fell out and you accidentally potted them. Gill tried to retrieve them and got her hand stuck in the pocket. Firemen had to rescue her (and your teeth) using washing-up liquid and a power saw. It might seem harsh for all this to lose out to a footpath, but it is an important footpath. One with political connections. HP has quite a few of those, actually, thanks largely to the part of it called Beaconsfield. The town saw Tony Blair's first crack at Parliament (1982 by-election – he lost his deposit), and in 1966 hosted the young Muammar Gaddafi, when as a Libyan military graduate he was sent to Beaconsfield's Army School of Education to learn English. He hated London, but loved the Buckinghamshire countryside. Further back, Benjamin Disraeli took the title 'Earl of Beaconsfield' on his elevation to the peerage, having been its MP for nearly 30 years. He was yet another nineteenth-century over-achiever, publishing several novels throughout his career, including *The Young Duke*, the book that gave us the term 'dark horse'.[2]

But today I'm heading for a political building near the village of Ellesborough. Parking opposite the church of St Peter and St Paul, I take the footpath leading into some heavily wooded hills. The shade those woods offer makes it perfect territory for jogging, as shown by a woman and her black Labrador heading in the opposite direction. The path crosses a quiet road, then after a while rejoins it for a few yards. It's at this point that the building first comes into view. A couple of fields away is the eastern elevation of a large red-brick country house. 'This is a protected site,' warns a sign, 'under Section 128 of the Serious Organised Crime and Police Act 2005.' Further on, and having recrossed the road, the footpath enters the grounds of the house. The front of the residence and its outbuildings are clearly visible to your right the whole time. Apart from when you cross its driveway, that is, which rises then dips so that the house disappears from view. But you've got something else to look at now: the two gatehouses a few yards to your left. Nearby is a ten-foot-high black metal pole, supporting several CCTV cameras pointing in different directions. You're reminded of another sign you saw a couple of minutes ago, stuck on a wooden pole in the middle of the field: 'The Chequers estate is monitored by security cameras. Thames Valley Police.'

---

[2] In the novel it's a horse-racing term for an animal that gamblers don't know about – its wider use came later.

We, or rather our Prime Minister, have Viscount Lee to thank for Chequers. The house itself dates from 1565, but was given to the nation by Lee in 1921. His thinking was that 'the better the health of our rulers the more sanely they will rule, and the inducement to spend two days a week in the high and pure air of the Chiltern hills and woods will, it is hoped, benefit the nation as well as its chosen leaders'. I'm reading the 'high and pure' bit when I nearly tread in something left by one of the cows grazing here today. Whether or not our rulers have ruled sanely is something I'll leave to you (we might ask whether Chequers could have saved Charles Leach), but it's undeniable that the house occupies a beautiful setting. This, of course, makes it ideal for entertaining world leaders:

HP (Hemel Hempstead): When German Chancellor Angela Merkel sat on the terrace at Chequers and commented, 'Your countryside is so lovely', David Cameron replied, 'Yes, Angela, and to think if things had turned out differently it could all have been yours.'

A not-entirely relaxed pause ensued, apparently, but finally Mrs Merkel laughed.

After crossing the drive the path climbs another hill into yet more woods on the house's west. Then it turns to the right, back towards Ellesborough. Circling the house like this takes the best part of an hour, with Chequers visible for much of the time. Today one of the fields is full of huge circular bails of hay, some lying on the recently harvested stubble, some stacked on a trailer awaiting collection. The vast expanse of yellow stretches to the green hills in the distance, with the red house balancing on the crease in between. It's crying out for John Constable to hop in a time machine bringing his easel and brushes with him. As it is the scene is recorded on an iPhone by a young American wearing a skull-and-crossbones T-shirt. He may well be reflecting on how different things would be back home. If by any miracle you managed to get this close to Camp David you would soon find yourself 'attended to' by several men wearing dark glasses and earpieces and curiously lacking in inter-personal skills. In Britain, we put a public footpath through the front garden.

Soon afterwards, I'm crossing the top of a seriously tall hill. You can no longer see Chequers, but you can see mile after mile after mile of Buckinghamshire and Oxfordshire. At this height the summer thermals are something else, and an enormous hawk soars directly overhead, wings outstretched and motionless. It holds the same position for so long, and the thoughts of security are so fresh in the memory, that for a second I suspect some sort of trickery, a fake bird radio-controlled by someone in the Chequers gatehouse. But then the wings fold, the hawk swoops away and I'm left with a refreshing sense of just how relaxed Britain can still be when it wants to.

The next area is OX. Although I'm not stopping in Oxford itself, the fact surely has to relate to the city's university. Nigh on a thousand years of history (no one's entirely sure of the exact figure) offer plenty to choose from. There was once a rule, for instance, which forbade students from bringing bows and arrows into class. Great Tom, the bell at Christ Church, still chimes 101 times every night to denote the college's original number of scholars. It used to be the signal for every college to lock its gates, and still happens at 9.05 p.m., this being nine o'clock in 'Oxford time' (sunrise there is five minutes later than in Greenwich). The same college had William Osler as a fellow. He was the early twentieth-century medic who during a lecture on diabetes demonstrated the importance of observation by dipping his finger in a urine sample, sucking it, then asking his students to do likewise. What, he wondered, was their observation? That the urine was very sweet, came the unanimous reply. 'Perhaps,' said Osler. 'But if you'd really been observant you would have noticed that I placed my middle finger in the urine but my index finger in my mouth.' As I head along the M40 today I wonder what Osler would have thought of the estate car in front of me, an ambulance owned by the NHS and forced to display a sign reading 'No drugs carried in this vehicle'.

Another Oxford academic was the Reverend Samuel Henshall, who in 1795 obtained a patent on the corkscrew. It's thought he was inspired by the gun worm, a tool used by soldiers to retrieve unspent charges from their musket barrels. Then there was J. R. R. Tolkien, who as well as creating Middle Earth was Oxford's Professor of Anglo-Saxon. His party trick was to take his class to the Eagle and Child pub (commonly known as the Bird and Baby), sit them round a table and ask them to speak one by one. Afterwards he would tell every student exactly where they came from. Except it wasn't only a party trick. 'The reason,' he would explain, 'is that I want you to believe me when I say *this* is how Anglo-Saxon sounded.'

Our fact, though, comes from the mid-1970s, and relates to the man who a decade or so later would invent the World Wide Web:

OX (Oxford): When he was a student at Oxford, Tim Berners-Lee was banned from using the university's computer.

He and a friend had been caught hacking on it.

After staying the night with my parents in Warwickshire, I head across to perhaps Britain's least trendy county, Shropshire.

Its unfashionable air could be because it gets lost in the border between England and Wales, or maybe because people are put off by the town whose postcode I'm investigating. Telford, according to Victor Lewis-Smith, 'is so dull that the bypass was built before the town'. But never judge a postcode area by the place that gives it its initials. Rather like Tim Berners-Lee, TF gifted the planet something that nearly everyone on it has heard of:

TF (Telford): The Shropshire town of Much Wenlock was the birthplace of the modern Olympic Games.

And there you were (if you're anything like me) thinking the International Olympic Committee had gone straight to the ancient Greeks for their inspiration. But no, William Penny Brookes was their man. He was the Much Wenlock doctor who founded his 'Olympian Games' to encourage a healthy lifestyle for 'all grades of man', after his work had shown him the problems caused by spending all your time down the pub. The first games were held at the town's racecourse in October 1850, and included athletics, football and cricket. The event became an annual fixture, with Brookes prepared to show he wasn't a complete health nut: additions included the Gimcrack Race, in which horse riders had to stop at several points to put on a pair of boots, have a drink and smoke a cigar. There was also the blindfold wheelbarrow race and the Balaclava Mêlée (named after the battle), in which men on horseback knocked the plumes off each other's helmets. Brookes was ahead of his time in inviting everyone to take part: a Mrs Gaskell objected that recreation for 'the working classes' made them lazy. Well, I say 'everyone' – Brookes didn't allow women into the serious events. They did have their own events, though. Choral singing, for instance. And knitting.

There were some precedents for the games. The Cotswold Olimpicks had started at Chipping Campden in 1612, and like the Wenlock version they continue to this day.[3] But it was Brookes who inspired the formation of the IOC. In 1994 the body's then president Juan Antonio Samaranch visited Much Wenlock to lay a wreath on Brookes's grave, saying: 'I came to pay homage and tribute to Doctor Brookes, who really was the founder of the modern Olympic Games.' The IOC's founder, Pierre de Coubertin, had come to the town in 1890, staying at the doctor's house for several days and watching the games. Four years later the IOC came into being, and two years after that the first official Olympics took place in Athens. Brookes couldn't quite hang on to see them, unfortunately, dying four months too soon. 'Now let us imagine ourselves a century and a half hence,' he'd once said. 'What might we behold? A stalwart, noble race, strong in body and mind.' A glance at Channel 5's documentary output would show Brookes that his dream hasn't quite come true, but the Olympics survive at international and Wenlockian level. In 1924 Harold Langley of Birmingham became the first person to compete in both, adding the long-jump in Paris to his Shropshire pentathlon the previous year.

It's no surprise that Much Wenlock's excellent little museum concentrates mainly on the Olympics. There are a couple of penny farthings bearing mannequins in Victorian athletic gear, the guy in the lead looking nervously round to check on his rival's progress. (I'd like to see Bradley Wiggins do his

---

[3] Still with the shin-kicking competition included. Though contestants no longer wear iron-tipped boots or prepare by hardening their shins with coal hammers.

stuff on a contraption like that.) There's a cuddly toy version of Wenlock, one of the mascots from London 2012. I read about Brookes and how he spread the word, for instance establishing the National Olympian Games in London in 1866. W. G. Grace was given time off from a cricket match to enter the 440-yard hurdles. God knows who the other competitors were, because Grace won. There's also mention of the 1900 Olympics (hosted, as in 1924, by Paris), where the shooting competition used live pigeons.

After the museum I explore the rest of Much Wenlock, starting with Brookes's grave at Holy Trinity Church. Some rather good organ-playing is emanating from the church, so I pop inside to enjoy a few bars. The organist's shoes are very pointy, almost at winklepicker level. When he breaks off I ask if that's to make hitting the right pedal easier. He confirms that it is.

'Are they specially made?'

'No. You can get them made.' He gives a doubtful look. 'But that's a bit pretentious.'

The town is a beauty. There are old-fashioned street names (The George Shut meets The Mutton Shut at right angles), while the second-hand shop is selling a vinyl collection catalogued with one of those handheld printers which churned out short lengths of stickable plastic tape. The previous owner's nerdish instincts might be a tad stronger than mine, but I nevertheless find them appealing. (So you know – Kate Bush's *Never for Ever* was number 1,216.) The Post Office shows how times have changed since Anthony Trollope's day: a sign advises 'Turkish Lira in stock now'. But most exciting of all is the freestanding pillar box outside the post office. Research for the FK (Falkirk) area later in the trip has included Carron, the ironworks named after the river on whose banks it was founded in 1759. As well as their military products – the

Duke of Wellington ordered that no other make of cannon was to be used by the British Army – Carron also took a hefty slice of the pillar-box market. Before reading this I'd never noticed that boxes have the manufacturer's name on the base, the bit painted black underneath the main red body. Since reading it, I've become addicted to spotting the names. This isn't something I've confessed to Jo, of course. A relationship can only bear so much strain. Nor did I tell her that, out on a bike ride the other day and sheltering from torrential rain in the portico of a village church, I'd read the noticeboard. Aside from wondering what the Women's Institute have been putting in their tea (a forthcoming talk was titled 'I Am a Tulip, What Are You?'), I was heartbroken by a Royal Mail message: 'Please note that this Church has no facility for receiving mail. It does not have a postcode.' Harsh of you, Royal Mail, harsh indeed. It's bad enough for the church that it lacks a letter box. Do you really have to rub it in by denying the poor thing a postcode?

Anyway, my straw poll has confirmed that yes, many pillar boxes do bear the words 'Carron Company Stirlingshire', including at least one in London's uber-hip enclave of Hoxton. This lunchtime, in the very different atmosphere of Much Wenlock, it's nice to add another Carron to the list. And to reflect on the workers who made them. Did they stop to think, as they poured metal into mould and wiped sweat from their brows, of the emotions that would drop into their creation over the years? The letters and cards telling of love and lust, anger and hate? The heartfelt truths, the downright lies? In the days before the internet, all human life could be found at the bottom of a pillar box. Bereavements were squashed up against births, condolences next to con tricks. Those hard-bitten men in Scottish ironworks allowed the nation to transmit its most intimate feelings.

Northwards now, heading for tonight's stopover of Blackpool. This means passing through another unticked area, CW. Crewe was the birthplace of Jimmy MacDonald, the man who voiced Mickey Mouse after Walt Disney became too hoarse from smoking. It's nice to note that Jimmy's mother's name was Minnie, but he left for the States as a baby, so doesn't really have a proper link with the area. Instead we turn to Crewe's most famous export:

CW (Crewe): In order to trick would-be forgers, the 'Winged B' emblem on Bentley cars has a different number of feathers on each side.

The logo has adorned the luxury vehicles since 1919, when designer F. Gordon Crosby had his cunning idea. So subtle is the trick that it takes quite a long time on Google images to confirm the fact, but yes, there are 10 feathers branching out to the left of the 'B', 11 to the right. Further motoring education comes as I look at the map and notice the town of Leyland, near Preston. Was this where the car company started? Indeed it was. Other place names that leap out are Vulcan Village (the name now given to the cottages inhabited by workers at the old Vulcan Foundry), Robin Hood (a hamlet, probably just cashing in on the legend) and Pleasington, settled centuries ago by someone called Plessa but which must now experience the opposite house-price effect to Minge Lane. My motorway (the M6) also goes near Margarine Corner, a bend in the A351 near Stoke-on-Trent where a lorry carrying Stork margarine overturned during the Second World War. People came from far and wide to help themselves. Rationing can test even the strictest moral code.

Finally I turn left on to the M55, crossing that section of the North-West known to the Royal Mail as FY. (Bolton had nabbed BL, so Blackpool and its environs are labelled after the Fylde, the coastal plain on which they lie.) At the motorway's end lies the mecca itself, the humming holiday hotspot which for generations of families has meant sun, sea and sand, all offered up with a cheeky grin and industrial quantities of ketchup. I've only been to Blackpool once before. That was seven years ago, during a political conference, and within minutes it's clear that the thronging delegates gave a false impression of how busy the town is these days. Tonight, at what must surely be the height of the holiday season, Blackpool is at best ticking over. Plenty of windows show vacancy signs, and the promenade is not what you'd call packed. As I search for my hotel, a few blocks back from the seafront, there's a perfect illustration of how Blackpool gets things that little bit wrong: a B&B aimed at gay customers displays the rainbow flag together with the slogan 'It's a gay thing!'

Or is that me being a metropolitan snob?[4] OK, the gay people I know wouldn't stay somewhere like that, but the place's very existence surely implies that there are other gay people who do. It's not the only misconception to get corrected: my memory of Blackpool's non-political clientele was that they were exclusively white, but tonight I see several Indian families. Fuel for my walk along the seafront comes from a chippy near the hotel. The owner reports that I wasn't totally mistaken about the town on my previous visit. 'It's definitely got quieter since then. Business has suffered. Part of the problem was a series they had on telly a couple of years back, following the emergency services around Blackpool. You follow the emergency services round any town, you're going to get some unpleasant sights.'

[4] If someone who lives in Suffolk can ever be a metropolitan snob.

Fair point. And I can only add that if there was a fly-on-the-wall series about this guy's chips, Blackpool would have to build 50 new hotels. I eat my dinner sitting on some concrete steps overlooking the beach, where one or two of the braver holidaymakers are still paddling and dawdling and trying to ignore the fact that at 8 p.m. in late July you really can struggle without a jumper. Soon a seagull positions itself ten yards away and eyeballs me unflinchingly, a look that says 'they're mine when you're finished, right?' Refusing to bow to its intimidation, I eat every last scrap, screw up the empty paper as tightly as possible, shove it deep into the nearest bin then walk away, not quite able to believe I've let a seagull wind me up. I recall the bird's cousins in Margate (huge) and Cardiff (aggressive): the project really is forming a clothes line of its own memories now. Another gust of sadness that it's nearly over blows in from the cold Irish Sea.

I'm halfway along the front here, between the North and South Shores, not far from the famous Tower. Hard to believe, as you gaze up at the famously populist structure – the top of which is for some reason illuminated a vibrant pink – that the inscription above the stage in its ballroom is from a Shakespearean sonnet: 'Bid me discourse, I will enchant thine ear.' The colour scheme continues down at ground level, where some of the horse-drawn carriages you can hire for a ride are pink Cinderella-like bubble-shaped affairs. No male would be seen dead in one of those, and quite a few females would think twice. I pass the Viking Hotel, 'Talk of the Coast' with its 'Premier Cabaret Show starring Buddy Lee'. Further along is the Cornhill Hotel, whose residents' lounge is visible through a large window. Onstage a singer is delivering a hearty 'Daydream Believer', deterred neither by having to adjust the karaoke backing track himself nor by his audience numbering precisely five. Over the road the Central

Pier offers a joint Elvis/Freddie Mercury tribute show called 'King and Queen'. There are gaps along the front these days, an empty hotel covered in scaffolding, even a hotel that's been completely demolished. But plenty of food is still available, very little of it salad. One establishment offers 'Dogs... Ribs... Wings... *and other things*'. Their italics, and ones that fill you with foreboding.

Still adorning the front is Gypsy Lavinia, the fortune-teller who's been around for so long that the photos outside her small wooden booth include one of her with a pre-nose job Tom Jones. 'Today only,' reads a sign, '£5, both palms.' Tempting as the offer is I carry on, using Lavinia instead as a cue for Blackpool's fact. The sort of people who form the customer base for fortune-tellers are, you would think, the same people responsible for this:

FY (Blackpool): Ernie, the computer that generates winning Premium Bond numbers, regularly receives gifts and cards from people hoping to increase their chances of winning.

The cards arrive at Premium Bonds HQ in Blackpool on Valentine's Day and at Christmas, while the gifts include holy water, castor oil and Epsom salts. You'd hope the last two, with their 'flushing out' effects, were meant to be ironic jokes from people wanting Ernie to produce their numbers. But if any of the senders really do think that some bizarre chemistry might be at work, they clearly haven't got their head round the way Ernie ('Electronic Random Number Indicating Equipment') does his stuff. Actually we're now on Ernie 4 (the first one having fired up in 1957), but like all his predecessors he shuns computer programs: precisely *because* programs are programmed they can never produce truly random numbers. Instead Ernie derives the numbers from 'thermal noise', the changes in voltage and heat given off by transistors. These really are random, and therefore totally unpredictable. Don't bother trying to hack Ernie, either. He's completely unconnected to any other computer.

Heading back to the hotel I pass signs of old Blackpool – including (I promise you) a man with a flat cap and a whippet – as well as signs that the place has changed. For instance someone at a bus stop is smoking something he definitely didn't buy at a tobacconist's. Then again the kids idling around on their bikes could have come from any of the last few decades. Overall you get the impression of somewhere that's dying, but very, very slowly. It's going to be a long time before Blackpool finally cashes in its chips.

The next morning offers up some biblical rain. I respond by heading to LA. Logical enough, were it not for the fact that this LA is the Lancaster postcode area, taking in the southern half of the Lake District. The northern half is covered by CA (Carlisle). Today I will visit one lake in each area. They have very different stories to tell.

The route is straight up the M6 again, then another left into the damply verdant terrain south of Kendal. The thing about the Lake District is that for all its wetness it still feels a decidedly cosy place. At least from inside a car it does. The narrow, winding roads are hemmed in by trees, and the hilliness means you're almost always in a valley. So you can never see that far, and what you can see is fairly dark, especially when you throw in the granite and slate from which most of the houses and drystone walls are built. Even when a vista does open up the rain does its best to close it back down pretty sharpish. Ignoring the turning for Windermere, I head instead to Coniston, the slightly smaller lake a few miles to the west.

Several people have decided that the current downpour isn't presenting them with quite enough water, so have taken their canoes and boats out on to the lake. Absurd as this seems, they are at least travelling at safe speeds. Unlike someone else here in 1967:

LA (Lancaster): Donald Campbell was killed during his second attempt at the world water speed record because he didn't refuel or wait for the wake from his first attempt to die down.

The story of what happened that January day is told in the village of Coniston itself, where a museum displays items of Campbell memorabilia. They even have part of his boat *Bluebird*, salvaged from the lake (along with Campbell's body) in 2001. Only a small part, mind you: while the rest is repaired, this battered and misshapen fragment has been left here as an illustration of what happens when a speedboat flips over at 300 mph. Not refuelling meant that the boat was lighter, so when it hit a wash from the first attempt it had even less chance of staying horizontal. The boat flew into the air, performed a perfect backward somersault and crashed into the lake. Only Campbell's helmet, shoes and oxygen mask floated to the surface, together with Mr Whoppit, the 'lucky' teddy bear who accompanied Campbell on all his record attempts. Mr Whoppit had been there the accident-free day in 1964 in Australia when his owner set the existing record of 276 mph. Yes, Campbell was only trying to claim the title from himself.

As you stand in the museum and contemplate his 1967 crash helmet, it's hard to decide whether he was mad or a hero. The standard answer with people like this is 'both'. Fair enough, I suppose. But Mr Whoppit now lives with Campbell's daughter Gina, who was 17 when her father died, and you have to ask whether she wouldn't have preferred a few more years with him rather than a lifetime with the bear. I gaze out of the window at the lashing rain and think of Campbell lying in the lake for over three decades, of the family disagreement about whether he should be disturbed (his sister opposed the 2001 retrieval). But further round the museum you read that Gina herself grew up to be a speed freak, racing power boats and even, at one point, holding the women's world water speed record. Like her father she insisted on taking Mr Whoppit with her. Like her father she tried to beat her own record and crashed. Unlike her father she survived, though did break both her collarbones. By this point Mr Whoppit must have been getting pretty pissed off.

Today's second lake lies the other side of Ambleside. In the town itself tourists vie with waterproofed walkers for pavement space while traffic snakes slowly through the streets. Crawling along in first I remember another lake, one that lost out to JCB's founder in ST: Lake Rudyard in Staffordshire. This was where a Mr Kipling met his future wife. They liked it so much they named their son after it. Finally the Ambleside bottleneck shoots me out, but there's still plenty of low-gear work to be done on the minor road cutting through to Ullswater. The hills overlooking its climbs and dips have clouds skimming their peaks, meaning each one looks like a volcano smouldering after an eruption. Finally I reach the lake itself, several miles long and also a host to Donald Campbell's record attempts. Its fact, though, is altogether calmer:

CA (Carlisle): So an advert based on Wordsworth's famous poem could be completed on schedule, Heineken paid for 6,000 daffodils to be driven from London to the Lake District.

It was 1982, 180 years after the yellow flowers at Ullswater's Glencoyne Bay inspired William and his sister Dorothy on one of their walks together (he wasn't wandering 'lonely as a cloud' after all). The brewing company had written another in its series of 'Heineken refreshes the parts other beers cannot reach' ads. This one would see the poet struggling with his stanzas until a sip of lager inspired him, at which point the tagline would appear, 'parts' replaced with 'poets' (ha ha). The ad agency were told that on 20 April they'd be guaranteed a veritable carpet of daffodils. But the crew arrived to find that after an unusually cold winter there wasn't a single one to be seen. No matter. Several calls to the capital's florists later, two huge lorries were on their way.

Today the lake's tranquillity is disturbed only by my attempts at stone-skimming (the rain having eased off enough to let me out of the car for a while). This is something I've been practising of late, having discovered a natural talent for it. It may not seem much of a talent, but trust me, when your sporting skills are as close to 'non-existent' as makes no difference, you take every chance you can. Today I'm on good form, even managing a few of those freak throws where the stone's second arc takes it further than the first. There's also a final bounce that splits itself up into several rapid-fire ones, making the throw an eleven-er, if I kept count correctly. I'm starting to consider a possible career change, but then look up the world record for stone-skimming and discover it's an astonishing 51 bounces.

The next stage of the journey brings memories of the project's very first trip, reading all that motorway trivia at Watford Gap. The M6, which I now rejoin, is Britain's longest motorway, only finishing after 232 miles because at (or actually just before) the Scottish border it changes identity and becomes the A74(M). Something else that happens at the border, I learn today, is the weather changes. Literally as I'm passing the huge 'Welcome to Scotland – *Fàilte gu Alba*' sign, the heavens close. Bright evening sunshine replaces the rain, and the sky turns from grisly grey to a blue that would make St Andrew proud. This part of the world didn't receive the longest shrift in my last book. Perhaps that was because I was slightly to the west, heading for Dumfries: scenery can, after all, change within a few miles. Perhaps I was tired and in a bad mood (as the bus doors opened at one rural stop the smell of cow dung filled the vehicle and stayed there for the rest of the journey). Whatever the reason, this evening, driving through the hills of South Lanarkshire, the sunset bathing everything blood-orange and a Burger King lorry in the inside lane proclaiming 'No Whoppers are left in this vehicle overnight', all seems for the best in the best of all possible border countries.

After a restful night in a farmhouse B&B outside Lanark, I'm primed for a busy Saturday that will knock off five of the remaining eight areas. Starting with the one I'm already in – ML (Motherwell). Up the road from Lanark is Hamilton, a small town whose graveyard glories in the name Bent Cemetery. It's a predominantly nineteenth-century affair, quite large and with paths you can drive along, which is a help as I look for the man I've come to visit:

ML (Motherwell): In order for the 10th Duke of Hamilton to fit inside his Egyptian sarcophagus, his legs had to be cut off.

The Duke had a strong interest in Egyptian mummies. Unlike Charles II, who collected dust from mummies and rubbed it on himself to acquire what he called 'ancient greatness', the Duke of Hamilton focused on what would happen to him after death. He became fascinated with the work of

Thomas Pettigrew, a surgeon who threw private parties in London at which he entertained guests by unrolling mummies and performing autopsies on them. (The British upper classes have always taken the phrase 'each to his own' that little bit further.) So impressed was the Duke that he arranged for his own body to be mummified by Pettigrew, then placed in an Egyptian sarcophagus of the Ptolemaic period. He'd bought this in Paris in 1836, supposedly for the British Museum. Whether he changed his mind or had always intended the stony vessel for himself isn't clear. Nor is it clear whether he'd actually tried the thing out for size. You would have thought this was a pretty basic first step, but when in 1852 the fateful day arrived, the sarcophagus proved too small. The Duke was over six feet tall, the Egyptian for whom the receptacle had been built wasn't. Off came several inches of the Duke's now mummified legs, and into the sarcophagus he went, before being interred in Hamilton Mausoleum. This building, by the way, used to have the longest echo of any man-made structure in the world, the sound of its slammed door lasting for a full 15 seconds. The record has gone now, however. It was stolen by ... well, we'll come to that.

The Duke has gone, too. In 1921 subsidence at the mausoleum meant he and several other members of the family had to be moved to Bent Cemetery, which is why I'm driving slowly around it this morning keeping an eye out for him. Having worked out roughly where he might be I complete the search on foot. The family have their own little hedged-off section. It's a pleasant spot, overlooked by an eight-foot-high rectangular monument bearing the names of the dukes and relatives buried there. A few feet from the entrance is a parked car, next to which stands a middle-aged man. He's scruffy verging on 'dosser', stubble several days old, tracksuit bottoms much older than that.

'D'yae need any help?' he asks. 'I noticed you looking round. I know a bit about the graves here.'

'Thanks,' I reply, 'but actually I'm all right.' I indicate the gap in the hedge.

'Ah, the Hamiltons,' he says.

Only now do I notice another man of similar appearance sitting in the driver's seat. 'Do you work here?' I ask the first man.

'Nae, nae. I'm just interested.'

'Right . . .' What sort of person hangs around a cemetery with his mate offering to help visitors? I like a graveyard myself – I am, after all, here – but something about this guy tells me conversation should be avoided. Giving the monument a quick once-over (it doesn't supply any more details about the truncated duke), I depart.

'Have a nice day,' calls the man. Looks like he's here for the duration.

Within minutes Motherwell has given way to the next area, Glasgow. The city itself was host, in June 1842, to the world's first bicycle accident. Kirkpatrick MacMillan, generally recognised as the bicycle's inventor, knocked over a small girl. She wasn't badly hurt, so when the case came to court the judge fined MacMillan a mere five shillings. In fact he seems to have taken quite a shine to the inventor: he got him to ride his bicycle in a figure-of-eight pattern around the courtroom, and even slipped him the money to pay the fine. Further out from Glasgow we find East Kilbride, one of the new towns built after the Second World War to relieve overcrowding in the city. Its location was chosen by Sir Patrick Abercrombie, who had very little time before getting the sleeper train back to London. He ordered his taxi driver to head five miles out from the city centre and turn right. They drove clockwise around this circle until Abercrombie saw a suitable place. 'There,' he said, then headed back to catch his train.

Neither of these, though, are the G fact. And a quirk of the Royal Mail's boundaries means that before reaching the fact I head into PA for a while, so let's deal with that first:

PA (Paisley): The leather for Lady Penelope's limousine in *Thunderbirds* came from the same company that upholsters the benches in the Houses of Parliament.

This is Bridge of Weir Leather (named after the village they inhabit), who have been turning cows into luxury coverings since 1905. Their clients have included not only Parliament (green leather for the House of Commons, red for the Lords) but also the Old Bailey, the Bank of England, the British Library and the Royal and Ancient Golf Club at St Andrews. Their leather has clad Concorde, Air Force One, the Orient Express and the *QE2*, and comforted the bottoms of those driving Rolls-Royces, Aston Martins (it takes about nine cows to do a Rapide), Lincolns and Henry Ford's Model T. To this day the company source 40 per cent of their hides from Scotland, the remainder coming from England and Ireland. Animals from fields with electric fences are preferred – barbed wire can mean scratched leather.

Crossing back into G territory, I continue towards Faslane Bay, a narrow stretch of water branching northwards off the Firth of Clyde. With the bay to my left I head through the small town of Helensburgh, then wait for the signs. Sure enough they appear: 'No unauthorised access'... 'This site is regulated by Military Lands Bylaws'... 'MOD Property – Keep Out'. All are pegged to the high fences and walls lining the left side of the road for much of the bay's length. But intimidating as the razor wire might look (God knows what it'd do to your leather), and momentous as it is to think that this is where Britain keeps its nuclear weapons (the submarines on the other side of that fence carry our Trident missiles), Faslane Naval Base does nothing to frighten me. This isn't because I'm emboldened by the peace camp over the road: its tatty multicoloured caravans and CND posters have, for the moment at least, been abandoned. No, it's because I know that:

G (Glasgow): The Royal Marines at Faslane Naval Base repel midges by wearing Avon's 'Skin So Soft' body lotion.

The tiny insects are a constant irritation in this part of Scotland. The navy's standard-issue mosquito repellent wasn't up to scratch (an apt phrase here, so thank you, John Chambers and your boxing regulations). We don't know which Marine first discovered that the beauty product – 'ensure your skin feels velvety soft, hour after hour' – also keeps midges away, or indeed what he was doing at the time, but ever since then the lads have been in love with the stuff. 'Some buy it online,' said an official spokesman. 'Others are ordering it through local Avon ladies.'

Morning turns into afternoon, and for a few miles I skirt a corner of the FK (Falkirk) area. This contains Doune, the town famous in the seventeenth century for making pistols, one of which fired the first shot in the American War of Independence. There's also Alloa, home to the brewery that developed Graham's Golden Lager in 1927 before renaming it 'Skol', this being the Scandinavian word for 'cheers'. As we saw earlier, the Carron Company gave Britain many of its pillar boxes, but it's to something originally made in Falkirk itself that we turn for our fact. The product is now such an icon that when the Museum of Scotland in Edinburgh asked celebrities to choose an exhibit which summed up the country, Sean Connery chose a crate of it. Like Skol, however, it was originally known by another name:

FK (Falkirk): The spelling of Irn-Bru was designed to get round new labelling regulations – before that it had been called 'Iron Brew', and although it contains iron it isn't brewed.

The change happened in 1946, the drink having been around since 1901. It's heartening, when you think about it, that the authorities still credit us with enough sense to realise that the firm's advertising slogan 'made in Scotland from girders' might not actually be true. Although I do wonder how many proud nationalists up here took notice back in 1922 when A. G. Barr and Co, makers of the legendary drink, changed the bottle's label. The picture of Adam Brown, a famous Highland athlete of the time, was replaced by one of a rower holding a glass of Iron Brew. Nothing there to offend Scottish sensibilities – except that the rower was from Cambridge University.

A late lunch is taken in Fort William (part of the Perth postal area, whose 'Strontian is the only place in Britain to have a chemical element named after it' fact featured earlier in the project). It's a disappointingly unpicturesque town, rescued only by the West Highland Museum. Here I read of a Model T Ford being driven to the top of nearby Ben Nevis in 1911, and reflect that the leather in it must have crossed the Atlantic twice. The ascent (a publicity stunt by an Edinburgh Ford dealer) took five days. Exactly 100 years later the feat was recreated, though because the mountain paths have been redesigned for walkers and include steps, the car could only be driven part of the way up. It was then disassembled so volunteers could carry the parts to the summit and put them back together, which seems even more impressive than the original stunt.

The museum's historical artefacts include a birching table, a fearsome-looking thing with two holes for the hands to go through and straps to hold the legs in place as the victim lay face down. This isn't quite as historical as you might assume: the last birching in Fort William was delivered in 1948, to a boy convicted of shop breaking.[5] Also on show is a nineteenth-century mail carrier from the remote island of St Kilda. This is nothing more nor less than a tin in a wooden box attached to a sheep's bladder. Letters were placed in the tin before being thrown into the sea, so the bladder could float them to the island of Lewis where they joined the regular mail. 'The carrier was surprisingly successful,' reads the note. 'Apparently two-thirds of the letters reached their destination.' I sense an email to Harry coming on...

From Fort William I head across country to the east coast, where today's final area awaits. 'Frustration causes accidents,' say the signs on the A82, and more than once I round a corner to see a car (sometimes two) heading towards me on my side of the road, their drivers refusing to stay trapped behind a dawdler for a single second longer. Far more relaxing is what happens when the road reaches the Caledonian Canal at Aberchalder: it swivels round. Red lights and a barrier bring me to a halt, then the swing bridge rotates a section of the road horizontally, thereby allowing a barge through. It's one of those solutions that seems obvious when you encounter it, but only when you encounter it. Soon afterwards Loch Ness appears on the right, and as it's over 20 miles long there's plenty of

---

[5] The museum's wi-fi takes a longer sweep of the past: its password is 'Jacobite'.

time to admire it. Plenty of room for a monster, too, though of course not even a loch is as big as the human imagination.

Eventually I reach Inverness. I'm turning right here to head south for the project's penultimate night of kip, but to the north, the other side of the Black Isle peninsula, is Invergordon. Buried there are the Inchindown oil tanks, used in the past to supply Royal Navy ships with fuel. The tanks were dug into a hillside to prevent them being attacked from the air. Some digging, too – each of the five main tanks (there's a slightly smaller sixth) is 260 yards (twice the length of a football pitch) by 30 feet wide by 44 feet high. Empty since 2002, they no longer serve any practical purpose. Oh, just the one – they take records away from Hamilton Mausoleum:

IV (Inverness): The Inchindown fuel tanks have the longest-lasting echo of any man-made structure in the world.

With its paltry 15 seconds the mausoleum can, I'm afraid, whistle. Not that you'll hear it above the noise of a pistol blank being fired inside one of the Inchindown tanks. This was how Trevor Cox, Professor of Acoustic Engineering at the University of Salford, tested the echo. An absence of doors meant he had to be pushed in via an 18-inch pipe ('I threw my clothes away when I got out'), but the squeeze was definitely worthwhile: 'My initial reaction was disbelief... I knew immediately we had a new world record.' Look in the *Guinness Book of Records* and you'll see the figure of 75 seconds. This is across all frequencies – the lower ones reverberated for 112 seconds. The mid-range frequencies used in normal speech managed 30. In your living room they'll last 0.4, in an opera house 1.2, while even St Paul's Cathedral only gives them a life of 9.2 seconds.

Talking of fuel tanks, today has been a long one in the car, so it's fitting it should end at a motorway hotel. Junction 6 services on the M90, to the west of Kinross, aren't as busy as Watford Gap, but then that makes their Travelodge all the more soothing a place to rest my head for the night. Breakfast coffee in the services is taken at the table next to a husband and wife biker couple. Her white crash helmet looks so much like a *Star Wars* stormtrooper's that I can't resist asking if it's deliberate. She says not, but that everyone thinks the same thing. Attached to the helmet is a mini walkie-talkie which allows her to talk to her husband on the road. May the force be with them.

Today is a relatively quiet one, simply moseying down to Yorkshire to tick off one more area before tomorrow accounts for the final two. This means heading past Edinburgh and across the border into Northumberland. I've never driven here before – the train to Aberdeen hugged the coast, of course, but this is inland. The border itself is done rather well: the road twists up to a summit where small car parks on either side allow you to get out and admire the view. There are two flagpoles, one for each country, although while the Scottish flag is cracking proudly in the wind the other pole is bare. Is this an attempt to influence the forthcoming independence referendum?

The map tells you that Northumberland is vast, but not until you've driven through the place can you really understand *how* vast. There is so much nothing round here it's almost intimidating, a bit like driving across the Australian outback, or possibly Mars. Admittedly neither of those have the astonishing number of trees to be found here, but in terms of human presence the effect is much the same. After a while, once you've got used to the beautiful emptiness, the hills get even steeper, producing so many blind summits that the drive becomes a rollercoaster ride. The car's brakes perform well, though my stomach gives faint hints that it might reprise events from the Shetland ferry. Eventually, however, the A68 stops the corrugated iron act, and all is smooth on the approach to the project's final hotel. The same could not be said, emotionally at least, for someone who stayed there in 1926:

HG (Harrogate): Agatha Christie, upset at her husband having an affair, signed into the Old Swan hotel in Harrogate using the name of his mistress.

The sort of touch you'd expect from a novelist, I suppose. Christie never talked about her eleven-day disappearance, so the full story will never be known. But what seems to have happened is that, already upset at her mother's recent death, she was told by Archibald that he was in love with another woman, Theresa Neale, and wanted a divorce. On Friday 3 December the couple quarrelled at their Berkshire home, Colonel Christie leaving to spend the weekend with Neale in Surrey. At 9.45 p.m. Agatha herself left the house. Her car was later found hanging over the edge of a chalk pit. It's thought that after crashing it she continued to London, catching a train from Waterloo to Harrogate. There she took a taxi to the Swan Hydro, as the hotel was then known (it offered the baths and water treatments popular in the spa town).

Arriving in the middle of a sunny Sunday afternoon, I find a much happier matrimonial picture. The Old Swan – a splendid great ivy-covered slab of a building that would scream 'Agatha Christie' even if she hadn't stayed here – is hosting a wedding. This accounts for most of the people in the bar and on the terrace. There are few more entertaining sights than a waistcoated five-year-old tearing across a hotel lawn, though heading for the bar I only just avoid treading on the bride's eight-foot train. Over my pint of bitter I read more about events in 1926. Christie's disappearance was of course a massive news story, with police and civilians scouring the area around the writer's home. It was the first search in Britain to use an aeroplane. Arthur Conan Doyle took a different approach, indulging his interest in the paranormal by taking one of Christie's gloves to a medium. The photos printed in the newspapers can't have been very good, because for 11 days Christie mingled unrecognised with other guests at the Swan, even joining in dances held in the ballroom. The cost of a week's stay at the time was £5.50. Eventually it was the hotel's banjo player, Bob Tappin, who realised her identity and alerted the authorities. Colonel Christie instantly journeyed to Harrogate to collect his wife. Agatha kept him waiting half an hour in the lounge while she finished dressing for dinner.

I think of that banjo player as strains of the wedding band's soundcheck drift out of the ballroom. Judging by their 'Blame it on the Boogie' the guests are in safe hands. The next morning, in the hotel's huge breakfast room, I think about the institution of marriage. Agatha Christie granted Archibald his divorce, later marrying the archaeologist Max Mallowan. His profession was an advantage, she said: 'The older I get, the more he appreciates me.' Among the other breakfasters are the newlyweds themselves, now in civvies rather than yesterday's finery.

At one point he heads out into the corridor to talk on his mobile phone, leaving his wife of a few hours eating on her own.

So this is it. The final day's travelling. A scoot round Harrogate on foot, then back into the car for the last two areas. Both lie a short distance off the M1, the very same motorway on which the project started.

'Genteel' is the word that occurs in virtually everything you read about Harrogate, usually harking back to its Victorian and Edwardian heyday. But there's still an air of gentility here today, albeit with respectable middle-aged ladies replaced by yummy mummies. A shop called Milk and Honey clothes their offspring exquisitely, while once the babysitter is in place they can head out to Jinnah, the smart Indian restaurant inhabiting an old Wesleyan school. The best shop name has to be Duttons for Buttons (were they ever going to pursue any other career?), though the most famous establishment is, of course, Bettys. The apostrophe is now officially discarded, though there never actually was a Betty – the tea room was started in 1919 by Frederick Belmont, a confectioner from Switzerland, and no one knows why he chose the name. This is as close to old-fashioned gentility as you'll get: the menu includes a request that 'you refrain from using your mobile phone to make telephone calls whilst in our café'. The dozens of tables inside are creaking under raspberry macaroons, engadine tortes and a tea blend 'from the Brahmaputra Valley's very best estates'. Even at eleven on a Monday morning the queue stretches out on to the pavement and needs a woman with a clipboard to manage it, so I continue savouring the sunshine instead. In the park over the road (beautifully kept, *d'accord*) I find two stone cherubs. The sign is another 'you wouldn't believe in a novel' specimen: 'This statue has been donated to Harrogate by Mrs Frainy Ardeshir in loving memory of her husband's sister Mrs Mehroo Jehangir.'

Eventually the motorway calls. It delivers me safely past Leeds and Sheffield to the southern extremities of the latter's postcode area. Here you find the village of Rhodesia (named after the owner of a nearby coalmine rather than Cecil, so they've felt no need to rebrand) as well as somewhere called Plumpington Rocks (who am I to argue?). Finally, occupying several thousand acres of Nottinghamshire, is the estate of Welbeck Abbey. This is where I've come for the fact. Not the Abbey itself – that's still the home of William Parente, descended from the Dukes of Portland – but rather the outbuildings that welcome the public. There's the Dukeries Garden Centre, the School of Artisan Food, the Harley Art Gallery and the Limehouse Café. The last of these gives a clue as to why I'm here, and so arming myself with a tea (bit of a queue, but nowhere near as bad as Bettys) I sit at an outside table to read the booklet found for me by the very helpful assistant in the Art Gallery.

It's called 'Tunnel Vision – The Enigmatic 5th Duke of Portland'. You just know that when a man's own estate calls him 'enigmatic' a truer verdict might be 'barking mad', and so it is here. William John Cavendish-Bentinck-Scott, born 1800, might have led a different life if his proposal of marriage to the distinguished soprano Adelaide Kemble had been accepted. But 'the intensity of his courting had alarmed her' (the booklet gives no further details), and anyway she was already married to someone else. The Duke, as he was to become, retreated into a life of seclusion. Some blamed his psoriasis, so bad that he slept between wet sheets and pinned instruction notes to his clothes such as 'things to go to the wash and be very slightly starched, scarcely perceptibly.'

Notes, you see, were a way of life for the Duke – he did 'seclusion' in a way that would have had Howard Hughes telling him to get out more. Even his own doctor wasn't allowed to see him. He had his bedroom door fitted with two letterboxes, one for incoming and the other for outgoing missives. His wide-ranging correspondence with everyone from his solicitor to Benjamin Disraeli was wonderful news for the Post Office, but his refusal to see people was a touch tricky for those on the estate. The Duke went out mainly at night, a servant walking

40 yards in front of him carrying a lantern. If he did venture out in daylight he wore two coats, a high upturned collar, a large hat and carried a huge umbrella. Employees were forbidden to acknowledge his presence. One workmen who saluted him was fired on the spot.

But the lowpoint of the Duke's madness – literally – was still to come:

S (Sheffield): The 5th Duke of Portland had a 15-mile network of tunnels built under his estate so he could tour it in total privacy.

The biggest tunnels were wide enough for two horse-drawn carriages to pass each other side-by-side. When the Duke travelled to London he had his carriage driven to Worksop station, loaded on to a train and then, when it reached the capital, taken to his residence, Harcourt House in Cavendish Square. Here the staff had to make themselves scarce until he'd walked through the front hall into his study. The tunnels at Welbeck were sometimes used to deliver the Duke's food on heated trucks (he ordered that a chicken be kept roasting at all times). The lamps lighting the tunnels were fed by the estate's own gasworks – now occupied by the art gallery – while the café stored the lime used in purifying that gas (hence its name).[6] How would the Duke react to the hoi polloi swarming over his land today, the toddler running round the open space between the café and the gallery, the plant-laden customers heading from the garden centre back to their cars? What would he make of the courses on offer in the food school – 'Artisan Butchery Fundamentals', 'French Baking', 'Introduction to Wild Yeast and Sourdoughs'?

---

[6] Back up the M1 a little way is Anston, the quarry that supplied the limestone from which the Palace of Westminster is built.

What, for that matter, would he make of 'Pulse and Cocktails', the roadside store I pass on the A1 (more convenient than the motorway for this final leg of the trip) between Grantham and Stamford? Formerly a McDonald's, it is now a bizarrely mainstream 'Sexy Superstore/Adult Shop'. Googling it later (very carefully), I'll find it boasts of being 'bright and modern with friendly, helpful staff' and offers 'a fantastic range of adult toys, bondage, lingerie, hosiery and sexy clothing', none of which, you have to say, would do your psoriasis any good. Shortly after the store I cross a postcode boundary for the last time, entering the project's one remaining area. It takes its LE code from Leicester, home to Adrian Mole and thousands of Asians ordered out of Uganda by Idi Amin in 1972. They only chose the city because its council had taken out adverts asking them not to, and they were 'curious to find out why'.

Walkers make their crisps in Leicester, getting through 800 tons of potatoes a day, while elsewhere the area offers us Joseph Hansom developing his famous cab in Hinckley, Barwell's Chris Kirkland earning his dad £10,000 by playing football for England before he was 30 (£100 at 100 to 1 when the boy was 11), and Taylor's of Loughborough casting the second-largest bell ever in Britain, Great Paul at St Paul's Cathedral. They'd still have the record if their tender for the 2012 Olympic Bell had been accepted: as it was the authorities chose a Dutch firm. Ask the Department of Transport about Leicestershire and they might, if they're consulting one of their 2014 press releases, tell you it's in the South-East. They also placed Manchester in the North-East and Plymouth in the North-West. A spokesman blamed a 'data source issue', insisting that staff 'were aware of the locations of places in England.'

Leaving the A1 I take the project's final B-road, the 668, prompting a personal memory of SW (Harrods staff lift, 1992:

'668 – Neighbour of the Beast'). The road winds through a couple of villages before landing me in the market town of Oakham. The market isn't on today, so there's plenty of room to park in the square and walk, in the hazy quiet of a Monday afternoon, through the passageway leading to the castle grounds. Quite a grand name for a pleasant grassy enclosure, about 200 yards across and surrounded by trees, with the 800-year-old castle over to one side. It isn't even a castle in the normal sense – in fact it looks exactly like a small parish church without the steeple. Inside it's one open space, stone arches supporting a timbered roof. Lining all four walls are horseshoes. Two hundred of them, ceremonial ones, from standard size up to three feet long, each bearing the name of a distinguished visitor: by tradition peers of the realm visiting Oakham for the first time have to present a horseshoe to the Lord of the Manor. It's thought that the custom arose after Henry de Ferrers took charge round here following the Norman conquest of 1066. His family emblem was a horseshoe ('ferrier' being French for farrier). The oldest shoe still on display is the one given by Edward IV in 1470 after his victory at the Battle of Losecoat Field. I'm scanning the wall for it when a voice says right in my ear: 'Welcome to Oakham Castle, sir.'

This makes me jump, especially as the delivery is a touch on the breathy side. I turn, taking a precautionary step backwards in the process, and see a man in his early twenties. His smile is that of a particularly enthusiastic meeter-and-greeter at an American theme park, though unlike such a person he isn't acting – you can tell from every fibre of his shirt, tie, light blue jacket and black trousers that working at Oakham Castle is all this man has ever dreamed of, all he *could* ever dream of. 'Are you looking for anything in particular?' he asks.

Clearly I am, but I don't want to admit this because it would mean a prolonged conversation, and facing that smile for too long might actually damage my eyesight. 'Just enjoying the horseshoes,' I reply.

'Yes,' he beams. 'They're lovely, aren't they?'

'Certainly are.'

He hands me a laminated sheet of A4 paper. 'This is some basic information. Do ask if you have any specific questions.'

'Thanks. Will do.'

I digest the sheet, my reading punctuated by the occasional 'welcome to Oakham Castle' in the background. Apparently Losecoat Field got its name from Edward's defeated opponents shrugging off their coats so they could run away more quickly. The horseshoes are iron, made by a local farrier, and the hall provides a 'beautiful and unusual setting for your marriage or civil partnership ceremony'. In fact as I'm reading I hear a couple telling Mr Smile that they themselves got married here 14 years ago.

'Oh, that must have been wonderful,' he replies.

They agree that it was.

The horseshoes in themselves don't merit a fact. The reason I'm here today is because of the way they're displayed, namely with the open end pointing downwards, something that is normally thought to bring bad luck. For the 124th and final time, I record an item of information:

LE (Leicester): The horseshoes at Oakham Castle are hung upside-down to stop the devil sitting in the hollow.

It's a Rutland thing. Look at the county council's arms and you'll see the same fate-tempting arrangement. Local brewers Ruddles, however, are more timid – the horseshoe on their labels has its open end pointing upwards. Examining the walls I see shoes presented by Princess Alexandra (2005) back through the Duke of Gloucester (1955) and the Duchess of Kent (1833) to Edward IV's 1470 specimen. It's massive, and less ornate than the modern ones, which are usually painted gold and embellished with the donor's crown. In 1899 someone called Julian, Lord Pauncefote left a shoe, not knowing that a century later people would take him for a character in *Blackadder*. 1969 saw a visit from Jeffery John Archer: you fear the worst, but no, the spelling's slightly different and this one's actually Earl Amherst.

By now, having done a lap of the place, I'm near Mr Smile again. I hand back the sheet, and, feeling a little braver, risk a conversation. He tells me it isn't only marriages that take place here. 'Every two years they carry on the tradition of holding a crown court here.'

'Real cases?'

'Oh yes. It happened last year – two or three cases were dealt with.' I look up the details later. One man was given 18 months for theft, another 20 months for the same offence. Sentencing of a third was adjourned when he pleaded guilty to GBH. All this after everyone had been greeted with a fanfare played by pupils at a local school and members of Uppingham Jazz and Soul Band.

We talk about the horseshoes. 'And the most recent one is Princess Alexandra?' I say, largely to reassure him that I read the notes.

'Oh,' he says, surprised. 'Didn't you know? About our visitor last week?'

'No – who was that?'

'The Duchess of Cornwall.' Saying the words ratchets up his smile another megawatt. I'm forced to momentarily avert my gaze again.

'Really?'

He points to a spot underneath Edward IV – looks like I've failed the observation test. 'We put her shoe next to that of her husband.' So they have – HRH Duchess of Cornwall (2014) hangs beside HRH The Prince of Wales (2003).

'How was she?'

'*Lovely.*' I wait a moment to see if there'll be any details of witticisms that fell from Camilla's lips. But there aren't. You get the impression Mr Smile doesn't want to let daylight in on the magic. Looking up the visit in the local newspaper I'll find confirmation from many eyewitnesses that both Camilla and Charles were indeed lovely.

As I'm leaving I overhear Mr Smile talking to an elderly woman about the horseshoe tradition.

'So they were an early form of autograph, really,' she says.

'Yes,' agrees Mr Smile. 'I suppose they were.'

They both stare up at the wall. The woman says: 'Now they do selfies.'

The codes are complete, the facts are filed, the project is over. I wander back to the main square, enjoying the sunshine and contrasting it with the rain and cold at Watford Gap all those months ago. I've been dreading this moment, the end of the road, the day when I finally revert to a life in which British travel no longer has as its subtext the first two letters of the final line of a location's address. And yet now the moment has arrived, all is fine. Instead of something closing down there's a sense of lots of other things opening up. The zipwire flight across a quarry with Barney will be just one of them. Underlying the whole feeling of possibility is the map itself, Blu-Tacked to Barney's wall (I checked those securing blobs underneath WR and KY the other day), a huge expanse of paper coated with inspiration. I love the thought that the map which will teach him about Britain is the one I used for this project. Already he's reminded me how easily our brains can accept absurd geographical complications. Hearing the Scottish independence referendum mentioned on the radio, he asked me if Scotland was a different country. 'Erm...' I replied. 'Yes and no...'

Actually, that's why I love the horseshoe fact being the one to round the project off: it's a reminder that so much of this big, important subject we call 'history' is actually very, very silly. Yes, there are wars and elections and constitutional crises, but so much of life in Britain is, at it always has been, delightful nonsense. Like the sign in my village's post office announcing that you don't have to be over 60 to join the Over 60s club. Even the things that are big and important are often made up of nonsense. RAF crews accidentally bombing Cambridgeshire. Royal wedding cables being put in place by ferrets. The country's grimmest prison giving us the toothbrush. Since my trip to Northern Ireland I've greeted media reports of angst about plummeting standards of behaviour with a smile, reflecting on how many people actually complained when that painter said of course his job was fucking boring.

The upside-down horseshoes are a reminder, too, that there's nothing as changeable as an eternal truth. British horseshoes are always hung the right way up, people will tell you – it's bad luck to do it the other way. Well, yes: unless you live in Rutland. These isles, according to the sort of people who always call them 'sceptred', are crammed full of glorious traditions going back centuries and centuries, which have never changed and never, God help us, will. Then all of a sudden one of them changes overnight and the sky stays exactly where it is and life carries on. The tradition of not using peers' first names, for instance. It was Alan Sugar, or Lord Sugar of Clapton, but most definitely *not* Lord Alan Sugar. Then in the mid-2000s everyone decided that didn't apply any more, first names are in, history's out. At least Sugar made his birthday card mistake when he was a mere 'Sir'. Imagine what his wife would have said if he'd signed it 'Lord'.

I end up sitting in the square for ages, thinking back on the project and where it has led me. Every trip was a reminder that you could spend the rest of your life mining this country for surprises and stories and still leave the reserves virtually intact. I've discovered people living in service stations for days at a time, hotel guests so famous they can't use the private entrance their money has bought them, sundials set an hour fast and bungalows that powered the Second World War. Even the disappointing bits weren't disappointing – you reach an age in life when a discovery is interesting simply because it's a discovery. So Southall and Swansea aren't places that I'll ever go back to, but they're places I'm glad I've been. At around the same age you realise that every step into the future takes you back into the past as well. Justin has experienced that at the Metropole Hotel. Four generations of his family have delivered the place into his care for a while. He's the fifth link in a chain – will one of his children become the sixth?

I end up sitting in the square for ages, to-do lists writing themselves in my brain: taking Barney on the Mail Rail, visiting the BPMA to savour more of *The Royal Mail, Its Curiosities and Romance*, climbing that mountain on the Isle of Man to look at all four UK countries simultaneously... So long am I here, in fact, that I see Mr Smile walking through on his way home from the castle. I can't help liking him. OK, so he stood a few inches closer than was totally comfortable, but his enthusiasm – for the castle, for the horseshoes, for history in general – was endearing. In a way he reminds me of Blackpool. He's a sign that for all we're constantly reading obituaries of Britain As She Used to Be, there's something very strong and determined in there that's going to take a very long time to die, if indeed it ever will. Blackpool is still making a living from the holidaymakers. Mr Smile – born, I'd wager, well over a decade after Johnny Rotten called the monarchy a 'fascist regime' – is still reduced to awestruck wonder in the presence of Charles and Camilla.

I'm not particularly bothered about either Blackpool or the monarchy, but that isn't the point. It's their link with history that's fascinating, the bridge they build between Britain's past and its future. A bit like the Royal Mail, really. The internet was going to kill the postie, we thought – but now it's given him a whole armful of Amazon packages to deliver. You can never predict what life is going to produce. Who knows, if you were to travel the UK's postcode areas a decade from now, what wonderful new facts you might collect?

For the time being, all that remains is to get in the car and head for home. I give one last imaginary tug of the forelock to Sir Rowland Hill, the father of the postcode, the Victorian whose idea inspired my twenty-first-century odyssey. That's at an end now. The mail is sorted, the obsession is over.

Guess I'll just have to find another one.

ACKNOWLEDGEMENTS

I'm hugely grateful to Alan Samson, Lucinda McNeile, Simon Wright, Margot Weale, Claire Brett, Graeme Williams, Anne O'Brien, Richard Collins and everyone else at Orion who has made working on this book so much fun. Thanks also to Charlie Viney: to misquote Sherlock Holmes on Irene Adler, he is always *the* agent.

If every press officer in the world did their job with even half the energy, imagination and wit of Harry Huskisson then researching books would be a hell of a lot easier. Thanks to him, and to his colleagues at the British Postal Museum and Archive, Chris Taft and Vicky Parkinson. The help of Jennifer Bird at the Royal Mail was also invaluable, as was that of Bruce Crossan and Michelle McCulloch in Shetland.

So many people assisted my research into the trivia and history and anecdote that make up the book's facts. I'd like to mention Ethan Thorpe at Lincolnshire County Council, Martin Wyatt at Lancashire Police, Nigel Chell at JCB, Marilyn Greene and Tim Shields at the London Transport Museum, David Gibson at Scottish Leather Group and Robert Massey at the Royal Astronomical Society. Thanks also to Mike Golding, Hugh and Sheila Sheer and Paul Johnson, as well as Nick Owen for his tales from the commentary box.

For their help in getting me round the country I'm grateful to Damien Henderson at Virgin Trains, Peter Meades at Abellio Greater Anglia, Richard Salkeld at East Coast Trains and Cheryl Kelday at NorthLink Ferries. Help in the 'roof over your head' department was graciously provided by Joanne Harvey at the Europa in Belfast, Scott Frankton at the Royal in Cardiff, Justin Baird-Murray at the Metropole in Llandrindod Wells, Tuanne Mac at the Great Northern in London, Kevin Healey at the Radisson Blu Edwardian in Manchester, Sophia Mead at the Travelodge in Kinross and everyone at the Old Swan in Harrogate. Thanks also to Anna Nash at the Rosewood in London and to Laura Jones at Zipworld.

For their help on various fronts I salute Dave Charleston, Andrew Harper, George Legendre, Andrew Martin, Kieran Meeke, George Pascoe-Watson, Laura Porter, Peter Rees, Camilla Swift and Caroline Williams. Catherine Bishop opened my eyes to the wonders of Dunkirk, while James Harkin and Emma Clarke struggled bravely with the problem that is Altrincham. As usual Travis Elborough, Paddy Hennessy, David Long and Richard Robinson were diamond mines of information. And this has been the book where I finally realised the truth about Chris Pollikett: there is no such thing as Google, it's just Chris with a very fast broadband connection.

The biggest thanks, though, go (as they always will) to Jo and Barney.

INDEX

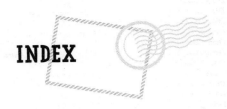

*References in italics are to the fact associated with a
particular postcode area*